Syncope

Syncope is a common condition related to transient loss of consciousness due to global cerebral hypoperfusion and caused by a variety of etiologies. Although it is self-limited, and usually benign, syncope can be the harbinger of life-threatening heart rhythm problems due to cardiac conditions. A multidisciplinary approach is practical for its evaluation and treatment, requiring the expertise of cardiologists, neurologists, emergency medicine specialists, and other clinicians. This book provides a detailed review of etiopathogenesis and a state-of-the-art update on therapeutic options offering recommendations based on the guidelines and experience of experts while discussing procedures and tests with their indications, methodology, interpretation, and limitations.

Key Features:

- Discusses new diagnostic tools, and therapeutic modalities including video monitoring.

- Provides up-to-date recommendations regarding the indications for and appropriate interpretation of noninvasive and invasive cardiac testing, for cardiologists and internists.

- Places particular emphasis on diagnosing and treating reflex and arrhythmic syncope.

Syncope
From Etiopathogenesis to
New Therapeutic Options

Edited by
Tolga Aksu, MD, FESC, FEHRA
and
Carlos A. Morillo, MD, FRCPC, FACC, FHRS, FESC

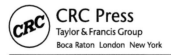

CRC Press
Taylor & Francis Group
Boca Raton London New York

CRC Press is an imprint of the
Taylor & Francis Group, an **informa** business

Designed cover image: www.shutterstock.com/image-photo/arm-supports-heart-concept-design-657615100

First edition published 2025
by CRC Press
2385 NW Executive Center Drive, Suite 320, Boca Raton FL 33431

and by CRC Press
4 Park Square, Milton Park, Abingdon, Oxon, OX14 4RN

CRC Press is an imprint of Taylor & Francis Group, LLC

© 2025 selection and editorial matter, Tolga Aksu and Carlos A. Morillo individual chapters, the contributors

Library of Congress Cataloging-in-Publication Data
Names: Aksu, Tolga, editor. | Morillo, Carlos A., editor.
Title: Syncope : from etiopathogenesis to new therapeutic options / edited by Tolga Aksu and Carlos A. Morillo.
Other titles: Syncope (Aksu)
Description: First edition. | Boca Raton : CRC Press, 2025. | Includes bibliographical references and index. | Summary: "Syncope is a common condition related to transient loss of consciousness due to global cerebral hypoperfusion and caused by a variety of aetiologies. Although it is self-limited, and usually benign, syncope can be the harbinger of life-threatening heart rhythm problems due to cardiac conditions. A multidisciplinary approach is practical for its evaluation and treatment, requiring the expertise of cardiologists, neurologists, emergency medicine specialists, and other clinicians. This book provides a detailed review of etiopathogenesis and a state-of-the art update on therapeutic options offering recommendations based on the guidelines and experience of experts while discussing procedures and tests with their indications, methodology, interpretation, and limitations"— Provided by publisher.
Identifiers: LCCN 2024022076 (print) | LCCN 2024022077 (ebook) | ISBN 9781032542348 (hbk) |
ISBN 9781032542331 (pbk) | ISBN 9781003415855 (ebk)
Subjects: MESH: Syncope—physiopathology | Syncope—therapy
Classification: LCC RB150.S9 (print) | LCC RB150.S9 (ebook) | NLM WB 182 | DDC 616/.047—dc23/eng/20240705
LC record available at https://lccn.loc.gov/2024022076
LC ebook record available at https://lccn.loc.gov/2024022077

ISBN: 9781032542348 (hbk)
ISBN: 9781032542331 (pbk)
ISBN: 9781003415855 (ebk)

DOI: 10.1201/9781003415855

Typeset in Palatino
by codeMantra

Dedicated to our children who bear the burden of accompanying us through this indefatigable journey toward the pursuit of knowledge and silently accept and support our endless hours of dedication to incomprehensible projects to their innocent minds.

T.A. and C.A.M.

Contents

Preface

"Syncope may arise due to a diseased condition of the heart itself. It usually occurs due to 'dyscrasia,' which is the unhealthy temperament of a person, or due to an inflammation or due to a tumour or due to 'erysipelas,' which is any disease that reddens the skins with diffuse purulent inflammations of internal organs, but also due to a sympathetic affection of the heart…" Galen. In *Hippocratis de victus acutorum commentaria iv*. In Kuhn CG, ed. Opera Omnia. Volume 15. Lipsiae: Libraria Car. Cnoblochii 1828: 600, 722, 775.

Fainting and transient loss of consciousness (TLOC) have fascinated physicians for centuries since the reportedly initial descriptions from Hippocrates. Galen, who was likely one of the most prolific authors on this topic, would be spellbound by the incredible advances over the past 40 years. The introduction of the head-up tilt-table test in 1986 by Kenny, Sutton, and collaborators provided a simple test that opened our minds to the diagnosis and understanding of the most frequent cause of syncope, namely, reflex "vasovagal" syncope. Almost 40 years after the introduction of this test that triggered an array of pathophysiologic and clinical trial studies from yoga to cardioneuroablation have forever changed our perception of the "common faint." Another transformational advance in our understanding and detection of this random event known as syncope is the development of the implantable loop recorded in the early 1990s by the Klein Group at the University of Western Ontario, in London, Canada. Capturing the ECG evidence during the actual episode of TLOC provided new insights and novel treatments for patients with recurrent syncope of unknown etiology.

Syncope, a symptom that can be due to many etiologies and a potential harbinger of sudden death, continues to be a challenge for the everyday physician who confronts these cases. In this comprehensive syncope textbook authored by world-renowned authorities in the field, we provide an updated pragmatic review of the state-of-the-art advances in the diagnosis, etiology, risk stratification, and management of syncope in the 21st century.

We anticipate that readers will find this textbook useful in the management of patients with syncope and will be provided with a widespread approach for the patient with syncope. We hope this textbook will also stimulate the upcoming generations of researchers in this field.

We would like to thank all the authors who have contributed chapters to this book and thank the publishers for all their assistance and patience at every stage of the publication. We would like to particularly thank Himani Dwivedi, Shivangi Pramanik, and Lavanya Sharma for their tireless efforts, for their constant reminders, and for putting up with us through the editorial process.

Acknowledgment

We would like to acknowledge our mentors, colleagues, trainees, and patients who have been the source of knowledge and inspiration.

About the Editors

Tolga Aksu, MD, FESC, FEHRA is a professor of cardiology. Currently, he is a member of the Department of Cardiology and Director of Clinical Electrophysiology at the Yeditepe University Hospital in Turkey. Dr. Aksu is clinically interested in invasive electrophysiology, device implantation, and catheter ablation therapies. Special interest areas include atrial fibrillation and cardioneuroablation, and he has been a pioneer and advocate in this field. Dr. Aksu has published more than 130 international scientific publications. He is an associate editor of *Journal of Electrocardiology* and SoMe Editor of JICE. He is also a member of the editorial board of *World Journal of Cardiology*, *Medicine Journal*, *Journal of Atrial Fibrillation*, and *Journal of Cardiac Arrhythmias*.

Carlos A. Morillo, MD, FRCPC, FACC, FHRS, FESC is a cardiac electrophysiologist, who served in the Chief Division of Cardiology (2015–2022) at the Libin Cardiovascular Institute, University of Calgary, Calgary, Alberta, Canada, and is currently on academic sabbatical leave at the Molecular and Novel Arrhythmia Mechanisms group at the Centro Nacional de Investigaciones Cardiovasculares (CNIC) in Madrid, Spain. He has been involved in syncope research since 1986 and has extensively investigated the mechanisms of neurally mediated syncope, and he has participated and led several landmark clinical trials related to the diagnosis and management of vasovagal syncope including the VPS, POST, and SPAIN trials. Prof. Morillo has published over 350 peer-reviewed articles and has also participated in several syncope guidelines from the ESC, ACC, AHA, HRS, and Canadian Society of Cardiology. Prof. Morillo's key research areas are related to the development of clinical trials in the areas of syncope, cardiac arrhythmias, AF ablation, screening and detection of AF in varied populations, and treatment of Chagas disease.

Contributors

Wayne O. Adkisson
Professor of Medicine, Cardiology Section
Veteran's Administration Medical Center
University of Minnesota Medical School
Minneapolis, Minnesota

Fares-Alexander Alken
Division of Cardiology, Angiology, Intensive
    Care Medicine
EVK Düsseldorf, cNEP
Cardiac Neuro-and Electrophysiology Research
    Consortium
Düsseldorf, Germany

Liane A. Arcinas
Department of Cardiac Sciences, Division of
    Cardiology
Libin Cardiovascular Institute
University of Calgary
Calgary, Alberta, Canada

Jacquie R. Baker
Department of Cardiac Sciences
Libin Cardiovascular Institute
Cumming School of Medicine
University of Calgary
Calgary, Alberta, Canada

David G. Benditt
Professor of Medicine, Cardiovascular
    Medicine
University of Minnesota Medical School
Minneapolis, Minnesota

Matthew T. Bennett
Division of Cardiology
University of British Columbia
Vancouver, British Columbia, Canada

Michele Brignole
Department of Cardiology
IRCCS Istituto Auxologico Italiano
San Luca Hospital
Milan, Italy

Leonardo Calò
Department of Cardiology
Policlinico Casilino
Rome, Italy

Mark W. Chapleau
University of Iowa Hospitals and Clinics
Iowa City, Iowa

Jean Claude Deharo
Centre for Cardiovascular and Nutrition,
    INSERM, INRAE
Aix Marseille University
and
Department of Cardiology, Syncope Unit
Timone Hospital
Marseille, France

Pietro Desimone
Tor Vergata University
Rome, Italy

Jeanne M. Du-Fay-de-Lavallaz
University of Basel
Basel, Switzerland

Artur Fedorowski
Department of Cardiology
Karolinska University Hospital
and
Department of Medicine
Karolinska Institute
Stockholm, Sweden

Jaume Francisco-Pascual
Unitat d'Arritmies, Servei de Cardiologia
Hospital Universitari Vall d'Hebron
Barcelona, Spain

Raffaello Furlan
Department of Biomedical Sciences
Humanitas University
Internal Medicine, IRCCS Humanitas Research
    Hospital
Milan, Italy

Domenico Giamundo
Tor Vergata University
Rome, Italy

Blair P. Grubb
Professor of Medicine
University of Toledo
Toledo, Ohio, USA

Régis Guieu
Centre for Cardiovascular and Nutrition,
    INSERM, INRAE
Aix Marseille University, France
Laboratory of Biochemistry
Timone Hospital
Marseille, France

Juan Camilo Guzmán
Syncope and Autonomic Disorder Unit,
    Arrhythmia Service, Cardiology Division
Department of Medicine, Faculty of Health
    Sciences
McMaster University
Hamilton, Ontario, Canada

Henry Huang
Division of Cardiology
Rush University Medical Center
Chicago, Illinois, USA

Ann-Kathrin Kahle
Division of Cardiology, Angiology, Intensive
    Care Medicine
EVK Düsseldorf, cNEP
Cardiac Neuro- and Electrophysiology
    Research Consortium
Düsseldorf, Germany

Khalil Kanjwal
Medical Director Cardiac Electrophysiology
Ascension Genesys Hospital
Grand Blanc, Michigan, USA

Rose Anne Kenny
Regius Professor of Physics
Trinity College, University of Dublin
Ireland

Asad Khan
Division of Cardiology
Rush University Medical Center
Chicago, Illinois, USA

Andrew D. Krahn
Division of Cardiology
University of British Columbia
Vancouver, British Columbia, Canada

Piotr Kulakowski
Centre of Postgraduate Medical Education
Department of Cardiology
Grochowski Hospital
Warsaw, Poland

Frederik de Lange
Amsterdam University Medical Centre
Amsterdam, Netherlands

Michael Liu
Department of Cardiology
Mayo Clinic, Arizona
Phoenix, Arizona, USA

Lina E. Lombo
Schulich School of Medicine and Dentistry
University of Western Ontario
London, Ontario, Canada

Christian Meyer
Division of Cardiology, Angiology, Intensive
    Care Medicine
EVK Düsseldorf
cNEP, Cardiac Neuro- and Electrophysiology
    Research Consortium
Düsseldorf, Germany
and
Institute of Neural and Sensory Physiology
cNEP, Cardiac Neuro- and Electrophysiology
    Research Consortium
Heinrich Heine University Düsseldorf
Medical Faculty, Düsseldorf, Germany

Angel Moya-Mitjans
Unitat d'Arritmies
Hospital Universitari Dexeus
Barcelona, Spain

Desmond O'Donnell
Specialist Registrar in Geriatric Medicine and
    Clinical Lecturer in Medical Gerontology
Trinity College
Dublin, Ireland

Brian Olshansky
University of Iowa Hospitals and Clinics
Iowa City, Iowa, USA

William H. Parker PhD, MD
University of Iowa Hospitals and Clinics
Iowa City, Iowa, USA

John A. Paydar
Department of Cardiac Sciences, Division of
    Cardiology
Libin Cardiovascular Institute
University of Calgary
Calgary, Alberta, Canada

Satish R. Raj
Division of Cardiology, Department of Cardiac
    Sciences, Libin Cardiovascular Institute,
University of Calgary
Calgary, Alberta, Canada
and
Autonomic Dysfunction Centre, Division of
    Clinical Pharmacology
Department of Medicine
Vanderbilt University Medical Center,
Nashville, Tennessess, USA

Wasim Rashid
Consultant Government Medical College
Srinagar Kashmir, India

Marco Rebecchi
Department of Cardiology, Policlinico Casilino
Rome, Italy

Giulia Rivasi
Division of Geriatric and Intensive Care
    Medicine
Careggi Hospital and University of Florence
Florence, Italy

Ermenegildo De Ruvo
Tor Vergata University
Rome, Italy

Roopinder Sandhu
Smidt Heart Institute, Cedars-Sinai Hospital
Los Angeles, California, USA
Division of Cardiology, University of Alberta
Edmonton, Alberta, Canada

Katharina Scherschel
Division of Cardiology, Angiology, Intensive
    Care Medicine
EVK Düsseldorf, cNEP
Cardiac Neuro- and Electrophysiology
    Research Consortium
Düsseldorf, Germany
and
Institute of Neural and Sensory Physiology,
    cNEP
Cardiac Neuro- and Electrophysiology
    Research Consortium
Heinrich Heine University Düsseldorf,
    Medical Faculty
Düsseldorf, Germany

Antonella Sette
Department of Cardiology, Policlinico Casilino
Rome, Italy

Robert S. Sheldon
Department of Cardiac Sciences, Division of
    Cardiology, Libin Cardiovascular Institute
University of Calgary
Calgary, Alberta, Canada

Dana Shiffer
Department of Biomedical Sciences
Humanitas University
Milan, Italy

Win-Kuang Shen
Mayo Clinic Arizona, Department of
    Cardiology
Phoenix, Arizona, USA

Dan Sorajja
Mayo Clinic Arizona, Department of Cardiolog
Phoenix, Arizona, USA

1 Syncope

Definition, Terminology and Classification

John A. Paydar, Liane A. Arcinas, Carlos A. Morillo,
Robert S. Sheldon, and Satish R. Raj

INTRODUCTION

Syncope is a common medical condition characterized by a transient and abrupt loss of consciousness (TLOC), typically caused by a temporary decrease in cerebral blood flow.[1,2] Studies have reported prevalence rates of up to 41%, with recurrent syncope occurring in approximately 13.5%.[1] While syncope is colloquially referred to as "fainting," it can have an array of underlying causes, some of which are life-threatening. This can make a proper diagnosis and optimal risk stratification in syncope patients difficult. Having a systematic approach to the classification of syncope can make this challenge more straightforward. Considering this complexity, this chapter aims to explore the definition, terminology, and classification of syncope (Table 1.1).

Table 1.1: Definitions of Syncope and Related Conditions

Term	Definition
Presyncope	A symptom presenting as an abrupt, transient, and complete loss of consciousness, often accompanied by the inability to maintain postural tone, with rapid and spontaneous recovery. The presumed mechanism is cerebral hypoperfusion. Importantly, presyncope should not exhibit clinical features of other non-syncope causes of loss of consciousness, such as seizures, antecedent head trauma, or apparent loss of consciousness (i.e., pseudosyncope) (AHA definition)
Syncope	An abrupt, transient, and complete loss of consciousness associated with the inability to maintain postural tone, often attributed to cerebral hypoperfusion. This definition excludes clinical features of other non-syncope causes of loss of consciousness (AHA definition)
Loss of consciousness	A cognitive state characterized by a lack of awareness of oneself and one's situation, with an inability to respond to stimuli (AHA definition)
Transient loss of consciousness (TLOC)	A self-limited loss of consciousness attributed to cerebral hypoperfusion, distinct from non-syncope conditions (AHA definition)
Non-transient loss of consciousness (non-TLOC)	An extended or prolonged loss of consciousness, usually related to different mechanisms than cerebral hypoperfusion (AHA definition)
Unexplained syncope (syncope of undetermined etiology)	Syncope for which the cause remains unknown following an initial evaluation, deemed appropriate by a healthcare provider. This evaluation typically includes a thorough history, physical examination, and ECG (AHA definition)
Orthostatic intolerance	A syndrome characterized by symptoms such as frequent, recurrent, or persistent light-headedness, palpitations, tremulousness, generalized weakness, blurred vision, exercise intolerance, and fatigue upon standing. These symptoms may occur with or without orthostatic tachycardia, orthostatic hypotension, or syncope (AHA definition)
Orthostatic tachycardia	A sustained increase in heart rate of at least 30 bpm within 10 minutes of transitioning from a recumbent to a quiet (non-exceptional) standing position (or at least 40 bpm in individuals aged 12–19) (AHA definition)
Orthostatic hypotension	A drop in systolic blood pressure of at least 20 mmHg or diastolic blood pressure of at least 10 mmHg upon assuming an upright posture (AHA definition)
- Initial (immediate) orthostatic hypotension	A transient blood pressure decrease occurring within 15 seconds after standing, often accompanied by presyncope or syncope (AHA definition)
- Classic orthostatic hypotension	A typical blood pressure drop upon standing (AHA definition)
- Delayed orthostatic hypotension	A gradual reduction in blood pressure that takes more than 3 minutes of upright posture to reach the threshold (AHA definition)

(Continued)

DOI: 10.1201/9781003415855-1

Table 1.1: (*Continued*) Definitions of Syncope and Related Conditions

Term	Definition
- Neurogenic orthostatic hypotension	Orthostatic hypotension due to autonomic nervous system dysfunction rather than environmental triggers like dehydration or drugs. It is often associated with lesions involving the central or peripheral autonomic nerves (AHA definition)
Cardiac (cardiovascular) syncope	Syncope caused by bradycardia, tachycardia, or hypotension due to low cardiac index, blood flow obstruction, vasodilatation, or acute vascular dissection (AHA definition)
Noncardiac syncope	Syncope due to noncardiac causes, including reflex syncope, orthostatic hypotension, volume depletion, dehydration, and blood loss (AHA definition)
Neurally mediated syncope	Syncope caused by a reflex that leads to vasodilation, bradycardia, or both (AHA definition)
- Vasovagal syncope	The most common form of reflex syncope mediated by the vasovagal reflex. It often occurs with an upright posture and is characterized by symptoms such as diaphoresis, warmth, nausea, and pallor, typically followed by fatigue (AHA definition)
- Carotid sinus syndrome	Reflex syncope associated with carotid sinus hypersensitivity, which is characterized by a pause of at least 3 seconds and/or a decrease in systolic pressure of at least 50 mmHg upon carotid sinus stimulation (AHA definition)
- Situational syncope	Reflex syncope is associated with specific actions such as coughing, laughing, swallowing, micturition, or defecation (AHA definition)
Postural orthostatic tachycardia syndrome	A clinical syndrome characterized by frequent symptoms upon standing, an increase in heart rate during positional changes, and the absence of orthostatic hypotension (AHA definition)
Psychogenic pseudosyncope	A syndrome characterized by apparent but not true loss of consciousness, which may occur without identifiable cardiac, reflex, neurological, or metabolic causes (AHA definition)

DOES MY PATIENT HAVE SYNCOPE?

When faced with a patient presenting with a potential syncopal episode, clinicians must begin by addressing several fundamental questions to determine whether the patient actually experienced syncope. TLOC is defined as a cognitive state in which an individual lacks self-awareness and awareness of their surroundings, rendering them unable to respond to stimuli.[1] An approach to potential causes of TLOC is outlined in Figure 1.1.

It is important to note that loss of consciousness can manifest as either transient or non-transient.[2] TLOC is a self-limited form of loss of consciousness and can be discerned by specific hallmarks, including amnesia for the period of unconsciousness, loss of responsiveness, and a brief duration.[2]

TLOC can further be categorized into traumatic and non-traumatic TLOC.[2] Traumatic TLOC typically occurs because of physical injury or head trauma, leading to a LOC.[2] On the other hand, non-traumatic TLOC encompasses a wide range of potential causes, with the added consideration that it can also lead to secondary trauma.

Within the spectrum of TLOC disorders, syncope represents a distinctive subset and is a key differential diagnosis. Syncope is considered a clinical diagnosis based on inferred physiology. The underlying mechanism is typically attributed to cerebral hypoperfusion, emphasizing the temporary decrease in blood flow to the brain. Notably, to meet the criteria for syncope, the episode should not exhibit clinical features indicative of other non-syncopal causes of loss of consciousness, such as seizures, antecedent head trauma, or apparent TLOC, often referred to as pseudosyncope.[1] This precise definition is crucial for distinguishing syncope from its myriad of mimicking conditions and guiding accurate diagnosis and treatment.

Non-Syncope TLOC

Neurological conditions, such as epileptic seizures, can manifest as non-syncope TLOC.[2] Epileptic seizures involve abnormal electrical activity in the brain and can lead to episodes of altered consciousness. Psychogenic causes also contribute to non-syncope TLOC and include conditions like non-hemodynamic faints (pseudosyncope) and psychogenic non-epileptic seizures.[2] Pseudosyncope mimics the clinical presentation of syncope but is not caused by cerebral

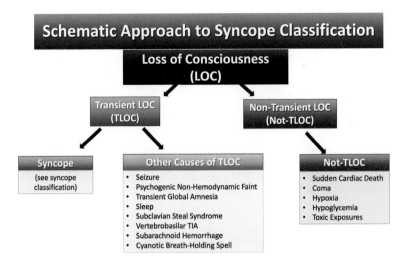

Figure 1.1 This figure provides a clear and systematic approach to comprehending the potential causes of loss of consciousness (LOC). It categorizes LOC into two main groups: transient LOC (TLOC) and non-transient LOC (non-TLOC), illustrating the overarching placement of syncope within these categories, while also highlighting the specific causes associated with both transient and non-transient episodes of LOC.

hypoperfusion, making it a distinct entity. Psychogenic non-epileptic seizures involve paroxysms of altered consciousness that are psychological rather than physiological in origin.[2]

Moreover, there are additional, albeit rare, causes of syncope, although delving into these specific causes exceeds the scope of this text. In brief, some examples encompass subclavian steal syndrome, vertebrobasilar transient ischemic attacks, subarachnoid hemorrhage, and cyanotic breath-holding spells.[2] These conditions, while sharing some similarities with syncope, have distinct underlying mechanisms and clinical characteristics that differentiate them. They may lead to cerebral hypoperfusion, which could be considered a variant of cerebral syncope, but they are not synonymous with classical syncope. Recognizing their existence is essential for distinguishing and arriving at an accurate diagnosis.

CLASSIFICATION OF SYNCOPE

The classification of syncope offers a systematic approach to diagnosing its underlying causes, which can vary in terms of prognosis and treatment strategies. A widely accepted classification system is based on the pathophysiology of syncope, centering on its defining feature: a reduction in cerebral blood flow that is usually due to a drop in systemic blood pressure (BP).[2] It is important to emphasize that while this decline in BP is a hallmark of syncope, clinical proof of this pathological mechanism is not usually clinically available. Instead, the diagnosis of syncope relies on the scenario being compatible with this mechanism.

Understanding whether a patient truly experienced syncope involves considering features that strongly suggest syncope while also recognizing factors that might lower suspicion. For instance, a prolonged loss of consciousness episode of 20 minutes generally precludes syncope, as syncope episodes are typically brief and followed by rapid recovery. One exception could exist when a head trauma results from a syncopal spell, where a prolonged LOC could result directly from the trauma. Additionally, syncope should not be accompanied by a true post-ictal period, which is a hallmark feature of seizures. These initial considerations serve as crucial starting points in the diagnostic journey, helping healthcare providers differentiate syncope from other conditions with similar presentations.

It is worth noting that the decline in BP triggering syncope can occur with a systolic BP as low as 50–60 mmHg at heart level or 30–45 mmHg at brain level while in an upright position.[3,4] It is essential, however, to understand that the relationship between systemic BP and cerebral blood flow is not absolute. Cerebral autoregulation mechanisms play a role in maintaining adequate blood flow to the brain, and syncope can manifest under various circumstances. Therefore, while

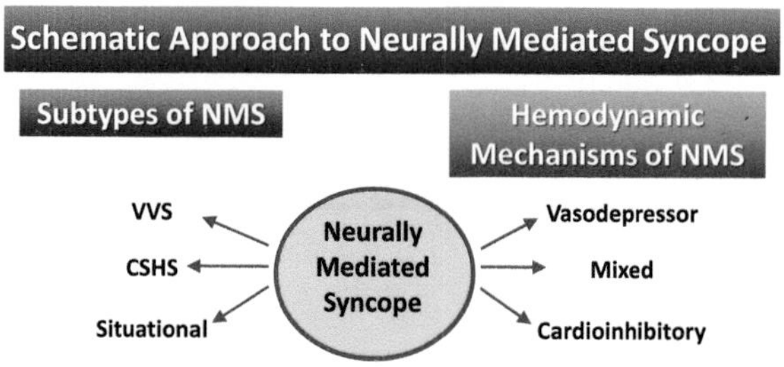

Schematic Approach to Neurally Mediated Syncope

Subtypes of NMS

Hemodynamic Mechanisms of NMS

VVS

CSHS

Situational

Neurally Mediated Syncope

Vasodepressor

Mixed

Cardioinhibitory

Figure 1.2 This diagram offers a clear framework for neurally mediated syncope (NMS) and its subtypes, including vasovagal syncope (VVS), carotid sinus hypersensitivity syndrome (CSHS), and situational syncope, as well as the hemodynamic mechanisms—vasodepressor, mixed, and cardioinhibitory.

very low systemic BP is a common trigger for syncope, it is not the sole factor, and syncope may occur even when BP is higher, depending on individual physiological responses. This highlights that syncope is primarily associated with a decrease in cerebral perfusion pressure, which can result from various causes and scenarios. "Cerebral syncope" is an example of this phenomenon, referring to a LOC associated with isolated cerebral vasoconstriction in the absence of systemic hypoperfusion.

BP hinges on the interplay between cardiac output (amount of blood flow) and total peripheral resistance (inverse to the size of vessels carrying blood).[2] A decrease in either of these components can precipitate hypotension and syncope. As a result, syncope is primarily categorized into three distinct pathophysiological groups: (1) neurally mediated syncope (NMS), (2) orthostatic hypotension (OH), and (3) cardiac syncope.[2] In this classification, we will begin with the most prevalent types and conclude with those posing potentially greater danger.

Neurally Mediated Syncope (NMS)

NMS, also referred to as reflex syncope, encompasses a spectrum of syncope initiated by reflexes originating in the autonomic nervous system. These reflexes can induce a sudden decrease in both BP and heart rate, ultimately resulting in a temporary LOC. NMS stands as the most prevalent form of syncope and can be further subcategorized into distinct subtypes, each based on the specific mechanisms that trigger these reflexes.[2,5]

Within NMS, two fundamental pathophysiological mechanisms are recognized (Figure 1.2).

The first is vasodepression, where inadequate sympathetic nervous system-mediated vasoconstriction leads to hypotension.[5,6] The second mechanism is cardioinhibition, in which bradycardia or asystole predominates, reflecting a sudden increase in parasympathetic nervous system tone.[5,6] Importantly, the specific hemodynamic pattern, whether it is cardioinhibitory, vasodepressor, or a combination of both, is independent of the trigger that initiates reflex syncope.[1] For example, both micturition syncope and orthostatic vasovagal syncope (VVS) can manifest as either cardioinhibitory syncope or vasodepressor syncope, irrespective of the specific triggering factor.[1] This emphasizes that various efferent mechanisms can underlie the different subtypes of NMS.

Hemodynamic Responses during NMS

Vasodepressor NMS: It is characterized hemodynamically by a sudden fall in total resistance due to excessive dilation of blood vessels with little change in cardiac output.[2]
Cardioinhibitory NMS: It is characterized by increased vagus nerve output, leading to a sudden decrease in heart rate.[7] This decrease in heart rate reduces cardiac output, causing an acute drop in BP, and a TLOC.[9]
Mixed NMS: Mixed NMS combines elements of both vasodepressor and cardioinhibitory mechanisms. This results in a combination of reduced BP and heart rate, leading to syncope.

CLINICAL CLASSIFICATIONS OF NMS

This classification emphasizes the triggering events that lead to NMS and provides a complementary perspective.

VVS: VVS is characterized by several key features: (1) It occurs when an individual maintains an upright posture for more than 30 seconds, faces emotional stress, experiences pain, or is in a medical setting[8]; (2) preceding symptoms include diaphoresis, warmth, nausea, and pallor[8]; (3) presents with relative bradycardia and hypotension when identifiable[8]; and (4) following the episode, individuals report a sensation of fatigue.[8] VVS can be further subdivided into orthostatic and cortical.

- **Orthostatic (Gravitational) VVS**: This subtype of VVS predominantly happens when a person is in an upright position. Most often, this occurs when standing up, although it can occur less frequently when they are seated.[2]

- **Cortical VVS**: This variant of VVS can be prompted by circumstances like experiencing fear, various types of pain (both physical and internal), medical procedures involving instruments, or a strong fear of blood.[2]

Carotid Sinus Hypersensitivity Syndrome (CSHS): CSHS is a specific subtype of NMS that occurs when there is an exaggerated response to stimulation of the carotid sinus.[2] The carotid sinus is a neurovascular structure located at the bifurcation of the common carotid artery into the internal and external carotid arteries. It contains baroreceptors, which are sensors that detect changes in pressure or stretching of the artery walls.[9] In particularly susceptible individuals, even mild stretching of the walls of the carotid sinus, such as with head rotation, neck masses, neck movement, or tight collars, could result in excessive stimulation of the carotid sinus leading to a sudden drop in BP and resulting syncope.[2]

CSHS is defined by specific criteria, including a pause in heart rate of equal to or greater than 3 seconds (sinus or atrioventricular (AV) block) and/or a systolic BP drop of equal to or greater than 50 mmHg during carotid sinus massage.[2] While carotid sinus massage is usually performed with the patient supine, it should also be repeated with the patient upright to optimize the detection of the hypotensive response. The prevalence of CSHS can vary depending on the method of evaluation and the population studied. It has been reported in up to 68% of elderly patients with syncope and approximately 35% of asymptomatic individuals who are over 65 years of age.[10]

Situational Syncope: Situational syncope is a subdivision of reflex syncope that encompasses syncope triggered by specific situations or actions, often related to autonomic reflexes. This category includes:

- **Micturition Syncope**: Syncope can occur during urination, often due to autonomic reflex responses.[2]

- **Defecation Syncope**: Syncope triggered during defecation.[2]

- **Swallowing Syncope**: Syncope triggered during swallowing.[2]

- **Sneeze Syncope**: Syncope triggered during sneezing. This is a phenomenon primarily characterized by increased intrathoracic pressure during vigorous sneezing, subsequently causing syncope.[2] While the dominant mechanism is related to elevated intrathoracic pressure, it can also occasionally result in vaguely mediated asystole or bradycardia.

- **Cough Syncope**: Syncope triggered during coughing. Similar to sneeze syncope, it is a condition primarily marked by syncope triggered by vigorous coughing, which elevates intrathoracic pressure.[2] Though the predominant mechanism is related to increased intrathoracic pressure, it can also, on occasion, lead to vaguely mediated asystole or bradycardia.

- **Post-Exercise Syncope**: Syncope can occur after intense physical activity. This is typically attributed to post-exercise vasodilation or a delayed recovery from exercise-induced vasodilation.[2]

- **Laugh Syncope**: Syncope triggered by a laugh. Excessive laughter, usually a "belly laugh," can involuntarily induce a Valsalva maneuver, leading to severely increased intrathoracic pressure and resulting in syncope.[2]

- **Brass Instrument Playing**: Syncope can occur during the act of playing brass instruments due to the specific breathing patterns involved, resembling a Valsalva maneuver, coupled with exertion.[2]

Understanding this classification of NMS, from both physiological and etiologic perspectives, is crucial for accurate diagnosis and appropriate management. The triggers for NMS and mechanisms of NMS may vary. Tailored treatment strategies can be implemented based on the specific NMS subtype encountered and ultimately improve patient care and outcomes.

Orthostatic Hypotension

OH, also referred to as postural hypotension, is a condition characterized by a significant drop in BP upon assuming an upright posture.[11] This phenomenon is objectively defined as a drop in systolic BP of ≥20 mmHg or a drop in diastolic BP of ≥10 mmHg when transitioning from a lying position to standing upright. Patients with an elevated BP, including those with supine hypertension, require a fall in systolic BP of ≥30 mmHg or a fall in diastolic BP of ≥15 mmHg.[11] OH can stem from a variety of underlying factors, which can be broadly categorized into neurogenic OH, drug-induced OH, and volume depletion.

Neurogenic OH: This category encompasses conditions characterized by dysfunction failure of the autonomic nervous system, specifically impairing its ability to appropriately regulate vasoconstriction.[2] Various conditions fall under this umbrella, including pure autonomic failure, multiple system atrophy, Parkinson's disease, dementia with Lewy bodies, autoimmune autonomic neuropathy, paraneoplastic autonomic neuropathy, and complications of diabetes mellitus, amyloidosis, and spinal cord injuries.[12] Additionally, the other two subtypes of OH, "drug-induced OH" and "volume depletion," can exacerbate neurogenic OH in affected patients, further compromising their orthostatic regulation.

Drug-Induced OH: This category is associated with the use of certain medications that can lead to vasodilation or affect fluid balance within the body. There are over 250 medications that have been linked to causing drug-induced OH.[13] Examples of such medications are diuretics, venodilators (e.g., nitrates and phosphodiesterase 5 inhibitors), vasodilators, central sympatholytics (e.g., clonidine, methyldopa, tizanidine), other antihypertensives, phenothiazines, and specific antidepressants, which are known culprits in inducing OH.[13]

Volume Depletion: OH can also result from conditions that cause a decrease in blood volume. These may include situations like severe hemorrhage, persistent diarrhea, or frequent vomiting, all of which can lead to a reduction in the overall blood volume within the circulatory system.

OH can be symptomatic or asymptomatic. While the diagnosis of OH does not depend on symptoms, the approach to its management depends both on the symptom burden and on the underlying cause. Accurate diagnosis and tailored treatment strategies are crucial to alleviate symptoms and improve a patient's overall quality of life.

Cardiac Syncope

Cardiac syncope warrants a careful examination within the realm of syncope, as it signifies a low cardiac output state typically stemming from heart-related issues. It can be further categorized into distinct subtypes, each characterized by unique mechanisms and clinical presentations.

Cardiac syncope, often indicative of a potentially fatal underlying disease process, is estimated to be the cause of syncope in 10% of syncopal events and carries a one-year mortality rate of 30%.[5,14] While less common than other forms of syncope, the potential life-threatening nature of cardiac syncope emphasizes the importance of this discussion.

Arrhythmia: Arrhythmias play a pivotal role in cardiac syncope among individuals with underlying heart conditions. They encompass a spectrum of abnormal heart rhythms, which can manifest as bradycardia or tachycardia, contributing to syncope episodes. In this context, it is essential to explore arrhythmias that are pertinent to cardiac syncope.

- **Bradycardia:** Syncope due to bradycardia often involves abnormalities in the heart's electrical conduction system. Conditions such as sinus node dysfunction, AV node disease, and distal conduction system disease can lead to dangerously slow heart rates, resulting in inadequate blood flow to the brain. Patients with bradycardia-related syncope may experience recurrent episodes of LOC, fatigue, and light-headedness.

- **Tachycardia:** Tachycardia-induced syncope can emerge from a spectrum of supraventricular and ventricular tachyarrhythmias, all of which can precipitate rapid, irregular heart rhythms that undermine effective cardiac output and lead to syncope.

  - **Supraventricular Tachycardias (SVTs):** SVTs comprise various rapid heart rhythms originating above the ventricles. SVTs can include atrial fibrillation (AF), atrial flutter, AV nodal re-entrant tachycardia (AVNRT), AV re-entrant tachycardia (AVRT), and atrial tachycardias (AT). While they are generally not a common cause of syncope, it is important to note their relevance in the context of cardiac syncope. SVTs are less likely to induce syncope compared to ventricular arrhythmias. While they can occasionally cause syncope directly due to the fast rate, they can also trigger a VVS episode that can lead to syncope. Ventricular arrhythmias pose a more significant risk of syncope due to their potential to severely impair the heart's pumping function, because they more commonly occur in patients with severe structural heart disease.

- **Ventricular Tachycardias (VTs):** Within the realm of VTs, several specific subtypes are noteworthy due to their association with various underlying conditions:

- **Monomorphic VT:** Often occurring in the presence of cardiac fibrosis, monomorphic VT often results from structural heart abnormalities. Episodes of this tachyarrhythmia may compromise cardiac output, potentially leading to syncope.

- **Polymorphic VT:** Conditions like long QT syndrome and Brugada syndrome are known to predispose individuals to polymorphic VT. These arrhythmias can be life-threatening and may lead to syncope episodes.

- **Bidirectional VT:** Bidirectional VT is associated with conditions such as catecholaminergic polymorphic VT and digoxin toxicity. It is characterized by ventricular beats occurring in two (or more) different directions in a repetitive pattern, which can lead to hemodynamic instability and syncope.

- **Other Ventricular Arrhythmias:** Various other ventricular arrhythmias, including those seen in arrhythmogenic cardiomyopathy and early repolarization syndromes, can also contribute to syncope. These tachyarrhythmias often indicate underlying structural heart disease and warrant careful evaluation and management.

Structural Cardiac Causes: Structural heart abnormalities can also precipitate cardiac syncope. These conditions often involve physical obstructions or damage to the heart's structure causing blood flow perturbations.

- **Obstructive:** Several obstructive cardiac conditions can lead to syncope. These include valvulopathies, such as aortic stenosis and mitral stenosis where abnormalities in heart valves result in improper functioning, causing blood flow obstructions. A massive pulmonary embolism (PE) can also restrict blood flow to the lungs, reducing oxygen supply and cardiac output. Pulmonary hypertension, which involves increased pressure in the pulmonary arteries, may result in right heart failure and syncope. Additionally, hypertrophic obstructive cardiomyopathy (HOCM) can lead to obstructed blood flow from the left ventricle to the aorta, causing symptoms such as chest pain, shortness of breath, and syncope. Cardiac tamponade, a condition where excess fluid accumulates in the pericardial sac, can significantly impede cardiac function, potentially leading to syncope.

- **Myocardial:** Conditions affecting the heart muscle itself can result in syncope, with two primary mechanisms at play.

  - **Mechanical Problems:** These can include issues like ventricular septal defects (VSD) or cardiac perforation leading to contained rupture. In these cases, the structural problems within the heart can directly affect cardiac output and lead to syncope.

  - **Arrhythmias due to Abnormal Myocardium:** Conditions such as hypertrophic cardiomyopathy (HCM), post-myocardial infarction (MI), and cardiac sarcoidosis can lead to abnormal myocardium. In these scenarios, the compromised myocardial tissue can trigger arrhythmias, potentially causing syncope.

  - **Ischemia Related:** While syncope is seldom the direct cause of MI, it is not uncommon as a consequence of an acute MI event.[15] One specific mechanism behind syncope associated with myocardial ischemia or acute MI, especially in cases involving an inferior MI, involves a reflex faint with both vasodepressor and cardioinhibitory components.[16] This phenomenon is presumed to be linked to the Bezold–Jarisch mechanism.[16] This reflex is triggered by an abundance of mechano- and chemo-sensitive receptors located in the infero-posterior region of the left ventricle, which is primarily supplied by the inferior coronary vessels.[16] These receptors activate afferent neural fibers, often referred to as C-fibers, within the vagus nerve, resulting in a predominantly vagal-mediated reflex.[16] Additionally, in the context of acute ischemia, new high-grade AV block on the electrocardiogram (ECG) or tachyarrhythmias such as paroxysmal monomorphic or non-sustained polymorphic VT can also serve as potential causes of syncope.[15]

■ **Diseases of the Aorta:** The aorta, the largest artery in the body, can be associated with various conditions that may lead to syncope. These include aortic dissection, aortic rupture (if self-contained), and aortic tumors with obstructive features. These aortic disorders can disrupt normal blood flow, weaken the aortic wall, or cause structural abnormalities, potentially resulting in syncope.

CONCLUSION

In conclusion, syncope is a multifaceted medical condition. Clinicians, medical students, and other healthcare professionals must be well-versed in the terminology associated with syncope to facilitate effective communication and diagnosis. A clear understanding of syncope classification is pivotal in guiding clinical decision-making and tailoring interventions to meet the unique needs of each patient.

REFERENCES

1. Shen WK, Sheldon RS, Benditt DG, et al. 2017 ACC/AHA/HRS guideline for the evaluation and management of patients with syncope: a report of the American College of Cardiology/American Heart Association Task Force on Clinical Practice Guidelines and the Heart Rhythm Society. *J Am Coll Cardiol.* 2017;70:e39–e110.

2. Brignole M, Moya A, De Lange FJ, et al. 2018 ESC guidelines for the diagnosis and management of syncope. *Eur Heart J.* 2018;39:1883–1948.

3. Wieling W, Thijs RD, Van Dijk N, Wilde AAM, Benditt DG, Van Dijk JG. Symptoms and signs of syncope: a review of the link between physiology and clinical clues. *Brain.* 2009;132:2630–2642.

4. Van Dijk JG, Thijs RD, Van Zwet E, et al. The semiology of tilt-induced reflex syncope in relation to electroencephalographic changes. *Brain.* 2014;137:576–585.

5. Mosqueda-Garcia R, Furlan R, Tank J, Fernandez-Violante R. The elusive pathophysiology of neurally mediated syncope. *Circulation.* 2000;102:2898–2906.

6. Morillo CA, Eckberg DL, Ellenbogen KA, et al. Vagal and sympathetic mechanisms in patients with orthostatic vasovagal syncope. *Circulation.* 1997;96:2509–2513.

7. Garcia A, Marquez MF, Fierro EF, Baez JJ, Rockbrand LP, Gomez-Flores J. Cardioinhibitory syncope: from pathophysiology to treatment-should we think on cardioneuroablation? *J Interv Cardiac Electrophysiol.* 2020;59:441–461.

8. Sheldon RS, Grubb BP, Olshansky B, et al. 2015 heart rhythm society expert consensus statement on the diagnosis and treatment of postural tachycardia syndrome, inappropriate sinus tachycardia, and vasovagal syncope. *Heart Rhythm.* 2015;12:e41–e63.

9. Wu TC. What is the real clinical significance of carotid sinus hypersensitivity in clinical practice? A dilemma still waiting for answers. *Arq Bras Cardiol.* 2020;114:254–255.

10. Seifer C. Carotid sinus syndrome. *Cardiol Clin.* 2013;31:111–121.

11. Freeman R, Wieling W, Axelrod FB, et al. Consensus statement on the definition of orthostatic hypotension, neurally mediated syncope and the postural tachycardia syndrome. *Clin Auton Res.* 2011;21:69–72.

12. Metzler M, Duerr S, Granata R, Krismer F, Robertson D, Wenning GK. Neurogenic orthostatic hypotension: pathophysiology, evaluation, and management. *J Neurol.* 2013;260:2212–2219.

13. Bhanu C, Nimmons D, Petersen I, et al. Drug-induced orthostatic hypotension: a systematic review and meta-analysis of randomised controlled trials. *PLoS Med.* 2021;18:e1003821.

14. Yasa E, Ricci F, Magnusson M, et al. Cardiovascular risk after hospitalisation for unexplained syncope and orthostatic hypotension. *Heart*. 2018;104:487–493.

15. Koene RJ, Adkisson WO, Benditt DG. Syncope and the risk of sudden cardiac death: evaluation, management, and prevention. *J Arrhythm*. 2017;33:533–544.

16. Wei JY, Markis JE, Malagold M, Braunwald E, Wei JY. Cardiovascular reflexes stimulated by reperfusion of ischemic myocardium in acute myocardial infarction. *Am J Physiol*. 1983;67:1621.

2 Epidemiology and Economics of Syncope

Dana Shiffer and Raffaello Furlan

INTRODUCTION

Syncope is a temporary loss of consciousness due to reduced blood flow to the brain followed by spontaneous recovery.[1–3] Around 40% of individuals have experienced at least one episode of syncope during their lives, making it a widely encountered clinical issue.[4–7] It shows a prevalence rate of 42% and an annual incidence of 6%, with episode rates ranging between 18.1 and 39.7 per 1,000 individuals.[8] Two age groups are particularly affected: teenagers around 15 years old, primarily due to vasovagal syncope, and those aged 70 or older, where the incident rate noticeably spikes.[9] For instance, the rate increases from 5.7 episodes per 1,000 men per year in the age group 60–69, to 11.1 episodes in the age group 70–79.[9]

In terms of causes, most syncopal episodes stem from non-threatening sources such as dehydration, vasovagal reactions, or medication side effects.[1,4] However, some are due to more alarming issues like abnormal heart rhythms or valve defects.[1] Vasovagal syncope is notably the most frequent cause in adults, making up over 85% of episodes in individuals below 40 and over 50% in the elderly.[9] The annual mortality rate in cardiac-related syncope ranges between 18% and 33%, whereas it is between 0% and 12% for non-cardiac cases.[8] However, identifying the cause of syncope is often complex since patients usually do not exhibit symptoms at the time they consult, and diagnostic tests have a low yield particularly when asymptomatic. After initial clinical evaluation, as many as one-third of syncope cases remain undetermined, and without diagnosis and treatment, the condition is prone to recur, exerting added pressure on both patients and caregivers.[1] Approximately one-third of general population patients will experience recurrent syncope, which is associated with a heightened risk of falls and injuries.[10] The quality of life for individuals with unresolved syncope is comparably impaired to those suffering from chronic illnesses such as terminal renal disease or structural cardiac anomalies.[11,12]

Furthermore, scientific research has demonstrated that even in people who are otherwise healthy, syncope episodes can be linked to heightened risks of other health issues and even death.[1,13] Specifically, cardiac-related syncope is believed to amplify the mortality risk twofold.[14,15] In terms of immediate physical dangers, almost one-third of patients experiencing syncope are found to sustain injuries or trauma upon arriving at emergency departments (EDs), with 5% of these instances being categorized as severe.[16,17]

The condition is responsible for approximately 1%–3% of ED visits and 1%–6% of hospital admissions, posing an urgent need to scrutinize the economic toll it takes.[18–24] Yet, beyond its clinical implications, syncope represents a sizable and often underestimated financial burden on healthcare systems.[25]

THE CHALLENGE OF DIAGNOSIS AND ADMISSION

One of the primary challenges in the healthcare system is the diagnosis and subsequent admission strategy for patients with syncope. Admission rates for syncope can vary dramatically, ranging from 13% to 83% depending on the institution and its protocols.[26–29] These figures reflect the inherent complexity of the condition. Even though numerous syncope guidelines have been introduced, there remains a significant variation in evaluation approaches and diagnostic outcomes across different physicians, medical facilities, and nations.[1,30–32] Healthcare providers are often cautious, admitting patients to the hospital for an extensive evaluation. This prudence stems from the difficulty in pinpointing the condition's root cause quickly and accurately. While some instances of syncope are relatively benign and do not necessitate in-depth evaluation, others could signify serious underlying conditions warranting further scrutiny. The resulting battery of tests can be costly and, ironically, might not even offer any definitive diagnostic clarity.[33]

THE ECONOMIC IMPLICATIONS

The financial ramifications of this diagnostic uncertainty are considerable. Syncope accounts for a significant share of emergency room visits and hospitalizations, causing the healthcare system to incur billions of dollars in costs annually. Although some local studies have tried to quantify the expenditures on a per-case basis, the figures can vary widely depending on geographical location and healthcare infrastructure.[34,35]

DOI: 10.1201/9781003415855-2

Various regional studies have highlighted the significant expenses related to hospital assessments for syncope.[36–38] When standardized to U.S. currency for comparison purposes, these costs have varied widely, from around $1,700 in the UK[36] to $4,534 in Canada[39] and to as much as $16,000 in Spain.[38] In Israel, the mean evaluation cost was 11,210±8,133 NIS, and the mean hospitalization cost accounted for 7,245±6,134 NIS of that sum.[40] The latest statistics indicate that the average cost of a hospital stay for syncope in the United States comes to approximately $5,300, accumulating to an estimated $2.4 billion in direct annual healthcare costs in the United States alone.[22,25] In Canada, despite having a lower rate of hospital admissions for syncope compared to other countries, falling within the 12%–15% range,[41,42] the overall spending is on the rise.[39] Research conducted in Alberta, Canada, has revealed that the biggest share of yearly expenses for patients with syncope is allocated to hospital stays, irrespective of whether they were discharged from the ED to their homes or admitted to the hospital.[41] Annual hospitalization costs in Canada were $66.6 million in 2004 and increased to $68.5 million in 2015.[39] Over a 10-year period, the financial burden of syncope-related hospital stays in Canada reached around $818.5 million, with a projected increase to $87.1 million annually by 2030.[39] The financial impact of syncope is notably high in Canada, even though only around 10,000 patients are hospitalized for this condition each year.[39] These numbers are alarming given that hospital admissions often result in additional tests extending the patient's hospital stay without frequently identifying a meaningful cause for the syncope.

OVERUTILIZATION OF DIAGNOSTIC TESTS

Extensive and pricey diagnostic tests are commonly conducted in EDs and during hospital stays to pinpoint the root cause of syncope.[43,44] One broad-based study observed that the median number of tests per patient with unexplained syncope was 13, with nearly half undergoing advanced imaging techniques.[34] This echoes a decade-long analysis that revealed the rate of computed tomography (CT) and magnetic resonance imaging (MRI) scans for syncope patients in EDs rose from 21% to 45% in recent times.[33] A recent systematic review examining the application and diagnostic value of head CT scans in patients with syncope found that 54.4% of ED patients with syncope underwent a head CT scan, which had a diagnostic yield of 3.8%, and that 44.8% of hospitalized syncope patients received a head CT scan, with a diagnostic yield of 1.2%.[45] In a more recent study, CT scans were performed on 42.5% of patients presenting with syncope to the ED with a diagnostic yield of only 0.82%.[35] Yet, both the Choosing Wisely initiatives in Canada and the United States advise against utilizing head CT scans for low-risk ED patients experiencing syncope.[46] Research indicates that such advanced imaging, when not clinically warranted, rarely affects diagnosis or management but significantly inflates costs.[40,44,45,47–51]

A comprehensive analysis of tests given to 10,036 patients presenting with syncope in the US ED found that only 9% yielded positive results. The most frequent tests were electrocardiogram (ECG) and stress tests, but they, along with other tests like CT scans and MRIs, had low positive findings. Financially, of the $43,347,332 spent on these tests, only $489,170 was for positive results, meaning $42,858,162 was spent without achieving definitive diagnoses, averaging a cost of $4,270 per patient.[35]

In light of the data, it is evident that while a significant number of patients undergo various diagnostic tests following syncope, a substantial majority of these tests yield negative findings. This underscores the importance of refining our diagnostic approach to syncope, aiming for more targeted and efficient testing strategies to optimize patient care and resource allocation.

Likewise, the prudent utilization of high-cost tests like invasive electrophysiological (EP) testing is crucial.[34] A multi-country observational study found that 25% of patients with recurrent, unexplained syncope underwent invasive EP testing with an estimated cost of £1,392 per test before receiving an implantable loop recorder.[34] However, strategies guided by implantable loop recorders have demonstrated a strong diagnostic yield and are considered financially sensible in comparison with traditional methods that include invasive EP tests.[52]

The frequent and sometimes needless employment of high-cost diagnostic tests, such as invasive EP studies, cardiac MRI, and CT scans, contributes significantly to these expenses. Such approaches, when not clinically indicated, rarely change patient management but inflate costs considerably. Alternative diagnostic tools like implantable loop recorders have proven to be cost-effective and provide significant diagnostic yields, questioning the utility of traditionally expensive methods.[52]

In contrast, studies have evaluated the diagnostic effectiveness of more budget-friendly methods like measuring orthostatic blood pressure, detailed history gathering, and basic ECG compared to other, more elaborate diagnostics for syncope.[53,54] Postural blood pressure measurements, recommended by the guidelines as one of the initial tests to perform for syncope evaluation,[1] are often overlooked despite being among the least expensive tests with the highest diagnostic yield.[44,53,55]

An example of the analytics accounting for the total costs of a tilt test procedure, a widely used test for assessing gravitational tolerance[56] in syncope work-up,[7] is provided in Table 2.1. Data were obtained from 117 tilt procedures that were carried out in 2022 at the Syncope and Orthostatic Disorder Unit, Humanitas Research Hospital, Rozzano, Italy. Please note that personnel accounts for 76% of total costs, being busy for about 1 hour during the test.

STRIVING FOR EFFICIENCY AND COST-EFFECTIVENESS

Efforts are being made to steer the management of syncope toward more cost-effective and efficient strategies. The workup of syncope and its economic costs have been the focus of several studies and initiatives. The "Choosing Wisely" campaign, a global initiative aimed at reducing unnecessary tests and treatments, has gained attention worldwide.[46] It encourages physicians and patients to discuss medical tests and procedures that may be unnecessary and potentially harmful.[57] In the evaluation of syncope, unnecessary testing and hospital admissions have been identified as common practices, leading to increased healthcare costs.[50] Studies have shown that extensive diagnostic testing, such as neuroimaging and cardiac monitoring, can contribute to the economic burden associated with syncope management.[58,59] The adoption of more systematic care pathways and the use of cost-effective diagnostic tools, such as implantable loop recorders, have been suggested to optimize the evaluation of syncope and reduce unnecessary costs.[60,61] Efforts to standardize clinical practice and reduce unnecessary services for syncope patients have been made through the development of guidelines and the implementation of integrated measurement frameworks.[1,2,54,62] These initiatives aim to improve the value and efficiency of care provided to syncope patients while minimizing unnecessary healthcare expenditures.

As healthcare systems put more focus on minimizing short-duration inpatient stays and hospital readmissions, Emergency Department Observation Units (EDOU) are increasingly emerging as a cost-effective substitute for full inpatient admission. While attempts to cut back on unnecessary and costly hospital stays have led to the formulation of clinical decision-making guidelines,[1,2]

Table 2.1: Cost Breakdown for a Tilt Table Test in Hospital Settings

Category	Cost in €	Percentage
Personnel costs		
Medical staff	€51	50.5%
Nursing staff	€26	25.5%
Material costs	€3.22	3.2%
Medical device costs	€1.04	1.0%
Maintenance	€0.07	0.1%
Indirect hospital operation costs	€10.19	10.2%
Management expenses	€8.89	–
General expenses	€1.30	–
Shared structural costs	€9.47	9.5%
Total	**€100.2**	**100.0%**

Note: Material costs group items such as electrodes, syringes, gloves, and masks.
Medical devices group costs related to the tilt bed, pulse oximeter, PC, ECG, and printer.
Management expenses group various services and administrative costs, from energy consumption to international marketing.
General expenses focus on more overarching costs, including communication and staff management.
Data were obtained from 117 tilt test procedures carried out during 2022 in the Syncope and Orthostatic Intolerance Unit at Humanitas Research Hospital, Rozzano, Italy. Costs were provided by courtesy of Dr. Elena Vanni, Humanitas Hospital Management Control Unit.

these have only scratched the surface in evaluating the effectiveness and utility of diagnostic tests in cases of syncope. Furthermore, the guidelines have not comprehensively explored the benefits of accelerated treatment within observation units.[63–65]

For patients considered to be at medium risk, recent suggestions have advocated for syncope unit (SU) management as a potential substitute for hospital admission.[66] This unit can be positioned within inpatient or outpatient environments, accepting referrals from EDs or local practitioners/cardiologists. Two clinical trials, which were randomized, assessed the efficiency of an ED-centric SU in contrast to regular care (meaning hospitalization).[67,68] These trials showcased a heightened diagnostic capability, diminished hospital admissions, cost savings, and no surge in negative patient outcomes for those assigned to the SU. An observational study found that the specialized SU significantly improved the diagnosis and management of patients with unexplained syncope, with 82% receiving a clear diagnosis after assessment.[69] Additionally, there was a marked reduction in associated costs, particularly an 85% drop in hospitalization costs during the nine-month follow-up after attending the unit.[69] Furthermore, another study estimated that the potential savings on a US national scale for handling intermediate-risk syncope patients in a specialized observation unit amount to $169 million dollars.[70]

Finally, emerging technologies like machine learning offer new avenues for cost-saving.[71] Recent studies found that machine learning algorithms could help to automatically identify syncope from an administrative database[72] and predict the length of stay for syncope patients in EDs with 80% accuracy, thus helping in more efficient triage and potentially lowering healthcare costs.[73]

CONCLUSION

Syncope represents a substantial economic burden on healthcare systems, exacerbated by diagnostic uncertainty and the subsequent overutilization of expensive tests and hospital admissions. Improved guidelines and innovative diagnostic approaches, potentially supplemented by technology, may offer paths to more cost-effective and efficient care. By focusing on targeted diagnostics and treatment, healthcare providers can not only improve patient outcomes but also substantially reduce the financial burden of this common yet enigmatic condition. The costs associated with diagnosing and treating syncope are exorbitant and are projected to rise if current practices continue. Addressing this will require a multipronged approach that involves creating standardized guidelines, adopting cost-effective diagnostic tools, and leveraging emerging technologies to optimize resource allocation. If we are successful in these endeavors, we can improve patient outcomes while significantly reducing the economic burden on healthcare systems.

REFERENCES

1. Brignole M, Moya A, De Lange FJ, et al. 2018 ESC guidelines for the diagnosis and management of syncope. *Eur Heart J.* 2018;39(21):1883–1948.

2. Shen WK, Sheldon RS, Benditt DG, et al. 2017 ACC/AHA/HRS guideline for the evaluation and management of patients with syncope: a report of the American College of Cardiology/American Heart Association Task Force on Clinical Practice Guidelines and the Heart Rhythm Society. *Heart Rhythm.* 2017;14(8):e155–e217.

3. Mosqueda-Garcia R, Furlan R, MD JT, Fernandez-Violante R. The elusive pathophysiology of neurally mediated syncope. *Circulation.* 2000;102(23):2898–2906.

4. Torabi P, Rivasi G, Hamrefors V, et al. Early and late-onset syncope: insight into mechanisms. *Eur Heart J.* 2022;43(22):2116–2123.

5. Solbiati M, Casazza G, Dipaola F, et al. Syncope recurrence and mortality: a systematic review. *Europace.* 2015;17(2):300–308.

6. Furlan R, Piazza S, Dell'Orto S, et al. Cardiac autonomic patterns preceding occasional vasovagal reactions in healthy humans. *Circulation.* 1998;98(17):1756–1761.

7. Furlan R, Heusser K, Minonzio M, et al. Cardiac and vascular sympathetic baroreflex control during orthostatic pre-syncope. *J Clin Med.* 2019;8(9):1434.

8. da Silva RM. Syncope: epidemiology, etiology, and prognosis. *Front Physiol*. 2014;5:471.

9. Blanc JJ. Syncope: definition, epidemiology, and classification. *Cardiol Clin*. 2015;33(3):341–345.

10. Ruwald MH, Olde Nordkamp LR. Is syncope a risk predictor in the general population? *Cardiol J*. 2014;21(6):631–636.

11. Barbic F, Dipaola F, Casazza G, et al. Syncope in a working-age population: recurrence risk and related risk factors. *J Clin Med*. 2019;8(2).

12. Van Dijk N, Sprangers MA, Colman N, Boer KR, Wieling W, Linzer M. Clinical factors associated with quality of life in patients with transient loss of consciousness. *J Cardiovasc Electrophysiol*. 2006;17(9):998–1003.

13. Toarta C, Mukarram M, Arcot K, et al. Syncope prognosis based on emergency department diagnosis: a prospective cohort study. *Acad Emerg Med*. 2018;25(4):388–396.

14. Soteriades ES, Evans JC, Larson MG, et al. Incidence and prognosis of syncope. *New Engl J Med*. 2002;347(12):878–885.

15. Moya A, Sutton R, Ammirati F, Blanc JJ, Brignole M, Dahm JB. Guidelines for the diagnosis and management of syncope (version 2009). *Eur Heart J*. 2009;30(21):2631–2671.

16. Kavi KS, Gall NP. Trauma and syncope: looking beyond the injury. *Trauma Surg Acute Care Open*. 2023;8(1):e001036.

17. Furlan L, Trombetta L, Casazza G, et al. Syncope time frames for adverse events after emergency department presentation: an individual patient data meta-analysis. *Medicina (Kaunas)*. 2021;57(11).

18. Grubb BP, Karabin B. Syncope: evaluation and management in the geriatric patient. *Clin Geriatr Med*. 2012;28(4):717–728.

19. Costantino G, Furlan R. Syncope risk stratification in the emergency department. *Cardiol Clin*. 2013;31(1):27–38.

20. Blanc JJ, L'her C, Touiza A, Garo B, L'her E, Mansourati J. Prospective evaluation and outcome of patients admitted for syncope over a 1 year period. *Eur Heart J*. 2002;23(10):815–820.

21. Suzuki M, Hori S, Nakamura I, Soejima K, Aikawa N. Long-term survival of Japanese patients transported to an emergency department because of syncope. *Ann Emerg Med*. 2004;44(3):215–221.

22. Sun BC, Emond JA, Camargo Jr CA. Direct medical costs of syncope-related hospitalizations in the United States. *Am J Cardiol*. 2005;95(5):668–671.

23. Costantino G, Perego F, Dipaola F, et al. Short- and long-term prognosis of syncope, risk factors, and role of hospital admission: results from the STePS (Short-Term Prognosis of Syncope) study. *J Am Coll Cardiol*. 2008;51(3):276–283.

24. Dipaola F, Costantino G, Perego F, et al. San Francisco Syncope Rule, Osservatorio Epidemiologico sulla Sincope nel Lazio risk score, and clinical judgment in the assessment of short-term outcome of syncope. *Am J Emerg Med*. 2010;28(4):432–439.

25. Sun BC. Quality-of-life, health service use, and costs associated with syncope. *Prog Cardiovasc Dis*. 2013;55(4):370–375.

26. Kenny RA, Bhangu J, King-Kallimanis BL. Epidemiology of syncope/collapse in younger and older western patient populations. *Prog Cardiovasc Dis*. 2013;55(4):357–363.

27. Garcia-Civera R, Ruiz-Granell R, Morell-Cabedo S, et al. Selective use of diagnostic tests inpatients with syncope of unknown cause. *J Am Coll Cardiol*. 2003;41(5):787–790.

28. Mitro P, Kirsch P, Valočik G, Murín P. A prospective study of the standardized diagnostic evaluation of syncope. *Europace*. 2011;13(4):566–571.

29. Abe H, Kohno R, Oginosawa Y. Characteristics of syncope in Japan and the Pacific rim. *Prog Cardiovasc Dis*. 2013;55(4):364–369.

30. Disertori M, Brignole M, Menozzi C, et al. Management of patients with syncope referred urgently to general hospitals. *Europace*. 2003;5(3):283–291.

31. Shen WK, Sheldon RS, Benditt DG, et al. 2017 ACC/AHA/HRS guideline for the evaluation and management of patients with syncope: a report of the American College of Cardiology/American Heart Association Task Force on Clinical Practice Guidelines and the Heart Rhythm Society. *J Am Coll Cardiol*. 2017;70(5):e39–e110.

32. Huff JS, Decker WW, Quinn JV, et al. Clinical policy: critical issues in the evaluation and management of adult patients presenting to the emergency department with syncope. *J Emerg Nurs*. 2007;33(6):e1–e17.

33. Probst MA, Kanzaria HK, Gbedemah M, Richardson LD, Sun BC. National trends in resource utilization associated with ED visits for syncope. *Am J Emerg Med*. 2015;33(8):998–1001.

34. Edvardsson N, Wolff C, Tsintzos S, Rieger G, Linker NJ. Costs of unstructured investigation of unexplained syncope: insights from a micro-costing analysis of the observational PICTURE registry. *Europace*. 2015;17(7):1141–1148.

35. Hatharasinghe AT, Etebar K, Wolsky R, Akhondi H, Ayutyanont N. An assessment of the diagnostic value in syncope workup: a retrospective study. *HCA Healthc J Med*. 2021;**2**.

36. Kenny RA, O'Shea D, Walker HF. Impact of a dedicated syncope and falls facility for older adults on emergency beds. *Age Ageing*. 2002;31(4):272–275.

37. Farwell DJ and Sulke AN. Does the use of a syncope diagnostic protocol improve the investigation and management of syncope? *Heart*. 2004;90(1):52–58.

38. Barón-Esquivias G, Moreno SG, Martínez Á, et al. Cost of diagnosis and treatment of syncope in patients admitted to a cardiology unit. *Europace*. 2006;8(2):122–127.

39. Tran DT, Sheldon RS, Kaul P, Sandhu RK. The current and future hospitalization cost burden of syncope in Canada. *CJC Open*. 2020;2(4):222–228.

40. Shiyovich A, Munchak I, Zelingher J, Grosbard A, Katz A. Admission for syncope: evaluation, cost and prognosis according to etiology. *Isr Med Assoc J*. 2008;10(2):104–108.

41. Sandhu RK, Tran DT, Sheldon RS, Kaul P. A population-based cohort study evaluating outcomes and costs for syncope presentations to the emergency department. *JACC Clin Electrophysiol*. 2018;4(2):265–273.

42. Thiruganasambandamoorthy V, Sivilotti ML, Le Sage N, et al. Multicenter emergency department validation of the Canadian syncope risk score. *JAMA Intern Med*. 2020;180(5):737–744.

43. Kapoor WN, Vorperian VR, Linzer M. Diagnosing syncope. Part 1: Value of history, physical examination, and electrocardiography. Clinical Efficacy Assessment Project of the American College of Physicians. *Ann Intern Med.* 1997;126(12):989–996.

44. Mendu ML, McAvay G, Lampert R, Stoehr J, Tinetti ME. Yield of diagnostic tests in evaluating syncopal episodes in older patients. *Arch Intern Med.* 2009;169(14):1299–1305.

45. Viau JA, Chaudry H, Hannigan A, Boutet M, Mukarram M, Thiruganasambandamoorthy V. The yield of computed tomography of the head among patients presenting with syncope: a systematic review. *Acad Emerg Med.* 2019;26(5):479–490.

46. Furlan L, Francesco PD, Costantino G, Montano N, et al. Choosing wisely in clinical practice: Embracing critical thinking, striving for safer care. *J Intern Med.* 2022;291(4):397–407.

47. Sheldon RS, Morillo CA, Krahn AD, et al. Standardized approaches to the investigation of syncope: Canadian Cardiovascular Society position paper. *Can J Cardiol.* 2011;27(2):246–253.

48. Goyal N, Donnino MW, Vachhani R, Bajwa R, Ahmad T, Otero R. The utility of head computed tomography in the emergency department evaluation of syncope. *Intern Emerg Med.* 2006;1(2):148–150.

49. Grossman SA, Fischer C, Bar JL, et al. The yield of head CT in syncope: a pilot study. *Intern Emerg Med.* 2007;2(1):46–49.

50. Lasam G, Dudhia J, Anghel S, Brensilver J. Utilization of echocardiogram, carotid ultrasound, and cranial imaging in the inpatient investigation of syncope: its impact on the diagnosis and the patient's length of hospitalization. *Cardiol Res.* 2018;9(4):197–203.

51. İdil H, Kılıç TY. Diagnostic yield of neuroimaging in syncope patients without high-risk symptoms indicating neurological syncope. *Am J Emerg Med.* 2019;37(2):228–230.

52. Krahn AD, Klein GJ, Yee R, Hoch JS, Skanes AC. Cost implications of testing strategy in patients with syncope: randomized assessment of syncope trial. *J Am Coll Cardiol.* 2003;42(3):495–501.

53. Saad Shaukat MH, Shabbir MA, Banerjee R, Desemone J, Lyubarova R. Is our initial evaluation of patients admitted for syncope guideline-directed and cost-effective? *Eur Heart J Case Rep.* 2020;4(2):1–4.

54. Angus S. The cost-effective evaluation of syncope. *Med Clin North Am*, 2016;100(5):1019–1032.

55. Johnson PC, Ammar H, Zohdy W, Fouda R, Govindu R. Yield of diagnostic tests and its impact on cost in adult patients with syncope presenting to a community hospital. *South Med J.* 2014;107(11):707–714.

56. Furlan R, Porta A, Costa F, et al. Oscillatory patterns in sympathetic neural discharge and cardiovascular variables during orthostatic stimulus. *Circulation.* 2000;101(8):886–892.

57. Levinson W, Kallewaard M, Bhatia RS, Wolfson D, Shortt S, Kerr EA. 'Choosing Wisely': a growing international campaign. *BMJ Qual Saf.* 2015;24(2):167–174.

58. Bhatia RS, Levinson W, Shortt S, et al. Measuring the effect of choosing Wisely: an integrated framework to assess campaign impact on low-value care. *BMJ Qual Saf.* 2015;24(8):523–531.

59. Frazier-Mills CG, Johnson LC, Xia Y, Rosemas SC, Franco NC, Pokorney SD. Syncope recurrence and downstream diagnostic testing after insertable cardiac monitor placement for syncope. *Diagnostics (Basel).* 2022;12(8).

60. Rogers JD, Higuera L, Rosemas SC, Cheng YJ, Ziegler PD. Diagnostic sensitivity and cost per diagnosis of ambulatory cardiac monitoring strategies in unexplained syncope patients. *PLoS One*. 2022;17(6):e0270398.

61. Providência R, Candeias R, Morais C, et al. Financial impact of adopting implantable loop recorder diagnostic for unexplained syncope compared with conventional diagnostic pathway in Portugal. *BMC Cardiovasc Disord*. 2014;14:63.

62. Born KB, Levinson W. Choosing wisely campaigns globally: a shared approach to tackling the problem of overuse in healthcare. *J Gen Fam Med*. 2019;20(1):9–12.

63. Grossman AM, Volz KA, Shapiro NI, et al. Comparison of 1-day emergency department observation and inpatient ward for 1-day admissions in syncope patients. *J Emerg Med*. 2016;50(2):217–222.

64. Mechanic OJ, Pascheles CY, Lopez GJ, et al. Using the Boston syncope observation management pathway to reduce hospital admission and adverse outcomes. *West J Emerg Med*. 2019;20(2):250–255.

65. Lin M, Wolfe RE, Shapiro NI, Novack V, Lior Y, Grossman SA. Observation vs admission in syncope: can we predict short length of stays? *Am J Emerg Med*. 2015;33(11):1684–1686.

66. Kenny RA, Brignole M, Dan GA, et al. Syncope unit: rationale and requirement – the European Heart Rhythm Association position statement endorsed by the Heart Rhythm Society. *Europace*. 2015;17(9):1325–1340.

67. Shen WK, Decker WW, Smars PA, et al. Syncope Evaluation in the Emergency Department Study (SEEDS): a multidisciplinary approach to syncope management. *Circulation*. 2004;110(24):3636–3645.

68. Sun BC, McCreath H, Liang LJ, et al. Randomized clinical trial of an emergency department observation syncope protocol versus routine inpatient admission. *Ann Emerg Med*. 2014;64(2):167–175.

69. Ammirati F, Colaceci R, Cesario A, et al. Management of syncope: clinical and economic impact of a Syncope Unit. *Europace*. 2008;10(4):471–476.

70. Sun BC, McCreath H, Liang LJ, et al. Randomized clinical trial of an emergency department observation syncope protocol versus routine inpatient admission. *Ann Emerg Med*. 2014;64(2):167–175.

71. Dipaola F, Shiffer D, Gatti M, Menè R, Solbiati M, Furlan R, et al. Machine learning and syncope management in the ED: the future is coming. *Medicina (Kaunas)*. 2021;57(4).

72. Dipaola F, Gatti M, Pacetti V, et al. Artificial intelligence algorithms and natural language processing for the recognition of syncope patients on emergency department medical records. *J Clin Med*. 2019;8(10).

73. Lee S, Reddy Mudireddy A, Kumar Pasupula D, et al. Novel machine learning approach to predict and personalize length of stay for patients admitted with syncope from the emergency department. *J Pers Med*. 2022;13(1).

3 Etiopathogenesis of Syncope

Lina E. Lombo and Juan Camilo Guzmán

INTRODUCTION

Syncope is not a disease but a symptom common to various conditions. It is defined as a transient loss of consciousness (TLOC) and loss of postural tone due to cerebral hypoperfusion character-ized by rapid onset, short duration, and spontaneous complete recovery. The etiologies of syncope include reflex-mediated, cardiogenic, orthostatic hypotension (OH), and other miscellaneous etiologies (Figure 3.1). Regardless of the cause of syncope, a drop in blood pressure (BP) and the temporary reversible global cerebral hypoperfusion are the final pathways leading to syncope. Although cerebral hypoperfusion causes TLOC, it does not result in neurological sequelae and typically lasts between 30 seconds and less than 5 minutes.[1]

It is critical to distinguish the causal condition of syncope and properly distinguish syncope from other causes of TLOC to ensure the proper prognosis and treatment of patients.

TRANSIENT LOSS OF CONSCIOUSNESS

TLOC is defined as a state of real or apparent loss of consciousness with loss of awareness, characterized by amnesia, abnormal motor control, unresponsiveness, and a short duration. The two major categories of TLOC are traumatic and non-traumatic. Traumatic TLOC is due to head trauma, and its cause is most often evident from obtaining a clinical history and imaging. Causes of nontraumatic TLOC include syncope, epileptic seizures, and psychogenic and rare causes. Distinguishing between nontraumatic causes of TLOC can prove challenging but essential to properly diagnose and treat patients (Figure 3.2).

Epileptic seizures causing TLOC include tonic, clonic, tonic-clonic, and atonic generalized sei-zures. They are characterized by abnormal or excessive brain electrical activity.[2]

Psychogenic TLOC can often be mistaken for epileptic seizures and syncope.[1] It is divided into two groups: psychogenic non-epileptic seizures (PNES) and psychogenic pseudosyncope (PPS). PNES resembles epileptic seizures with abnormal movements and normal brain activity, and PPS resembles syncope without gross movements. Triggers of PNES and PPS can include traumatic life events, mental stimuli, or pain.[3] Reports of patients experiencing both PPS and syncopal episodes have been reported,[4] which can make the distinction between PPS and syncope even more chal-lenging. Additionally, the duration of the apparent TLOC in PSS is long, more than 5 minutes, and may have a high frequency of episodes—several times per day or year.

Rare causes of TLOC have distinct clinical presentations. These causes include intracerebral or subarachnoid hemorrhage, vertebrobasilar and carotid transient ischemic attack, and metabolic disorders such as hypoglycemia, hypoxia, and hyperventilation with hypocapnia.[1]

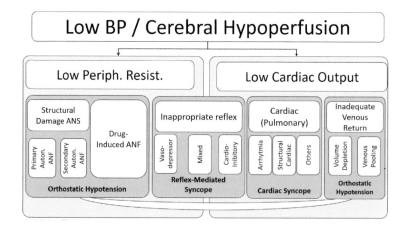

Figure 3.1   Major causes of syncope.

DOI: 10.1201/9781003415855-3

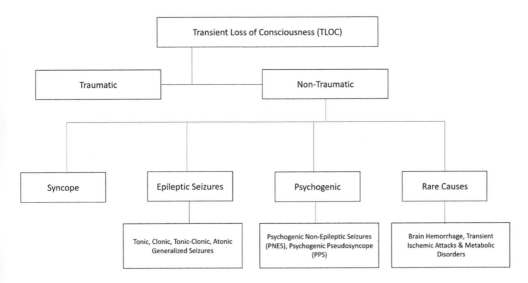

Figure 3.2   Causes of transient loss of consciousness (TLOC).

CEREBRAL PERFUSION AND SYSTEMIC HYPOTENSION

During consciousness, the normal cerebral blood flow (CBF) is about 50 mL/100 g/min, while hypoperfusion occurs when the CBF is below 22 mL/100 g/min. TLOC occurs after 10 seconds of cerebral hypoperfusion. Multiple mechanisms regulate CBF to prevent brain injury. A mean arterial BP (MAP) between 50 and 150 mmHg can maintain a constant CBF.[6] The failure to maintain systemic arterial BP is a central mechanism by which cerebral hypoperfusion occurs in syncope. By definition, the MAP is determined by cardiac output (CO) and total peripheral resistance (TPR). CO is determined by the heart rate (HR) and stroke volume (SV). TPR is determined by the vascular tone of the systemic circulation, vascular structure, and mechanics.[7] A decrease in any of these parameters can lead to syncope.

$$MAP = CO \times TPR$$

$$CO = HR \times SV$$

Etiologies for syncope are divided into three major categories: reflex-mediated, cardiac, and OH. Other miscellaneous causes of syncope include iatrogenic causes (Figure 3.1).

Reflex-Mediated Syncope

Reflex-mediated syncope (RMS), also known as vasovagal syncope (VVS) and neurally mediated syncope, is the most common form of syncope in adults. RMS is a general term used to describe types of syncope resulting in abnormal BP and HR autoregulation and cerebral perfusion, leading to TLOC.

BAROREFLEX AUTONOMIC REGULATION

Normally, the baroreflex regulates BP and CBF. Baroreceptors are stretch-sensitive receptors that respond to changes in BP by increasing or decreasing CO and TPR. These receptors are in the aortic arch and carotid sinus and are connected to the nucleus of the solitary tract (NTS) in the medulla oblongata by the vagus nerve and the glossopharyngeal nerve, respectively. At the NTS, efferent pathways are integrated with the cardioinhibitory and vasomotor centers. These efferent fibers include parasympathetic and sympathetic fibers that pass through the cardiac plexus before synapsing at the heart. During an increase in BP, the NTS stimulates the cardioinhibitory center, resulting in the stimulation of the parasympathetic afferent, the vagus nerve, to decrease HR and SV by activating postganglionic parasympathetic neurons at the sinoatrial node. Conversely, a decrease in BP triggers a decrease in parasympathetic activity, while increasing sympathetic activity increases HR and SV. Additionally, sympathetic innervation of peripheral blood vessels increases vasoconstriction to increase TPR, resulting in an overall increase in BP (Figure 3.3).

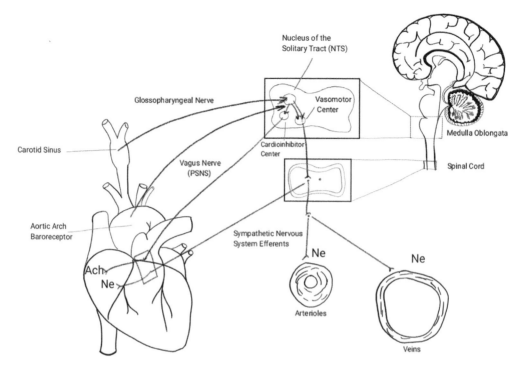

Figure 3.3 Baroreflex.

PATHOPHYSIOLOGY OF RMS

Although the autonomic nervous system mediates RMS, pathophysiological mechanisms are not completely understood. The afferent limb of the baroreflex arc begins with a trigger. Although this trigger may be emotional stress or pain, it is often unidentifiable. It is believed that this trigger, usually in combination with central hypovolemia (from upright posture or dehydration), results in increased cardiac contractility in the setting of a relatively underfilled left ventricle. This may trigger mechanoreceptors in the ventricle that signal via vagal afferents to the central nervous system. This increases the parasympathetic efferent firing at the sinus node and the atrioventricular nodes, leading to bradycardia. The decrease in HR can be profound, with asystole that can last several seconds. Simultaneously, decreased sympathetic activity results in decreased vascular tone in both the arterioles and venules. This results in decreased preload, venous return, ventricular volume, and, subsequently, the MAP, leading to CBF hypoperfusion and syncope. Typically, if the patient falls or is laid supine, the increase in circulating blood volume from the lower extremities, combined with the decreased work necessary to get cerebral hypoperfusion, will cause the patient to regain consciousness rapidly.[8]

Further, subclassifications of RMS pertain to a precise trigger. These include VVS, situational syncope, and syncope due to carotid sinus syndrome. VVS can be triggered by emotional, hemodynamic, or sensory stimuli.[9] Reflex syncope in carotid sinus hypersensitivity syndrome patients is triggered by pressure on the carotid area generally when turning the neck.[9] Situational syncope may be triggered by coughing, micturition, and defecation (see Chapter 2).[10] How each trigger specifically causes syncope is complex and will be expanded upon in Chapter 6.

Cardiac Syncope

Cardiac syncope stems from distinct conditions that lower CO. As previously mentioned, dysregulation and drops in CO will lead to a drop in BP, which can trigger a syncopal episode. There are two major etiological branches in cardiac syncope: structural and electrical. Electrical causes of cardiac syncope include bradyarrhythmia, tachyarrhythmia, inherited channelopathies, and drug-induced arrhythmias (Figure 3.4). During bradyarrhythmia, the decrease in HR is not enough to sustain adequate CO. Conversely, in tachyarrhythmias, the exaggerated increase in HR

Medication Class	Offending drugs
Alpha-1 Antagonists	Doxazosin, Prazosin, Tamsulosin, Terazosin
Alpha-2 Agonists	Clonidine, Guanfacine
Diuretics	Furosemide, Torsemide, Hydrochlorothiazide, Acetazolamide, Spironolactone
Nitrates	Nitroprusside, Isosorbide Dinitrate, Nitroglycerin
Beta-blockers	Propranolol, Metoprolol, Atenolol, Bisoprolol, Carvedilol, Labetalol
Tricyclic Antidepressants	Amitriptyline, Nortriptyline, Imipramine, Desipramine
Phosphodiesterase Inhibitors	Sildenafil, Vardenafil, Tadalafil

Figure 3.4 Medications that may promote orthostatic hypotension.

leads to insufficient ventricular filling, lowering CO.[10] Inherited channelopathies are disorders that affect cardiac ion channels, causing life-threatening arrhythmias that affect CO.[11]

Structural conditions altering CO include ischemic cardiomyopathy, valvular abnormalities (commonly aortic stenosis), nonischemic/dilated cardiomyopathy, hypertrophic obstructive cardiomyopathy (HOCM), and pulmonary emboli.[12] These structural conditions can pertain to the heart or other major vasculature. The mechanism by which structural abnormalities impair CO may be through ventricular filling impairment and arrhythmias.[12,13] Thus, electrical cardiac syncope and structural cardiac syncope are interrelated.

Orthostatic Hypotension

OH is a drop in BP (>20 mmHg systolic and/or >10 mmHg diastolic) that occurs within 3 minutes of standing, is associated with symptoms of orthostatic intolerance, and can lead to syncope. OH is divided into two etiological groups: non-neurogenic OH and neurogenic OH (nOH). Non-neurogenic OH is caused by reduced CO and/or impaired vasoconstriction without a primary autonomic disorder. Conversely, nOH typically results from inadequate vasomotor sympathetic release of norepinephrine due to autonomic dysfunction. This reduction in sympathetic innervation also blunts HR's response less than expected. nOH can be classified into primary and secondary autonomic dysfunction. Among the primary causes of nOH are a group of neurodegenerative diseases characterized pathologically by the deposition of protein alpha-synuclein in the central and peripheral nervous systems, including Parkinson's disease (PD), multiple system atrophy (MSA), pure autonomic failure (PAF), and Lewy body dementia. Secondary autonomic dysfunction includes metabolic conditions, pulmonary hypertension, renal failure, amyloidosis, multiple myeloma, and multiple sclerosis, among other conditions. There are also a variety of metabolic, autoimmune, infiltrative, and paraneoplastic conditions that cause secondary autonomic dysfunction. Among these, diabetes is the most common cause, and about 8% of diabetics develop nOH.

Non-neurogenic causes of OH can include hypovolemia, cardiac pump failure, and venous pooling. Several conditions, including dehydration, chronic bleeding, adrenal insufficiency, diabetes insipidus, diarrhea, and chronic vomiting, can cause hypovolemia. Finally, a common cause of OH leading to syncope is medication side effects, interactions, and polypharmacy. Over 250 medications are associated with OH.[14] The use of diuretics, antihypertensives, antipsychotics, and antidepressants can trigger OH, leading to syncope (Figure 3.4).[15,16]

Other Causes of Syncope

Syncope can be caused by vascular abnormalities that can result in patient morbidity and mortality. These conditions include pulmonary embolism, subclavian steal, aortic dissection, cerebrovascular disease, intracerebral hemorrhage, carotid/vertebral dissection, and abdominal aortic aneurysm.[17]

CONCLUSION

Syncope remains a complex clinical phenomenon that has challenged practitioners for generations. This chapter has delved into the multifaceted etiopathogenesis of syncope, including reflex-mediated, cardiac, and OH. Moreover, since syncope is a symptom of many causes and resembles non-syncopal conditions, a thorough investigation of clinical history, diagnostic tests, and proper differential diagnosis are essential to managing patients with syncope. As the understanding of syncope's etiopathogenesis expands, it is becoming increasingly apparent that a multidisciplinary approach involving collaboration between cardiologists, neurologists, and other specialists is crucial in ensuring diagnosis and effective management. This knowledge will lead to more tailored and effective interventions for patients who experience syncope, ultimately improving the quality of life and reducing the risk associated with TLOC.

REFERENCES

1. Wardrope A, Newberry E, Reuber M. Diagnostic criteria to aid the differential diagnosis of patients presenting with transient loss of consciousness: A systematic review. *Seizure*. 2018 Oct:61:139–148. doi: 10.1016/j.seizure.2018.08.012. Epub 2018 Aug 16.

2. Brignole M, Moya A, de Lange FJ, et al; ESC Scientific Document Group. 2018 ESC Guidelines for the diagnosis and management of syncope. *Eur Heart J*. 2018 Jun 1;39(21):1883–1948. doi: 10.1093/eurheartj/ehy037.

3. Liao Y, Du J, Benditt DG, Jin H. Vasovagal syncope or psychogenic pseudosyncope: a major issue in the differential diagnosis of apparent transient loss of consciousness in children. *Sci Bull* (Beijing). 2022 Aug 31;67(16):1618–1620. doi: 10.1016/j.scib.2022.07.024. Epub 2022 Jul 19.

4. Saal DP, Overdijk MJ, Thijs RD, van Vliet IM, van Dijk JG. Long-term follow-up of psychogenic pseudosyncope. *Neurology*. 2016 Nov 22;87(21):2214–2219. doi: 10.1212/WNL.0000000000003361.

5. Brignole M, Moya A, De Lange FJ, et al. *Eur Heart J*. 2018: 29562304.

6. Ruland S, Aiyagari V. *Hypertension*. 2007: 17353508.

7. Fu Q, Levine BD. *Auton Neurosci*. 2015.

8. Jeanmonod R, Sahni D, Silberman M. *Vasovagal Episode*. StatPearls Publishing, 2023.

9. Mohamed HA. *Libyan J Med*. 2008.

10. Kaufmann H, Norcliffe-Kaufmann L, Palma JA. *N Engl J Med*. 2020: 31914243.

11. Mizrachi EM, Sitammagari KK. *Cardiac Syncope*. StatPearls Publishing, 2023.

12. Van Dijk JG, Wieling W. *Prog Cardiovasc Dis*. 2013: 23472770.

13. Fernández-Falgueras A, Sarquella-Brugada G, Brugada J, Brugada R, Campuzano O. *Biology*. 2017.

14. Suwanwongse K, Shabarek N. *Cureus*. 2020.

15. Bhangu JS, King-Kallimanis B, Cunningham C, Kenny RA. *Age Ageing*. 2014: 24496179.

16. Merck & Co. (2023). www.merckmanuals.com/professional/multimedia/table/some-drug-causes-of-syncope

17. Long B, Koyfman A. *J Emerg Med*. 2017: 28662832.

4 Initial Evaluation and Risk Stratification in Syncope

Robert S. Sheldon, Liane A. Arcinas, Frederik de Lange, and Roopinder Sandhu

THE EPIDEMIOLOGY OF SYNCOPE

The epidemiology of syncope, although seemingly simple, underlies all our efforts toward wrist ratification diagnosis and prediction, and is quite dependent on the setting. In the general population, syncope occurs over a lifetime in at least 40% of people[1,2] and possibly more. The problem arises in that in population-based studies almost all of syncope is quite benign,[3] due to either vasovagal syncope, initial orthostatic hypertension,[4] or hypotension due to drug effects or dehydration. However, much of the literature and our concerns about the diagnosis and risk ratification evaluation of syncope are based on emergency department populations, and these patients are different. There is universal agreement[5,6] that the initial assessment of the patient with syncope should include both an attempt at diagnosis and a risk assessment that should be done even in the absence of a firm diagnosis.

Prevalence versus Cumulative Incidence: Syncope has many causes and clinical presentations, and the incidence depends on the population being evaluated. Estimates of isolated or recurrent syncope may be inaccurate and underestimated because epidemiological data have not been collected in a consistent fashion or because a consistent definition has not been used. Interpretation of the symptoms varies among patients, observers, and healthcare providers. The evaluation is further obscured by the inaccuracy of data collection and by improper diagnosis. Syncope prevalence is a misnomer for an event that occurs intermittently and very briefly, and the term "lifetime cumulative incidence" captures the intended meaning better.[2] Two actuarial time-dependent studies from Canada[1] and the Netherlands[2] both estimated the cumulative incidence of syncope by age 60 to be about 36%, with most cases due to vasovagal syncope. Above this age, the cumulative incidence continues to rise,[7] and although vasovagal syncope continues to be common, various types of cardiac syncope also occur. It seems likely that over a lifetime most people faint at least once.

Community Syncope Populations: The ascribed causes of syncope depend on the setting and population and can vary markedly. An academic outpatient syncope clinic in Amsterdam[3] reported rigorously determined final diagnoses in 264 syncope patients. Patients provided a detailed, structured history and, if necessary, received subsequent investigation and were then followed carefully for a mean of 430 days. Almost all patients were found to have reflex syncope, initial orthostatic hypotension, or syncope with presumed psychological causes. Cardiac syncope was present in only 3%, and fully 17/18 patients with a baseline diagnosis of cardiac syncope suggested by the referring physician were found to have other causes. In observational and randomized studies of VVS[8–11], the median number of historical syncope spells is in the range of 10–20 faints, and the likelihood of fainting again in the next 1–2 years is 30–60%. The strongest predictor of syncope recurrence is the number of faints in the year before specialist assessment.[12] The high number of lifetime spells and high likelihood of recurrence is not generally appreciated, and they are associated with injury, poor quality of life, anxiety, and depression.[13–16] Therefore, in community-based populations, evaluation might focus on the diagnosis of these common, often benign causes and the likelihood of syncope recurrence and its impact on quality of life.

Acute Care Syncope Populations: The issues in the emergency department are quite different. Depending on the country, the admission rate through emergency departments to inpatient hospital beds ranges from 10% to 80%, despite the lack of evidence that hospital admissions reduce mortality.[17,18] Although VVS is not associated with an increased risk of mortality, it remains a significant cause of emergency department visits, costs, morbidities, and reduced quality of life.[5,6] Internationally, the most common apparent cause of syncope in all age groups is reflex syncope, and cardiac syncope becomes more common with advancing age. In the acute care sector, as with community-based syncope clinics, there are surprising findings. The likelihood of death in the first year of follow-up is no longer 25% in patients with apparent cardiac syncope, as reported in the seminal study by Kapoor et al.[19] Solbiati et al.[20] reported a meta-analysis that showed that the 10-day rate of major adverse events was 9%, with death constituting 1%. Even by one year, the risk of death is only 8%. The causes of death over the first year of follow-up as reported in administrative datasets[17] included chronic ischemic heart disease, acute myocardial infarction, lung cancer, chronic obstructive pulmonary disease, cerebrovascular accidents, and heart failure.

DOI: 10.1201/9781003415855-4

Two propensity analyses[17,18] reported that hospital admission is associated with increased mortality[21] when accounting for baseline factors. A large, detailed, prospective observational study of arrhythmic outcomes by[21] reported an extremely low incidence of sudden death, with most causes due to benign and treatable arrhythmias.[22,23]

TAKING A VALUABLE HISTORY

As with almost any clinical entity, the first step in the evaluation of syncope is careful history-taking.[5,6] Gathering a comprehensive history is crucial in identifying (1) if the patient did have a true transient loss of consciousness with the syncopal origin, (2) its potential cause, and (3) high-risk features that warrant further investigation.[5,6]

Establishing Syncope and its Potential Cause: The initial evaluation begins with establishing if the patient experienced a true syncopal episode.[5,6] In approximately 60% of cases, syncope can be identified and differentiated from other causes of transient loss of consciousness through careful history-taking alone in 60% of cases, rising to 90% if performed in an expert syncope unit,[4,6] a definition first proposed in 1992.[24] Most often, patients could provide a history that can confidently identify syncope. Gathering information from witnesses or family members can also provide crucial insights into the nature of the event.

Diagnosing the Cause of Syncope: Once syncope is suspected, the rest of the history-taking process should help delineate the potential cause of the event, which then can direct the diagnostic and therapeutic pathway for syncope.

Important features in history directing the diagnostic pathway include[5,6,25]:

Timing and Circumstances Surrounding the Syncope: A syncope that occurs after pain, an unpleasant sight, micturition, or head rotation is suggestive of a reflex-mediated cause. Syncope occurs with exertion or while supine points to a potential cardiac cause of syncope.

Prodrome: Prodromal symptoms such as pallor, sweating, tunnel vision, nausea, or vomiting typically precede reflex syncope.

Number of Previous Similar Events: A longstanding history of recurrent syncope before the age of 40 years is also usually seen in patients with reflex syncope.

Medical History: Patients with known or suspected structural heart disease, arrhythmias, or previous cardiac events are at higher risk of cardiac causes for syncope.

Medications and Recreational Drugs: Medications and recreational substances, particularly those that can affect the cardiovascular system, should be reviewed. New or increased doses of vasoactive medications can lead to orthostatic hypotension.

Family History: A family history of sudden cardiac death, inheritable arrhythmias, or cardiomyopathy.

Risk Evaluation Features in History: Certain high-risk evidence-based features in the patient's history can indicate a potentially serious underlying cardiovascular condition, necessitating a more in-depth evaluation of syncope.[5,6,25,26] These critical factors should flag a high-risk patient, regardless of initial diagnostic evaluation.

- Loss of consciousness without prodrome, or only with a brief prodrome.
- New onset of chest pain, dyspnea, abdominal pain, headache, and/or neurological deficits.
- Syncope during exertion.
- Syncope during the supine position.
- Presence of known structural heart disease, ischemic heart disease, or previous arrhythmias.
- Family history of inheritable cardiac or arrhythmic conditions, or sudden cardiac death.

CONDUCTING AN INFORMATIVE PHYSICAL EXAMINATION

Physical examination should include[27] supine and standing vitals at 1 minute, 3 minutes, 5 minutes, and 10 minutes of upright posture to identify orthostatic changes in blood pressure and/or heart rate. Bilateral upper arm blood pressure should be used to screen for aortic dissection in selected patients.

A focused physical examination should be done to rule out acute and/or life-threatening conditions, as well as to look for potential etiologies for syncope. These critical factors should flag a high-risk patient, regardless of initial diagnostic evaluation.

High-Risk Features in Physical Examination[5,6,25]

- Evidence of bleeding

- Unexplained systolic blood pressure of <90 mmHg

- Persistent bradycardia (<40 bpm) in an awake state and without physical training

- Undiagnosed systolic murmur

- Discrepant blood pressure in upper limbs

- Focal neurological signs

Electrocardiogram

A resting electrocardiogram (ECG) is recommended for the initial evaluation of all patients with syncope.[5,6]

Features on the ECG that are suggestive of a cardiac origin of syncope include[5,6,28,29]: These critical factors should flag a high-risk patient, regardless of initial diagnostic evaluation.

- Acute ischemic changes

- Mobitz II second degree, high grade, and complete heart block

- Sustained or non-sustained ventricular tachycardia

- Type 1 Brugada pattern

- Prolonged QT

- Persistent inappropriate sinus bradycardia (<40 bpm) or (spontaneous) slow AF (<40 bpm)

- Bundle branch block, intraventricular conduction disturbance, or pathologic q waves suggestive of ischemic heart disease or cardiomyopathy

- Dysfunction of a cardiac implantable electronic device

- Pre-excited QRS complex

- Negative T waves in right precordial leads and/or epsilon wave suspicious for arrhythmogenic cardiomyopathy

USE OF CLINICAL DECISION RULES AND RISK SCORES

Approximately 50% of patients who present to the ED with syncope are admitted (although the rate varies between 12% and 86%).[5,6] The decision for admission is complicated by varying resources available for immediate testing, a lack of consensus on acceptable short-term risk of serious outcomes, varying availability, and the lack of data demonstrating that hospital-based evaluation improves outcomes and expertise of outpatient diagnostic clinics. All studies so far show that the most prevalent cause of syncope in all age groups and all settings [general population,[30] emergency departments,[30] dedicated syncope units[3,4]] is reflex syncope, which is a benign phenomenon. In patients with a presumptive cause of reflex-mediated syncope and no other dangerous medical conditions identified, in-hospital evaluation is unlikely to provide benefit. Unnecessary admission in low-risk patients can even be harmful.[31] The use of clinical decision rules and standardized protocols has not changed this rate significantly until now. Clinical judgment has always been a better tool to predict risk than the clinical decision rules tested so far.[32] The composite estimate of outcomes of these decision rules is that in the next 7–30 days, only 0.8% die and 6.9% have a non-fatal severe outcome while in the emergency departments, while another 3.6% have a post-ED serious outcome,[33] whereas it is crucial to identify these high-risk patients to ensure early, rapid, and intensive investigation, by far not all patients at high-risk need hospitalization (Table 4.1).

Clinical Decision Rules and Risk Scores in Real Life: Individual risk factors and risk scores (Table 4.2) are correlated with short- and long-term clinical outcomes but may not be primary determinants for admission to the hospital. In a recent comparison of different syncope risk scores in a small prospective observational case series, the Canadian Syncope Risk Score (CSRS) may be

Table 4.1: Factors Identifying Risk of Adverse Outcomes in Patients with Syncope

Syncope: High-Risk Features

History	Physical Exam	Electrocardiogram
• No prodrome or only with a brief prodrome	• Unexplained systolic blood pressure <90 or >180 mmHg	• Acute ischemic
• During exertion	• Undiagnosed systolic murmur	• Mobitz II second degree, high grade, and complete heart block
• During supine position	• Persistent bradycardia (<40 bpm) awake and without physical training	• Sustained or non-sustained ventricular tachycardia
• New chest pain, dyspnea, abdominal pain, headache, and/or neurological deficits		• Type 1 Brugada pattern
		• Prolonged QT
• Known structural heart disease or previous arrhythmias	• Discrepant upper limb blood pressures	• Persistent inappropriate sinus bradycardia (<40 bpm) or slow AF (<40 bpm)
• Family history of inheritable cardiac or arrhythmic conditions or sudden cardiac death	• Focal neurological signs	• Bundle branch block, intraventricular conduction disturbance, or pathologic q waves suggestive of ischemic heart disease or cardiomyopathy
		• Dysfunction of a cardiac implantable electronic device
		• Pre-excited QRS complex
		• Negative T waves in right precordial leads and/or epsilon waves

used as a safety risk score for a 30-day risk of major adverse cardiac events (MACE) and mortality after discharge from the emergency department.[34] Although we have to realize that none of these rules are used widely in EDs due to poor sensitivity and specificity reported from external validation, or due to a lack of external validation.[34,35]

Overviewing these clinical decision rules and risk scores shows that older age, history of worrisome cardiac events, syncope with serious heart conditions, e.g., valvular heart disease, and any abnormal ECG, are the features that should be addressed in the clinical work-up of a patient with T-LOC.[5,6,25] The guideline-based initial evaluation as the standard structured approach in the previous chapters consists of thorough history-taking, complete physical examination (including supine and standing BP measurement), and a 12-lead ECG and addresses most of these items properly. Three prospective studies[4,36,37] confirmed the safety and feasibility of the guideline-based structural approach in the ED.

The Canadian Syncope Risk Score: To address the limitations of prior risk scores, the (CSRS) was developed[38] as a tool to identify which patients presenting to the ED with syncope were at risk for serious short-term adverse events (death, myocardial infarction, arrhythmia, structural heart disease, pulmonary embolism, serious hemorrhage, and procedural interventions) within 30 days following ED discharge. A prospective multicenter cohort of new syncope patients was used to validate the CSRS,[39] and no differences were found between observed and predicted risk. The area under the receiver operating characteristic curve was 0.91 (95% CI, 0.88–0.93).

International external validation of the CSRS demonstrated good performance for identifying patients at low risk for serious outcomes and superior performance compared to Osservatorio Epidemiologico della Sincope nel Lazio (OESIL) score.[40] However, this finding was mainly driven by the clinician's presumed initial diagnosis of syncope. The CSRS has also been used[22,23] to identify patients at risk for a serious arrhythmia (arrhythmias, interventions for arrhythmia, and unexplained death) to help inform decisions regarding cardiac monitoring duration. A serious arrhythmic outcome was experienced by 3.7% of syncope patients within 30 days. According to CSRS risk categories, half of arrhythmic outcomes were identified within 2 hours of ED arrival in low-risk patients and within 6 hours in medium- and high-risk patients. Among the medium- and high-risk patients, 91.7% of arrhythmic outcomes occurred within 15 days.[22,23] There were no ventricular arrhythmias or unexplained deaths in the low-risk patients, whereas 0.9% of medium-risk patients, and 6.3% of high-risk patients had experienced an outcome.

Questionable Benefit of Admission: Following an initial evaluation consisting of detailed history, focused physical exam, and 12-lead ECG, one of the roles of risk stratification is to aid

Table 4.2: Risk Scores for Adverse Outcomes in Patients with Syncope

Study	Risk Factors	Outcomes
Martin et al.[42]	Abnormal ECG Age>45 years Heart failure Ventricular arrhythmias	One-year arrhythmic death/severe arrhythmia
Sarasin[43]	Abnormal ECG Age>65 years Heart failure	Arrhythmia
Oesil[44]	Abnormal ECG Age>65 years No prodromes Cardiac history	One-year total mortality
San Francisco Rule[45]	Abnormal ECG Heart failure Dyspnea Hematocrit Systolic BP<90 mmHg	Serious events at seven days
Boston Syncope Rule[46]	Symptoms of acute coronary syndrome Worrisome cardiac history Family history of SCD Valvular heart disease Signs of conduction disease Volume depletion Persistent abnormal vital signs Primary central nervous system event	Reduction of admission 30-day serious events
Del Rosso (EGSYS)[47]	Abnormal ECG/heart disease Palpitations Exertional or supine Precipitant (low-risk factor) Autonomic prodrome (low-risk factors)	Two-year total mortality Cardiac syncope
STePS[28]	Abnormal ECG Trauma No prodrome Male sex	10-day serious events
Syncope risk score[48]	Abnormal ECG: +1 >90 years of age: +1 Male sex: +1 Positive troponin: +1 History of arrhythmia: +1 Systolic BP>160 mm H: +1 Near syncope (a low-risk factor): −1	30-day serious events
Reed et al.[29]	Chest pain associated with syncope Abnormal ECG: HR≤50 bpm/Q waves B-natriuretic peptide≥300 pg/mL Hemoglobin≤90 g/L O_2Sat≤94% on room air Fecal occult blood	One-month serious events
Thiruganasambandamoorthy et al.[38]	Predisposition to vasovagal symptoms: −1 History of heart disease: +1 SBP<90 or >180 mmHg: +2 Elevated troponin: +2 QRS axis<−30 or >100: +1 QRS duration>130 ms (+1) QTc interval>480 ms (+2) Diagnosis of VVS in ED: −2 Diagnosis of cardiac syncope in ED: +2	30-day serious events

decision-making regarding the need for hospital admission. There is consensus among both the U.S. and European guidelines[5,6] that in patients without a serious condition (i.e., possible reflex syncope or low-risk features), hospitalization is unlikely to improve short- and long-term outcomes and these patients should be managed in an outpatient setting. The approach for intermediate-risk patients remains unclear. A structured ED observation protocol (time-limited observation, i.e., 6 to <48 hours and expedited access to cardiac testing/consultation) may be one potential strategy yet is based on sparse data from randomized clinical studies.[41]

The length of stay in the hospital will vary depending on the time it takes to treat an identifiable cause or the diagnostic work-up needed to be performed when syncope at the time of admission is unexplained. The diagnostic work-up should be focused and based on a clear differential diagnosis.

ECG MONITORING

When a syncope patient is admitted to the hospital for further evaluation, guidelines recommend the use of continuous ECG monitoring for those with a suspected cardiac etiology.[5,6] In the absence of high suspicion of an arrhythmic cause for syncope, the diagnostic yield for inpatient telemetry is low and not cost-effective; however, guidelines do not specify when to discharge these patients. In patients with high-risk features and recurrent yet infrequent syncope that remains unexplained after a comprehensive inpatient evaluation, an implantable cardiac monitor may be warranted.[5,6]

The CSRS has also been used to identify patients at risk for arrhythmic outcomes to help inform decisions regarding cardiac monitoring duration and patient disposition.[23] A serious arrhythmic outcome was experienced by 3.7% of syncope patients within 30 days. Very few of these were fatal or potentially fatal. According to the CSRS risk categories, half of the arrhythmic outcomes were identified within 2 hours of ED arrival in low-risk patients and within 6 hours in medium- and high-risk patients. Among the medium- and high-risk patients, 91.7% of arrhythmic outcomes occurred within 15 days. There were no ventricular arrhythmias or unexplained deaths in the low-risk patients, whereas 0.9% of medium-risk patients and 6.3% of high-risk patients had experienced an outcome. Identifying which patients are at high risk for a serious arrhythmia not identified during the ED evaluation and would benefit from further outpatient ECG monitoring remains unclear.

In a second study from the CSRS investigators, the Canadian Arrhythmia Risk Score was developed and comprised of the following variables: lack of vasovagal predisposition, heart disease, any ED systolic blood pressure <90 or >180 mmHg, troponin (>99th percentile), QRS duration >130 ms, QTc interval >480 ms, and ED diagnosis of cardiac/vasovagal syncope. It accurately predicted the diagnosis and treatment of arrhythmias and death within 30 days after ED disposition (C-statistic 0.90 [95% CI=0.87–0.93]).[22] In the overall cohort of 5,010 syncope patients, 2.1% suffered a 30-day arrhythmia/death after ED disposition. A score of ≤0 was associated with <1% risk, scores of 1–3 were associated with 1.9%–7.5% risk, and scores of 4–8 were associated with 14.3%–22.2% risk of arrhythmia or death within 30 days of ED disposition. These data suggest (1) ECG monitoring in the ED for 6 hours and (2) ECG monitoring for 14 days as an outpatient. Serious arrhythmic events are low and further risk stratification with the Canadian Syncope Arrhythmia Score can be performed to safely conduct outpatient rhythm monitoring.

CONCLUSION

These findings prompt three unexpected observations. First, syncope and its direct etiologies are rare causes of death: syncope is safe. Second, to be efficient and economical, searching for an arrhythmic cause requires[22,23] careful patient and test selection and the benefit of hospital admission for this purpose is dubious. Third, the high rate of non-arrhythmic causes of death suggests that syncope may simply be a risk marker that happens to bring a risk-laden patient to medical attention,[17,18] and evaluating all other morbidities may provide optimal patient-oriented care.

Therefore, syncope may not be as complex as it seems. Patients in community-based ambulatory clinics require assessment and care targeting the common causes of reflex syncope, initial orthostatic hypotension, classic orthostatic hypotension, and a gentle search for psychological causes.[3] Patients in acute care settings require an efficient and economic assessment of remediable arrhythmic causes[22,23] and a thorough assessment and management of their co-morbidities.[17,18] Given this accumulating evidence, system research and implementation are needed to improve pre-hospital triage of syncope patients to reduce admission of syncope patients to and through our internationally overcrowded emergency departments.

REFERENCES

1. Serletis A, Rose S, Sheldon AG, Sheldon RS. Vasovagal syncope in medical students and their first-degree relatives. *Eur Heart J.* 2006;27:1965–1970.

2. Ganzeboom KS, Mairuhu G, Reitsma JB, Linzer M, Wieling W, van Dijk N. Lifetime cumulative incidence of syncope in the general population: a study of 549 Dutch subjects aged 35–60 years. *J Cardiovasc Electrophysiol.* 2006;17:1172–1176.

3. de Jong JSY, van Zanten S, Thijs RD, et al. Syncope diagnosis at referral to a tertiary syncope unit: an in-depth analysis of the FAST II. *J Clin Med.* 2023;12:2562.

4. de Jong JSY, Blok MRS, Thijs RD, et al. Diagnostic yield and accuracy in a tertiary referral syncope unit validating the ESC guideline on syncope: a prospective cohort study. *Europace.* 2021;23:797–805.

5. Brignole M, Moya A, de Lange FJ, et al. 2018 ESC guidelines for the diagnosis and management of syncope. *Eur Heart J.* 2018;39:1883–1948.

6. Shen WK, Sheldon RS, Benditt DG, et al. ACC/AHA/HRS guideline for the evaluation and management of patients with syncope: executive summary: A report of the American College of Cardiology/American Heart Association Task Force on Clinical Practice Guidelines and the Heart Rhythm Society. *J Am Coll Cardiol.* 2017;70:620–663.

7. Torabi P, Rivasi G, Hamrefors V, et al. Early and late-onset syncope: insight into mechanisms. *Eur Heart J.* 2022;43:2116–2123.

8. Lei LY, Raj SR, Sheldon RS. Midodrine for the prevention of vasovagal syncope: a systematic review and meta-analysis. *Europace.* 2022;24:1171–1178.

9. Sheldon R, Faris P, Tang A, et al. Midodrine for the prevention of vasovagal syncope: a randomized clinical trial. *Ann Intern Med.* 2021;174:1349–1356.

10. Pournazari P, Sahota I, Sheldon R. High remission rates in vasovagal syncope. *JACC: Clin Electrophysiol.* 2017;3:384–392.

11. Sahota IS, Maxey C, Pournazari P, Sheldon RS. Clusters, gaps, and randomness: vasovagal syncope recurrence patterns. *JACC Clin Electrophysiol.* 2017;3:1046–1053.

12. Sumner GL, Rose MS, Koshman ML, Ritchie D, Sheldon RS. Recent history of vasovagal syncope in a young, referral-based population is a stronger predictor of recurrent syncope than lifetime syncope burden. *J Cardiovasc Electrophysiol.* 2010;21:1375–1380.

13. Jorge J, Raj S, Liang Z, Sheldon R. Quality of life and injury due to vasovagal syncope. *Clin Auton Res.* 2022;32:147–149.

14. Jorge JG, Raj SR, Teixeira PS, Teixeira JAC, Sheldon RS. Likelihood of injury due to vasovagal syncope: a systematic review and meta-analysis. *Europace.* 2021;23:1092–1099.

15. Jorge JG, Pournazari P, Raj SR, Maxey C, Sheldon RS. Frequency of injuries associated with syncope in the prevention of syncope trials. *Europace.* 2020;22:1896–1903.

16. Ng J, Sheldon RS, Ritchie D, Raj V, Raj SR. Reduced quality of life and greater psychological distress in vasovagal syncope patients compared to healthy individuals. *Pacing Clin Electrophysiol.* 2019;42:180–188.

17. Kaul P, Tran DT, Sandhu RK, Solbiati M, Costantino G, Sheldon RS. Lack of benefit from hospitalization in patients with syncope: a propensity analysis. *J Am Coll Emerg Phys Open.* 2020;1:716–722.

18. Probst MA, Su E, Weiss RE, et al. Clinical benefit of hospitalization for older adults with unexplained syncope: a propensity-matched analysis. *Ann Emerg Med.* 2019;74:260–269.

19. Kapoor WN, Karpf M, Wieand S, Peterson JR, Levey GS. A prospective evaluation and follow-up of patients with syncope. *N Engl J Med.* 1983;309:197–204.

20. Solbiati M, Casazza G, Dipaola F, et al. Syncope recurrence and mortality: a systematic review. *Europace.* 2015;17:300–308.

21. Thiruganasambandamoorthy V, Wells GA, Hess EP, Turko E, Perry JJ, Stiell IG. Derivation of a risk scale and quantification of risk factors for serious adverse events in adult emergency department syncope patients. *CJEM*. 2014;16:120–130.

22. Thiruganasambandamoorthy V, Stiell IG, Sivilotti MLA, et al. Predicting short-term risk of arrhythmia among patients with syncope: the Canadian syncope arrhythmia risk score. *Acad Emerg Med*. 2017;24:1315–1326.

23. Thiruganasambandamoorthy V, Rowe BH, Sivilotti MLA, et al. Duration of electrocardiographic monitoring of emergency department patients with syncope. *Circulation*. 2019;139:1396–1406.

24. Sheldon R, Killam S. Methodology of isoproterenol-tilt table testing in patients with syncope. *J Am Coll Cardiol*. 1992;19:773–779.

25. Berecki-Gisolf J, Sheldon A, Wieling W, et al. Identifying cardiac syncope based on clinical history: a literature-based model tested in four independent datasets. *PLoS One*. 2013;8:e75255.

26. Priori SG, Blomström-Lundqvist C, Mazzanti A, et al. 2015 ESC guidelines for the management of patients with ventricular arrhythmias and the prevention of sudden cardiac death: The Task Force for the Management of Patients with Ventricular Arrhythmias and the Prevention of Sudden Cardiac Death of the European Society of Cardiology (ESC). Endorsed by: Association for European Paediatric and Congenital Cardiology (AEPC). *Eur Heart J*. 2015;36:2793–2867.

27. Raj SR, Guzman JC, Harvey P, et al. Canadian Cardiovascular Society position statement on Postural Orthostatic Tachycardia Syndrome (POTS) and related disorders of chronic orthostatic intolerance. *Can J Cardiol*. 2020;36:357–372.

28. Costantino G, Perego F, Dipaola F, et al. Short- and long-term prognosis of syncope, risk factors, and role of hospital admission: results from the STePS (short-term prognosis of syncope) study. *J Am Coll Cardiol*. 2008;51:276–283.

29. Reed MJ, Newby DE, Coull AJ, Prescott RJ, Jacques KG, Gray AJ. The ROSE (risk stratification of syncope in the emergency department) study. *J Am Coll Cardiol*. 2010;55:713–721.

30. Olde Nordkamp LR, van Dijk N, Ganzeboom KS, et al. Syncope prevalence in the ED compared to general practice and population: a strong selection process. *Am J Emerg Med*. 2009;27:271–279.

31. Canzoniero JV, Afshar E, Hedian H, Koch C, Morgan DJ. Unnecessary hospitalization and related harm for patients with low-risk syncope. *JAMA Intern Med*. 2015;175:1065–1067.

32. Costantino G, Sun BC, Barbic F, et al. Syncope clinical management in the emergency department: a consensus from the first international workshop on syncope risk stratification in the emergency department. *Eur Heart J*. 2016;37:1493–1498.

33. Solbiati M, Casazza G, Dipaola F, et al. Syncope recurrence and mortality: a systematic review. *Europace*. 2015;17:300–308.

34. Thiruganasambandamoorthy V, Sivilotti MLA, Le Sage N, et al. Multicenter emergency department validation of the Canadian syncope risk score. *JAMA Intern Med*. 2020;180:737–744.

35. Serrano LA, Hess EP, Bellolio MF, et al. Accuracy and quality of clinical decision rules for syncope in the emergency department: a systematic review and meta-analysis. *Ann Emerg Med*. 2010;56:362–373.e1.

36. van Wijnen VK, Gans ROB, Wieling W, Ter Maaten JC, Harms MPM. Diagnostic accuracy of evaluation of suspected syncope in the emergency department: usual practice vs. ESC guidelines. *BMC Emerg Med*. 2020;20:59.

37. Ghariq M, van den Hout WB, Dekkers OM, et al. Diagnostic and societal impact of implementing the syncope guidelines of the European Society of Cardiology (SYNERGY study). *BMC Med*. 2023;21:365.

38. Thiruganasambandamoorthy V, Kwong K, Wells GA, et al. Development of the Canadian Syncope Risk Score to predict serious adverse events after emergency department assessment of syncope. *CMAJ*. 2016;188:E289–E298.

39. Thiruganasambandamoorthy V, Sivilotti MLA, Le Sage N, et al. Multicenter emergency department validation of the Canadian syncope risk score. *JAMA Intern Med*. 2020;180:737–744.

40. Zimmermann T, du Fay de Lavallaz J, Nestelberger T, et al. International validation of the Canadian syncope risk score: a cohort study. *Ann Intern Med*. 2022;175:783–794.

41. Sun BC, McCreath H, Liang LJ, et al. Randomized clinical trial of an emergency department observation syncope protocol versus routine inpatient admission. *Ann Emerg Med*. 2014;64:167–175.

42. Martin TP, Hanusa BH, Kapoor WN. Risk stratification of patients with syncope. *Ann Emerg Med*. 1997;29:459–466.

43. Sarasin FP. A risk score to predict arrhythmias in patients with unexplained syncope. *Acad Emerg Med*. 2003;10:1312–1317.

44. Colivicchi F, Ammirati F, Melina D, Guido V, Imperoli G, Santini M. Development and prospective validation of a risk stratification system for patients with syncope in the emergency department: the OESIL risk score. *Eur Heart J*. 2003;24:811–819.

45. Quinn JV, Stiell IG, McDermott DA, Sellers KL, Kohn MA, Wells GA. Derivation of the San Francisco Syncope Rule to predict patients with short-term serious outcomes. *Ann Emerg Med*. 2004;43:224–232.

46. Grossman SA, Fischer C, Lipsitz LA, et al. Predicting adverse outcomes in syncope. *J Emerg Med*. 2007;33:233–239.

47. Del Rosso A, Ungar A, Maggi R, et al. Clinical predictors of cardiac syncope at initial evaluation in patients referred urgently to a general hospital: the EGSYS score. *Heart*. 2008;94:1620–1626.

48. Sun BC, Derose SF, Liang LJ, et al. Predictors of 30-day serious events in older patients with syncope. *Ann Emerg Med*. 2009;54:769–778.e1.

5 Diagnostic Tests in Syncope

5A Diagnostic Tests in Syncope

Tilt-Table Testing, Autonomic Tests, and Electrophysiological Study

Wayne O. Adkisson and David G. Benditt

INTRODUCTION

Transient loss of consciousness (TLOC) is a common presenting complaint. The differential diagnosis in such cases may include syncope (i.e., TLOC due to transient self-limited cerebral hypoperfusion), but the clinician must also consider other causes such as seizures, intoxication, accidental falls with a concussion, and metabolic disturbances among other possibilities. Consequently, the first step is determining whether the patient's symptoms are due to syncope or another cause. In this regard, the key available tools are clinical assessment by an experienced practitioner and if necessary selective use of diagnostic tests.

The initial evaluation of the patient with syncope (which typically includes a detailed medical history incorporating eyewitness accounts, when possible, an ECG, and active standing for 3 minutes during a clinic visit) results in a presumptive diagnosis in approximately 50%–60% of cases.[1,2] The diagnostic evaluation for patients *without* a diagnosis after the initial evaluation consists of either trying to formulate a diagnosis by employing selected ancillary tests or the use of long-term ECG monitoring or both. Ancillary testing may provide a satisfactory explanation by presumably mimicking spontaneous events (e.g., vasovagal syncope on tilt-table testing), but sensitivity and specificity are potential problems. On the other hand, ambulatory ECG monitoring requires waiting until there is a recurrence of the clinical event; this entails some concern due to fear of an uncertain outcome but generally has proved safe and effective.

In this chapter, we discuss diagnostic tests commonly used for determining the etiology of syncope when the diagnosis remains in doubt after the initial evaluation. In the EGSYS-2 report, the most common diagnosis after additional diagnostic testing in the group of patients who did not have a diagnosis established after the initial evaluation was reflex syncope (i.e., vasovagal syncope, carotid sinus syndrome, and various situational faints). In addition, of the additional diagnostic tests performed, a tilt-table study had the highest diagnostic yield.[3] Given these observations, we begin with a discussion of tilt-table testing but also include the active standing test as it has greater sensitivity for documenting initial/immediate orthostatic hypotension.

Tilt-Table Testing and Active Standing Test

Changing from a supine to an upright posture causes a large gravitational shift of blood from the chest to the venous capacitance system below the diaphragm. This orthostatic stress may result in two different abnormal responses; the first is a vasovagal reaction which is an expression of a neural reflex susceptibility leading to varying degrees of hypotension and bradycardia. The second response is progressive hypotension, which is an expression of the failure of the compensatory autonomic reflexes to provide appropriate vasoconstriction withstanding. Orthostatic hypotension (OH) has been categorized as initial/immediate, classic, and delayed (Table 5.1).

Table 5.1: Orthostatic Hypotension Consensus Definitions (Freeman R et al, Clin Autonom Res 2011 and Torabi P et al Front Cardiovasc Med 2020)

Orthostatic Hypotension	Timing	BP/HR DiagnosticThreshold
Initial/Immediate	Shortly following movement to upright posture. BP nadir approximately at 10 seconds and typically complete by 20–30 seconds	Transient systolic BP decrease >40 mmHg and/or diastolic >20mmHg
Classic	Occurs 30 sec to 3 min after assuming upright posture	Sustained decrease in systolic BP >20 mmHg and/or diastolic BP >10 mmHg
Delayed	After 3 min of upright posture	Less well defined

DOI: 10.1201/9781003415855-5

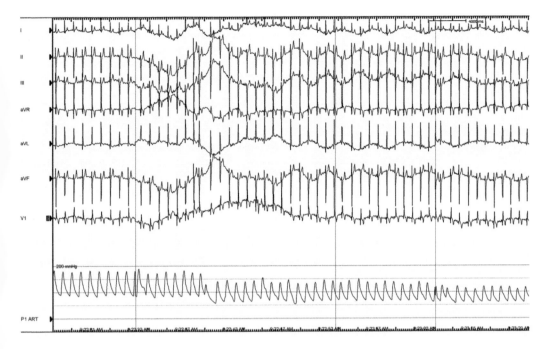

Figure 5.1 Active standing test in an older male with falls. With movement to upright posture (indicated at left by baseline ECG artifact as patient moves from seated to standing) there is a subsequent and persistent fall in BP, compatible with classic Orthostatic hypotension.

Active Standing Test

Prior to the tilt study, some laboratories may include a more formalized active standing test utilizing beat-to-beat BP monitoring, often with a longer duration of active standing than is typically used in the clinic. Active standing is more sensitive in particular for the diagnosis of initial/immediate OH and postural tachycardia syndrome (POTS). In our laboratory, active standing is initiated by movement from a seated position which is easier than moving from a supine position for older or frail individuals. The duration is typically 10 minutes with a chair immediately behind the patient and ongoing close supervision by a nurse or physician to prevent falls (Figure 5.1).

Tilt-Table Testing

Tilt-table testing is indicated soon after the initial evaluation in patients with uncertain syncope when syncope is suspected to be related to a vasovagal mechanism or delayed OH.[4] Tilt testing may not be helpful in other forms of reflex syncope, such as carotid sinus syndrome, cough syncope, post-micturition syncope. In some such cases, specialized evaluation testing may prove helpful (e.g., carotid sinus massage, cough testing, stretch testing).

Tilt testing is not needed in patients whose reflex syncope is already diagnosed by clinical history and in patients with single or rare syncope unless justified by special situations (e.g., injury, anxiety, occupational implications such as aircraft pilots). However, tilt-table testing may be used to help patients recognize symptoms of impending syncope, in order to facilitate their initiation of protective steps such as sitting or lying down, or physical counter-maneuvers (leg muscle tensing, leg crossing, forearm muscle tensing, etc.).[5]

Tilt-table testing has been used to diagnose syncope in elderly patients with unexplained falls. In such cases, the history provided by the patient may be unclear and testing may elicit a reflex faint or orthostatic hypotensive faint. In any case, the patient should be queried to determine whether the test resulted in symptoms similar to spontaneous events.

Tilt-table testing may be useful in distinguishing syncope with abnormal movements from seizures and similarly has been used in patients who fail to respond to anti-seizure medications. In these circumstances, EEG monitoring has been used in conjunction with tilt-table testing.[6] Tilt-table testing (in conjunction with EEG) has been used to distinguish psychogenic pseudo-syncope from VVS.[7]

A variety of protocols have been used for tilt-table testing. In general, the degree of head-up tilt should be between 60° and 80°. When tilt-table testing was first introduced for the syncope evaluation, the head-up tilt duration was 45–60 minutes. Subsequently, modifications to the protocol have resulted in progressive shortening of the test. Currently, the most widely accepted duration of the drug-free baseline tilt is 20 minutes. Noninvasive beat-to-beat blood pressure (BP) monitoring and continuous ECG monitoring are required.

The test is best performed in the morning and in a fasting state (for approximately 3 hours). However, to avoid the confounding issue of fasting-related hypovolemia, IV hydration with 100 mL of normal saline (or lactated Ringer's) per hour of fasting should be provided prior to the tilt-table study.

The use of provocative medications has declined in recent years. Nitroglycerin (0.3–0.4 mg sublingual) is currently the most frequently used agent. Nitroglycerin, especially in the absence of IV volume replacement, frequently results in progressive hypotension leading to symptoms. This should be considered a pharmacologic effect of the medication. If there is an abrupt drop in BP and HR after the administration of NTG, then the observation can be considered a positive, vasovagal, response.

In some laboratories, isoproterenol may still be employed as a provocative agent. However, isoproterenol protocols require more time than those using nitroglycerin, and recently, isoproterenol has become very expensive. If used at all, isoproterenol should be used with caution in patients with known ischemic heart disease or arrhythmias.

Tilt-table testing is safe. There have been no reported deaths during the test. Atrial fibrillation can be induced during or after a positive tilt test and is usually self-limited.

Responses to Tilt Testing

The endpoint of tilt-table testing is the induction of either reflex hypotension/bradycardia or delayed orthostatic hypotension, associated with syncope or severe presyncope. The positive responses have been classified by the Vasovagal Syncope International Study (VASIS) group into three main categories according to the various patterns of blood pressure and heart rate observed during the test.

The *vasovagal* pattern is characterized by an initial phase of rapid and full compensatory reflex adaptation to the upright position resulting in a stabilization of blood pressure and heart rate (HR tends to rise initially and patient may complain of palpitations) and may last for several minutes. The onset of the syncopal vasovagal reaction leads to an abrupt fall in blood pressure and heart rate. The BP fall tends to occur much earlier than the HR but may be subtle and only detected in retrospect. Vasovagal symptoms coincide with this phase. Once the vasovagal reaction starts, it leads to syncope or at least severe near-syncope within a few minutes (in general <3 minutes) (Figure 5.2).

Prodromal symptoms are present in virtually all cases of tilt-induced vasovagal syncope. Syncope typically occurs within 1 minute of the onset of prodromal symptoms. During the prodromal phase, blood pressure falls markedly; this fall frequently precedes a decrease in heart rate, which may be absent at least at the beginning of this phase. When reflex syncope is induced, according to the

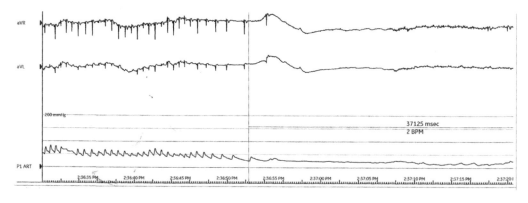

Figure 5.2 Induction of prolonged asystole (approx. 37sec) leading to syncope during a tilt-test in a patient suspected of vasovagal faints. ECG leads aVR and aVL are preset along with beat-0to-beat non-invasive blood pressure tracing. Recovery of heart rate and blood pressure was slow but is seen at far right of tracings. The positive finding helped to convince the patient that the diagnosis was now established, and that she should follow the treatment recommendations.

Table 5.2: VASIS Classification of Tilt-table Responses (Sutton R et al, Eur J Cardiac Pacing & Electrophysiol 1992, Schroeder C, et al, PLoS One 2011)

Class	Description	Typical Occurrence Frequency
VASIS 1	Mixed HR slowing and BP decrease without severe bradycardia	60%
VASIS 2A	Cardioinhibition without asystole	6%
VASIS 2B	Severe cardioinhibition in which asystole is present	2%
VASIS 3	Vasodepression	30%

predominance of hypotension versus bradycardia, the responses are classified as cardioinhibitory, vasodepressor, or mixed and may be further subdivided as in the VASIS classification (Table 5.2).

Orthostatic hypotensive responses are usually distinctly different than the vasovagal response. As noted earlier, the initial/immediate OH response is better detected by the active standing test. The pattern of *delayed (sometimes termed "progressive") orthostatic hypotension* is characterized by an inability to obtain a steady-state adaptation to the upright position, and therefore, there is a slow progressive decrease of blood pressure until symptoms occur. In contrast to a vasovagal event, abrupt bradycardia is absent. Further, in delayed OH there is a gradual decline in BP as opposed to an abrupt drop in BP seen with a vagal vasodepressor event.

The pattern of *delayed orthostatic hypotension plus vasovagal reaction* combines the previous two patterns. Initially, the behavior of blood pressure and heart rate is similar to that of delayed orthostatic hypotension, but later a clear vasovagal reaction develops with the typical fall in heart rate of variable magnitude determining a cardioinhibitory or a mixed response. Syncope occurs at the time of maximum bradycardia.

Autonomic Tests

When there is a suspicion that syncope may be related to OH or severe otherwise unexplained chronotropic incompetence testing of **autonomic function** is often an essential part of the patient's evaluation and may be carried out in the same facility as the tilt-table test. Although we are discussing autonomic testing *after* the review of tilt-table testing, when **autonomic tests** are included as part of the tilt evaluation they are done *prior* to the tilt, usually with the patient sitting.

There are three basic tests of autonomic function that can be performed without the need for specialized equipment: *Valsalva maneuver (VM) and deep breathing,* sometimes referred to as *respiratory sinus arrhythmia.* As with a tilt-table study, beat-to-beat BP and continuous ECG monitoring are required. While it is often considered separately, *carotid sinus massage (CSM)* is a test of autonomic function but is rarely helpful in patients <55 years of age. Other tests such as the quantitative sudomotor axon reflex test (QSART) or the thermoregulatory sweat test or nerve conduction studies are generally the purview of specialized neurology laboratories and are not discussed here.

1. *Valsalva Maneuver*

The Valsalva maneuver (VM) is a forced expiration targeting a pressure of 40 mmHg and maintained for 15 seconds. The glottis should remain open (there needs to be a "leak" in the system which is usually provided by a small hole in the mouthpiece). Patients should be instructed not to take a deep inspiration before starting the VM; the VM should begin after a normal inhalation. The primary weakness of the VM is it is dependent on patient effort. The inability to achieve 40 mmHg and maintain it for 15 seconds impairs the interpretability of the test.

A detailed discussion of the physiologic response to the VM is beyond the scope of this discussion. The interested reader is referred to the explanation in Looga.[8] In brief, the response to VM has been divided into four phases (Figures 5.3 and 5.4). In phase 1, there is an increase in BP related to the rise in intrathoracic pressure due to forced exhalation. Phase two has been subdivided into phase 2a (early) and phase 2b (late).

In phase 2a, as forced exhalation continues the increase in intrathoracic pressure leads to a decline in venous return to the right heart. Of necessity, underfilling of the right ventricular leads to underfilling of the left ventricle, which results in a drop in cardiac output and a drop in BP. In late phase 2, phase 2b, the drop in BP during phase 2a leads to a reflex increase in sympathetic tone. Systemic vascular resistance and HR both increase in healthy responders resulting in correction of the hypotension seen in phase 2b.

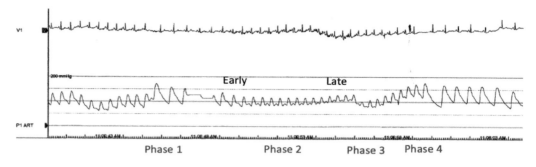

Figure 5.3 The 4 phases of VM are illustrated. Phase 1 blood pressure (BP) rise is due to initiation of increased intrathoracic pressure when subject blows against a 40 mmHg resistance. Phase 2 shows diminution of pulse pressure and increase in heart rate (HR) as venous return is impaired due to high intrathoracic pressure. Note that in this healthy patient the terminal portion of Phase 2 shows an increase in mean BP as a result of increased sympathetic. Phase 3 fall in BP is the result of termination of the forced expiratory resistance. Phase 4 shows a BP overshoot as normal venous return and cardiac output resume with consequent baroreceptor slowing of HR.

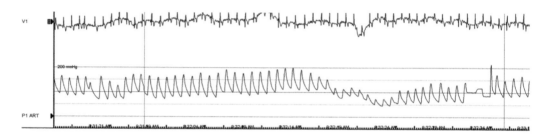

Figure 5.4 Valsalva maneuver recordings in an older male with known autonomic failure. Note that as forced expiration begins there is a moderate increase in BP, but thereafter (Phase 2) the pressure falls dramatically. The test was terminated and BP slowly recovered without overshoot. Additionally, despite hypotension there is no evident chronotropic response.

Phase 3 occurs when forced exhalation ceases. The sudden drop in intrathoracic pressure results in a transient drop in BP. As with phase 1, the change in BP in phase 3 is mechanical—the decrease in intrathoracic pressure is transmitted to the great vessels. The changes in BP seen in phase 1 and phase 3 are not due to changes in autonomic tone.

In phase 4, with normalization of venous return in the face of increased sympathetic tone in healthy individuals there is a dramatic rise in BP that exceeds the baseline BP. The rise in BP triggers, via the baroreceptor reflex, an increase in vagal tone with subsequent slowing of the HR.

There have been multiple methods proposed for analyzing the cardiovascular response to the VM.[9] The most commonly used is the Valsalva Ratio (VR), which is the ratio of the maximal tachycardia (phase 2b or phase 3) and maximal bradycardia in phase 4. Normal values for the VR have been determined for age and gender.[10] However, in the context of syncope due to autonomic dysfunction qualitative interpretation of the VM is sufficient.

2. *Deep Breathing (Respiratory Sinus Arrhythmia)*

Respiration is associated with cyclical HR changes, so-called respiratory sinus arrhythmia. Deep breathing attempts to formalize and quantify the HR response to respiration. As with the VM, deep breathing is dependent on adequate patient effort. The test is performed by having the patient breathe in for 5 seconds and then out for 5 seconds. A variety of phone-based apps intended for stress reduction can be used to assist the patient in the timing of inspiration and expiration. Deep breathing is performed for one minute—six cycles. The difference between the fastest and slowest heart rate during each inspiration and expiration cycle is calculated and then averaged. Age and gender-adjusted normative values are available in the literature. In brief, a difference of ≥15 is normal. A difference of <5–7 is abnormal at any age.

3. *Carotid sinus massage*

Carotid sinus massage (CSM) is generally only recommended in patients >40 years of age in whom the initial evaluation fails to disclose a diagnosis. Occasionally, it may be helpful in syncope patients of any age who had undergone prior neck surgery or irradiation.

To distinguish between cardioinhibitory, vasodepressor, or mixed responses to CSM, the test should be done with beat-to-beat BP monitoring.[11] Additionally, the test is best undertaken with the patient upright but safe, such as in an armchair or secured on a tilt table.

CSM resulting in a ventricular pause of >3 seconds and/or a drop in systolic blood pressure of >50 mmHg defines carotid sinus *hypersensitivity* (CSH). Carotid sinus hypersensitivity is not an infrequent finding in asymptomatic older patients. Therefore, such a finding must be interpreted with caution and not automatically assumed to be diagnostic of the cause of syncope. Importantly, CSH rarely results in syncope in asymptomatic patients undergoing CSM.[12] When an abnormal response to CSM does result in the reproduction of a patient's clinical syncopal episode(s), this is considered to be carotid sinus *syndrome* (CSS). In these circumstances, it is usually necessary to conduct CSM with the patient in an upright position (see above) and the symptom-inducing maneuver is often associated with a ventricular asystole >6 seconds.[13]

Understanding the relationship between CSS and spontaneous, otherwise unexplained, syncope is crucial. This relationship has been studied by comparing the recurrence rate of syncope in patients with and without pacemaker therapy. Two randomized studies demonstrated fewer recurrences at follow-up in patients implanted with pacemakers than in patients without pacing.[14,15] In two other randomized trials, patients with CSS were monitored using implanted devices. The implanted devices commonly record long spontaneous pauses.[16,17] These findings suggest that cardioinhibitory CSS is a strong predictor of future asystolic events.

Electrophysiological Study (EPS)

In the evaluation of the causes of syncope, a positive electrophysiology study (EPS) is most frequently seen in patients with structural heart disease.[18] There are four scenarios when EPS testing might be considered in the evaluation of syncope patients: suspected sinus node disease, bifascicular bundle branch block (impending high-degree AV block), suspected supraventricular tachycardia, and suspected ventricular tachycardia. Indications for EPS and level of evidence are summarized in Table 5.3.

Suspected Sinus Node Disease (SND)

The role of EPS in the evaluation of suspected sinus node dysfunction (SND) is limited. A prolonged sinus node recovery time (SNRT) induced by periods of relatively rapid atrial pacing is associated with a higher likelihood of syncope due to sinus arrest or exit block. In the presence of a prolonged SNRT (SNRT >2 seconds or corrected SNRT >800 ms), sinus node dysfunction may be the cause of syncope. However, while uncontrolled observational reports suggest that pacing may

Table 3: Indications for Electrophysiological Testing in Suspected Syncope (Modified after 2018 ESC Guidelines for Diagnosis and management of Syncope; Syncope Task Force, Eur Heart J 2018;39:1883–1948)

Recommendation	Class	Level of Evidence
EPS is indicated when syncope remains unexplained after initial evaluation in patients…		
….with syncope and previous myocardial infarction or other scar-related conditions	I	B
….with bifasicular block (see text)	IIa	B
….when sinus or other bradycardia is present but ambulatory ECG recordings have failed to document a correlation between symptoms and bradycardia or ambulatory ECG recording is not deemed safe given particular patient circumstances	IIb	B
….with palpitations preceding syncope but initial evaluation including ambulatory ECG have been non-diagnostic	IIB	C

be beneficial in such circumstances, the prognostic value of a prolonged SNRT is at best debatable. In any case, EPS for the detection of SND has largely been supplanted by prolonged electrocardiographic monitoring.

Bundle Branch Block

In patients with syncope and bifascicular bundle branch block, documentation of a prolonged HV interval (i.e., >55 ms) denotes a conduction defect localized in the His-Purkinje system and predicts a higher likelihood of progression to a high-degree AV block. However, only very prolonged HV intervals (i.e., ≥70 ms) are considered diagnostic, whereas intermediate values have a low specificity usually considered insufficient for diagnosis.[19] Documentation of block below the His bundle is also considered pathologic. The number of abnormal results is increased either by stressing the conduction system pharmacologically (infusion of type 1 antiarrhythmic drugs) or by pacing.[20] However, the negative predictive value remains low with as many of a third of patients with a negative EPS for infra-Hisian conduction disease later identified as having significant AV block.[21] As with SND, EPS in patients with syncope and evidence of conduction system disease has largely given way to the use of long-term electrocardiographic monitoring. Recent studies (PRESS, SPRITELY) have not shown a clear benefit of empiric cardiac pacing for the prevention of syncope recurrence, and consequently, in such cases, further diagnostic evaluation is needed.

Suspected Supraventricular Tachycardia

In patients with syncope preceded by sudden and brief palpitations, the induction during EPS of a rapid supraventricular arrhythmia reproducing hypotensive or spontaneous symptoms is usually considered diagnostic. Symptom reproduction may require induction of the arrhythmia with the patient in an upright posture on a tilt table. However, with modern ambulatory ECG monitoring, EPS is rarely necessary for diagnosis. EPS is primarily indicated if a therapeutic procedure, i.e., catheter ablation of the suspected culprit arrhythmia, is being planned during the same session. Further, "palpitations" or "rapid heart beating" as a prodromal symptom in syncope are not definitive for an underlying tachyarrhythmia, as patients with vasovagal syncope may offer the same complaints.

Suspected Ventricular Tachycardia

Spontaneous or inducible sustained monomorphic ventricular tachycardia and/or severely depressed systolic function are the two strongest predictors of a life-threatening arrhythmia being the cause of syncope and, conversely, their absence suggests a more favorable etiology (e.g., vasovagal faint).

EPS with programmed electrical stimulation to unmask ventricular tachyarrhythmias is an effective diagnostic test in patients with prior myocardial infarction (or other cardiomyopathies that result in myocardial scarring) and unexplained syncope.[22] The induction of monomorphic ventricular tachycardia at EPS is thought to be a specific event that should guide therapy; conversely, non-inducibility predicts a low risk of sudden death and ventricular arrhythmias. The induction of polymorphic ventricular tachycardia and/or ventricular fibrillation has low specificity and is of no value in risk stratification and therapeutic decisions (Figure 5.5).

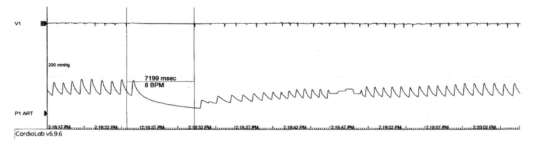

Figure 5.5 Right side carotid sinus massage (CSM) in a seated patient with history of recurrent collapse events. The maneuver resulted in a 7.1 second pause, followed by slow recovery of BP even after return of a reasonable heart rate. These findings are consistent with both cardioinhibitory and vasodepressor physiology, and was supportive of a diagnosis of Carotid Sinus Syndrome in this individual.

It is important to note that patients with heart failure and an indication for ICD therapy according to current guidelines should receive this therapy before and independently of the evaluation of the mechanism of syncope.

In conclusion, programmed ventricular stimulation is indicated only in patients with syncope of unknown etiology and prior myocardial infarction or other disorders resulting in myocardial scar. In these patients, the inducibility of sustained monomorphic ventricular tachycardia is diagnostic of the cause of the syncope; conversely, the non-induction predicts a more favorable outcome.

Exercise Testing

Exercise testing is indicated in patients who experience syncope during or shortly after exertion. The following two situations may be responsible for exercise-related syncope and should be considered separately.

Syncope occurring during active exercise in the presence of structural heart disease is likely to have a cardiac cause. Tachycardia-related exercise-induced second- and third-degree AV block is an ominous finding with frequent progression to chronic AV block. The resting ECG frequently shows an intraventricular conduction abnormality. Hypertrophic cardiomyopathy, anomalous coronary artery origin, and many of the channelopathies may also present with syncope during active exercise. Thus, syncope during active exercise is considered to be high risk. An exception is patients with significant autonomic dysfunction. These patients may also present with syncope during active exercise.

By contrast, post-exertional syncope (either purely hypotensive or hypotensive and bradycardic) is almost invariably due to autonomic failure or a reflex mechanism. In the absence of evident structural heart disease, syncope occurring immediately after exercise in athletes is a benign condition, with a good long-term outcome.

Syncope during active exercise is infrequent. As a consequence, exercise testing is only seldom needed in the evaluation of syncope. However, in patients with chest pain suggestive of ischemia, stress testing (and eventually coronary angiography) is recommended as the first evaluation step soon after the initial evaluation as part of the evaluation of the underlying comorbidities. In this situation, exercise testing (as well as coronary angiography) is not being used as a means of diagnosing the cause of syncope. Overall, exercise testing is appropriate in <10% of patients with uncertain syncope.

Video Recording

Video recording in conjunction with tilt and EEG monitoring has been used in some laboratories. Video recording, along with EEG, aids in the diagnosis of psychogenic pseudo-syncope (PPS) and psychogenic non-epileptic seizures (PNES).

Home video recording of spontaneous events using ubiquitous and widely available "smartphones" may also be useful. This is especially true in patients with PPS or PNES since patients with these conditions tend to have more frequent episodes and a longer duration of episodes.

Other Tests

Echocardiography

While echocardiography is an excellent modality for confirming or refuting, the clinical suspicion of underlying structural heart disease and is invaluable for risk stratification echocardiography rarely identifies the etiology of syncope. Intracardiac masses (e.g., atrial myxoma) may be the best example of an echocardiographic diagnosis in this category but are very rare. Transesophageal echocardiography, computed tomography, magnetic resonance imaging, and pulmonary scintigraphy may be performed in selected cases, when aortic dissection and hematoma, pulmonary embolism, cardiac masses, pericardial and myocardial diseases are suspected, and echocardiography alone has not been diagnostic. None of these studies are indicated in the routine evaluation of a patient with syncope. They should be used to confirm (or refute) the presence of underlying structural heart disease when the initial evaluation raises concerns for structural heart disease.

Blood Pressure Monitoring

Twenty-four-hour ambulatory BP monitoring (ABPM) and home BP monitoring (HBPM) both have a role, albeit limited, in establishing the etiology of syncope. They are most often used in patients suspected of syncope related to orthostatic hypotension. These modalities do not allow for direct correlation with syncope.

An unconscious patient will not be able to obtain a home BP measurement. Home BP monitoring may allow for confirmation that a patient's symptom of near syncope is associated with hypotension. Even then, orthostatic hypotension in this circumstance may be transient. By the time the patient is able to obtain a BP reading, their symptoms may have resolved and the BP may well have returned to normal.

Testing not Indicated in the Evaluation of Syncope

Unnecessary testing adds greatly to the cost of taking care of patients with suspected syncope. In the absence of head trauma, abnormal findings on neurologic or vascular examination, or a high suspicion of a seizure disorder, patients being evaluated for syncope do not need to undergo brain imaging with CT or MRI, ultrasound, or angiographic evaluation of the carotids or vertebral arteries, routine EEG (see special circumstances noted above), or CT evaluation of the aorta or pulmonary vasculature.

Summary of Key Points

- The initial evaluation, including standing BP and an ECG, will establish the diagnosis in most patients.

- Blood tests should be selective and only obtained when clinically indicated.

- Patients deemed at high risk for life-threatening arrhythmias, or falls and injury, should be admitted to the hospital for ECG monitoring and evaluation.

- Tilt-table testing is not needed for diagnosis in patients with typical vasovagal syncope but may be useful to educate the patient regarding the recognition of spells and convince the patient that the clinician's diagnosis is correct.

- Tilt-table testing may be useful for diagnosing classic or delayed orthostatic hypotension (OH), but active standing is better for recognition of initial/immediate OH.

- CSM in patients over 40 years of age may be useful but is to be interpreted with caution as many older individuals exhibit carotid sinus hypersensitivity that is unrelated to their syncope.

- EPS has a limited role but may be considered in patients with underlying structural heart disease or ECG evidence of significant conduction system disease, though extended monitoring with an ICM has been shown to be safe and cost-effective.

- Use of an ICM early in the evaluation is recommended.

REFERENCES

1. van Dijk N, Boer KR, Colman N, et al. High diagnostic yield and accuracy of history, physical examination, and ECG in patients with transient loss of consciousness in FAST: the Fainting Assessment study. *J Cardiovasc Electrophysiol*. 2008;19(1):48–55. https://doi.org/10.1111/j.1540-8167.2007.00984.x.

2. Brignole M, Menozzi C, Bartoletti A, et al. A new management of syncope: prospective systematic guideline-based evaluation of patients referred urgently to general hospitals. *Eur Heart J*. 2006;27(1):76–82. https://doi.org/10.1093/eurheartj/ehi647.

3. Ungar A, Del Rosso A, Giada F, et al. Evaluation of Guidelines in Syncope Study 2 Group. Early and late outcome of treated patients referred for syncope to emergency department: the EGSYS 2 follow-up study. *Eur Heart J*. 2010;31(16):2021–2026. https://doi.org/10.1093/eurheartj/ehq017.

4. Benditt DG, Ferguson DW, Grubb BP, et al. Tilt table testing for assessing syncope. *J Am Coll Cardiol*. 1996;28(1):263–275. https://doi.org/10.1016/0735-1097(96)00236-7.

5. van Dijk N, Quartieri F, Blanc JJ, et al. PC-Trial Investigators. Effectiveness of physical counterpressure maneuvers in preventing vasovagal syncope: the Physical Counterpressure Manoeuvres Trial (PC-Trial). *J Am Coll Cardiol*. 2006;48(8):1652–1657. https://doi.org/10.1016/j.jacc.2006.06.059.

6. Zaidi A, Clough P, Cooper P, Scheepers B, Fitzpatrick AP. Misdiagnosis of epilepsy: many seizure-like attacks have a cardiovascular cause. *J Am Coll Cardiol*. 2000;36(1):181–184. https://doi.org/10.1016/s0735-1097(00)00700-2.

7. Blad H, Lamberts RJ, van Dijk GJ, Thijs RD. Tilt-induced vasovagal syncope and psychogenic pseudosyncope: overlapping clinical entities. *Neurology*. 2015;85(23):2006–2010. https://doi.org/10.1212/WNL.0000000000002184. Erratum in: *Neurology*. 2017;88(3):335.

8. Looga R. The Valsalva manoeuvre--cardiovascular effects and performance technique: a critical review. *Respir Physiol Neurobiol*. 2005;147(1):39–49. https://doi.org/10.1016/j.resp.2005.01.003.

9. Pstras L, Thomaseth K, Waniewski J, Balzani I, Bellavere F. The Valsalva manoeuvre: physiology and clinical examples. *Acta Physiol (Oxf)*. 2016;217(2):103–119. https://doi.org/10.1111/apha.12639.

10. Low PA, Denq JC, Opfer-Gehrking TL, Dyck PJ, O'Brien PC, Slezak JM. Effect of age and gender on sudomotor and cardiovagal function and blood pressure response to tilt in normal subjects. *Muscle Nerve*. 1997;20(12):1561–1568. https://doi.org/10.1002/(SICI)1097-4598(199712)20:12<1561::AID-MUS11>3.0.CO;2-3.

11. Brignole M, Moya A, de Lange FJ, et al. ESC Scientific Document Group. 2018 ESC guidelines for the diagnosis and management of syncope. *Eur Heart J*. 2018;39(21):1883–1948. https://doi.org/10.1093/eurheartj/ehy037.

12. Kerr SR, Pearce MS, Brayne C, Davis RJ, Kenny RA. Carotid sinus hypersensitivity in asymptomatic older persons: implications for diagnosis of syncope and falls. *Arch Intern Med*. 2006;166(5):515–520. https://doi.org/10.1001/archinte.166.5.515.

13. Wieling W, Krediet CT, Solari D, et al. At the heart of the arterial baroreflex: a physiological basis for a new classification of carotid sinus hypersensitivity. *J Intern Med*. 2013;273(4):345–358. https://doi.org/10.1111/joim.12042.

14. Brignole M, Menozzi C, Lolli G, Bottoni N, Gaggioli G. Long-term outcome of paced and nonpaced patients with severe carotid sinus syndrome. *Am J Cardiol*. 1992;69(12):1039–1043. https://doi.org/10.1016/0002-9149(92)90860-2.

15. Claesson JE, Kristensson BE, Edvardsson N, Währborg P. Less syncope and milder symptoms in patients treated with pacing for induced cardioinhibitory carotid sinus syndrome: a randomized study. *Europace*. 2007;9(10):932–936. https://doi.org/10.1093/europace/eum180.

16. Menozzi C, Brignole M, Lolli G, et al. Follow-up of asystolic episodes in patients with cardioinhibitory, neurally mediated syncope and VVI pacemaker. *Am J Cardiol*. 1993;72(15):1152–1155. https://doi.org/10.1016/0002-9149(93)90985-l.

17. Maggi R, Menozzi C, Brignole M, et al. Cardioinhibitory carotid sinus hypersensitivity predicts an asystolic mechanism of spontaneous neurally mediated syncope. *Europace*. 2007;9(8):563–567. https://doi.org/10.1093/europace/eum092.

18. Linzer M, Yang EH, Estes NA 3rd, Wang P, Vorperian VR, Kapoor WN. Diagnosing syncope. Part 2: Unexplained syncope. Clinical efficacy assessment project of the American College of Physicians. *Ann Intern Med*. 1997;127(1):76–86. https://doi.org/10.7326/0003-4819-127-1-199707010-00014.

19. Kalscheur MM, Donateo P, Wenzke KE, Aste M, Oddone D, Solano A, et al. Long-term outcome of patients with bifascicular block and unexplained syncope following cardiac pacing. *Pacing Clin Electrophysiol.* 2016;39(10):1126–1131. https://doi.org/10.1111/pace.12946.

20. Kaul U, Dev V, Narula J, Malhotra AK, Talwar KK, Bhatia ML. Evaluation of patients with bundle branch block and "unexplained" syncope: a study based on comprehensive electrophysiologic testing and ajmaline stress. *Pacing Clin Electrophysiol.* 1988;11(3):289–297. https://doi.org/10.1111/j.1540-8159.1988.tb05006.x.

21. Brignole M, Menozzi C, Moya A, et al. International Study on Syncope of Uncertain Etiology (ISSUE) Investigators. Mechanism of syncope in patients with bundle branch block and negative electrophysiological test. *Circulation.* 2001;104(17):2045–2050. https://doi.org/10.1161/hc4201.097837.

22. Olshansky B, Hahn EA, Hartz VL, Prater SP, Mason JW. Clinical significance of syncope in the electrophysiologic study versus electrocardiographic monitoring (ESVEM) trial. The ESVEM Investigators. *Am Heart J.* 1999;137(5):878–886. https://doi.org/10.1016/s0002-8703(99)70412-6.

5B Diagnostic Tests in Syncope

ECG, Prolonged Ambulatory Monitoring, and Exercise Stress Testing

Matthew T. Bennett and Andrew D. Krahn

BACKGROUND

Syncope is common, affecting more than 35% of the general population at least once in their lifetime, with many of these people having recurrent syncope.[1] Syncope is the resultant symptom from many conditions including those that are malignant, such as ventricular tachycardia (VT), and those that are benign, such as vasovagal syncope (VVS).[2] Furthermore, the treatment of syncope-associated conditions varies widely from invasive devices such as an implantable cardiac defibrillator (ICD) in the case of VT, to simple lifestyle measures in the case of VVS. Given such disparity in prognosis and treatment recommendations, the evaluation of a patient who has had syncope must have a high diagnostic accuracy. In addition, given the financial pressures on many medical systems and the potential impact on patients while awaiting evaluation (anxiety and occupation/driving restrictions), a syncope evaluation must be cost-effective and efficient.

The causes of syncope can be categorized into non-cardiac syncopes such as reflex syncope (vasovagal, situational, and carotid sinus syndrome), orthostatic intolerance (dehydration, medication-related, neurogenic, postural orthostatic tachycardia, and initial orthostatic hypotension), or cardiac syncope (arrhythmic, structural, or cardiopulmonary).[3] The initial syncope evaluation includes a comprehensive history and physical examination that pays particular attention to features supporting or refuting one of these diagnoses (see Chapter 4). In addition, dependent on the clinical suspicion based on the history and physical examination, the diagnostic strategy in the evaluation of syncope may include an assessment of structural heart disease, ischemia, provocative testing, and rhythm monitoring. A comprehensive understanding of how to evaluate a patient who has had syncope will allow the clinician to diagnose, risk stratify, and initiate treatment accurately in a cost-effective and efficient manner. This chapter will focus on the diagnostic tests used in the evaluation of the patient with syncope and dovetail with Chapter 4 which describes the initial evaluation and risk stratification in syncope.

Electrocardiogram (ECG)

The performance of a 12-lead electrocardiogram is recommended for all patients who have had syncope.[3] Although the diagnostic yield of an ECG is fairly low (<5%–12%),[4–6] it is rapid, inexpensive, and widely available. The presence of a high-risk ECG finding (see Table 5.1; Figures 5.1–5.3) can prompt the decision to pursue and direct further evaluation.

Table 5.1: High-Risk Electrocardiogram Features

High-Risk ECG Features

Bradycardia-related	Tachycardia-related
Bifascicular block	Atrial fibrillation, supraventricular tachycardia, or ventricular tachycardia
Intraventricular conduction abnormality (QRS≥120 ms)	Long or short QT interval
Mobitz 1 second-degree AV block with PR prolongation, Mobitz 2 second-degree AV block, complete heart block	Early repolarization
Asymptomatic inappropriate sinus bradycardia (<50 bpm), sinoatrial block, or sinus pause of ≥3 seconds in the absence of negatively chronotropic medications	Brugada pattern
	Features of ARVC (negative T waves in the right precordial leads, epsilon waves, or ventricular late potentials)
	Q waves suggestive of prior myocardial infarction
	Left ventricular hypertrophy
	Ventricular pre-excitation

DOI: 10.1201/9781003415855-6

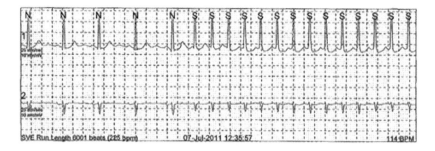

Figure 5.1 Holter monitor tracing showing supraventricular tachycardia.

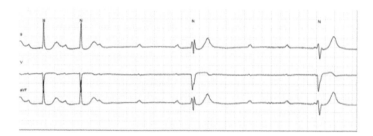

Figure 5.2 Event monitor tracing showing paroxysmal complete heart block.

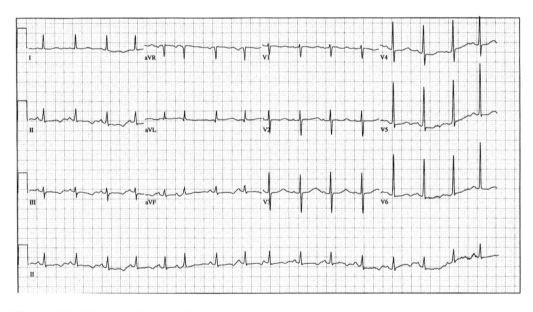

Figure 5.3 Electrocardiogram showing sinus rhythm with prolonged QT interval.

Cardiac Rhythm Monitoring

Extended cardiac rhythm monitoring is used for patients where the cause of syncope is suspected to be due to tachyarrhythmias or bradyarrhythmias where empiric treatment has not been initiated, or where excluding an arrhythmic cause of syncope is necessary. The type and duration of this monitoring are dictated by the frequency and severity of syncope, and the index of suspicion that the primary cause is arrhythmia.[3,7,8]

Holter Monitoring

The Holter monitor is a portable, battery-operated electronic rhythm-recording device that connects to the patient through bipolar electrodes. Data from up to 12 electrocardiographic leads are stored and subsequently analyzed. Additional markers for patient-activated events and time correlates are included to allow greater diagnostic accuracy. Continuous electrocardiographic monitoring is possible for 24–72 hours with conventional Holter monitors.

Holter monitoring has several drawbacks. In patients with syncope, the low likelihood of recurrence during the monitoring period is the major limiting factor. In addition, the physical size of the device may disrupt sleep or discourage participation in activities that precipitate symptoms. Furthermore, Holter monitors must be removed while showering. Lastly, although there are some emerging Holter technologies/data centers that provide real-time monitoring with prescribed notifications, the majority of current Holter monitors have a delay in rhythm analysis and notification.

Patch Recording Devices

Multiple manufacturers produce a single-lead patch cardiac rhythm-recording device that provides minimally invasive intermediate-term (7–14 days) monitoring without the electrodes and battery systems associated with Holter monitors. These patches either record and store the data to be subsequently analyzed, or communicate in real-time via smartphone to a rhythm analysis center. One major advantage is ease of use and patient acceptance, since they are a low-profile single patch like a large dressing, and can get wet, so do not need to be removed. One minor drawback is a single-lead, in contrast to multi-lead, Holter monitors, which aid in morphology and p-wave detection.

Hand Held and Wrist Recorders

Wrist and mobile phone-based recording devices have emerged as minimally invasive technologies with the ability to both record the heart rhythm and identify the absence of a pulse. It must be remembered when considering that the rhythm-recording devices must not solely rely on the patient for activation, as the patient who has had syncope will be incapacitated during the recording time of interest. Having said that, pause or bradycardia/tachycardia notification may provide indirect information, but does not record a rhythm strip.

External Loop Recorders

External loop recorders continuously record and store a single external modified limb lead electrogram with a memory buffer of up to 60 minutes. Following syncope, the patient activates the device which then stores the recorded information for several minutes before and after activation. The captured rhythm strip is then uploaded and analyzed. The recording device is connected to skin electrodes on the patient's chest wall that need to be removed for bathing or showering, require weekly battery changes, and can be uncomfortable during sleep. Although this system could theoretically be used indefinitely, it is commonly used for up to three to four weeks and has largely been supplanted by extended patch monitors.

Vest Technology

Several vendors currently offer wearable monitoring systems that have the potential to acquire and transmit multiple physiologic parameters including the ECG and respiratory parameters.[9–11] Many of these technologies fall within the direct-to-consumer health and fitness sector and have not pursued approval to be used in day-to-day clinical care.

Insertable Cardiac Monitors

The insertable cardiac monitor (ICM, formerly implantable loop recorder) permits prolonged monitoring without external electrodes (Figure 5.4). An ICM is preferred for the evaluation of infrequent recurrent syncope or for syncope suspected to be due to tachy or bradyarrhythmia, when empiric treatment has not been initiated. Similar to the external loop recorder, it is designed to detect arrhythmia and specifically correlate symptoms with recorded cardiac rhythms. The implanted device obviates surface electrodes and accompanying compliance issues. ICMs are much smaller than a conventional pacemaker generator and are typically implanted in the left parasternal pre-pectoral region under a local anesthetic through a minor surgical procedure.[12] These devices use an overwritable memory buffer that continuously monitors and can record the patient's one-lead ECG over a three-year period. Events can be permanently stored on the device through an autoactivation feature (triggered by preprogrammed parameters for tachycardia or

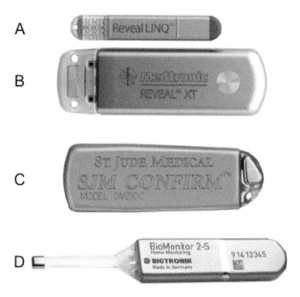

A

B

C

D

Figure 5.4 Examples of currently available insertable cardiac monitors. A: Reveal LINQ (Medtronic), B: Reveal XT (Medtronic), C: Confirm (Abbott, formerly St. Jude Medical), D: BioMonitor 2-S (Biotronik).

bradycardia) or through patient activation, or the device can be programmed to overwrite old events with newly acquired events if memory capacity is needed.[12] These devices are typically connected to remote monitoring, which facilitates memory access when automatic or patient-activated events are stored.

Diagnostic Yield of Prolonged Rhythm Monitoring in Unexplained Syncope

Overall, the diagnostic yield for unexplained syncope depends on the frequency of symptoms, duration of monitoring, and modality of prolonged rhythm recording. For frequent symptoms that occur at least once per week, 24–48 hours of Holter monitoring may be adequate. When symptoms are less frequent symptoms (<1 episode per week but ≥1 episode per month), a patch monitor or cardiac event recorder is preferred. For very infrequent symptoms (<1 episode per month), an ICM should be considered.[13,14]

Although the 24-hour Holter monitor is commonly performed due to its availability, its diagnostic yield is extremely low, and symptom-rhythm correlation is only identified in 2–6%.[15–17] It likely plays a role in primary care as a rule-out test when frequent symptoms correlate with normal rhythm and provide reassurance. Increasing the Holter surveillance duration to 72 hours increases the diagnostic yield to 16%.[18] A head-to-head comparison demonstrated clear incremental benefit to extending monitoring to 14 days, and 81% of patients preferred the patch to Holter monitoring.[19] External cardiac event recorders and ICMs are superior and more cost-effective than conventional Holter monitoring and provide a diagnostic yield of 20%–56% and 42%–87%, respectively.[20–25]

In addition to identifying whether syncope is attributed to arrhythmia, an ICM can also determine whether patients with neurocardiogenic syncope have a cardioinhibitory or solely vasodepressor component and whether they may benefit from a pacemaker. The Second Vasovagal Pacemaker Study randomized 100 patients with a typical history of VVS and a positive tilt table test to a dual-chamber pacemaker programmed DDD with rate drop or ODO.[26] There was no difference in the risk of recurrent syncope within 6 months or enrollment. Presumably, this was due to the dilution of the benefit of pacing for the cohort with a cardioinhibitory component by the cohort with a vasodepressor component. In the ISSUE-3 study, 77 patients who had ICM-documented cardioinhibitory response (syncope with asystole ≥3 seconds or asystole ≥6 seconds not associated with syncope) were randomized to a dual-chamber pacemaker programmed ON vs OFF. During the two-year follow-up, there was a reduction in the rates of syncope from 57% to 25% when the pacemaker was ON.[27]

ECG with High Lead Placement

A type 1 Brugada ECG pattern is characterized by a complete or incomplete right bundle-branch block pattern, with coved ST-segment morphology with at least 2 mm of ST elevation in the right precordial leads (V1–3). In patients suspected to have Brugada syndrome, altering the electrode lead placement from standard to high leads placed 2 intercostal spaces above the standard positions (see Figure 5.5) can expose a type 1 pattern in susceptible patients. The presence of a type 1 Brugada ECG pattern with high electrode lead placement appears to portend a similar prognosis to that of individuals with a type 1 ECG pattern recorded with electrodes in the standard position.[28]

Provocative Testing

The use of provocative testing through intravenous drug infusions may be helpful in making the diagnosis of a hereditary arrhythmia syndrome such as Long QT syndrome (LQTS), Brugada syndrome (BrS), and catecholaminergic ventricular tachycardia (CPVT). These tests are performed in a setting with continuous ECG monitoring and resuscitation capability (both resuscitation equipment and trained personnel). The common medications infused are flecainide, ajmaline, procainamide, or pilsicainide for uncovering a Brugada ECG pattern, epinephrine or adenosine for an LQTS pattern, and epinephrine for CPVT. During testing, 12 lead ECGs are performed before and at regular intervals during medication infusion.[29]

For LQTS and CPVT, exercise is typically preferred for provocation, but may not be feasible for some patients. For LQTS, a provocative epinephrine infusion test is deemed positive if there is a paradoxical QT/QTc response or if there is an increase in the absolute QT interval by 30ms at an epinephrine infusion rate of 0.05 µg/kg/minute,[30] an increase in the absolute QT interval by 35 ms[31] or QTc prolongation by 30 ms[32] at an epinephrine infusion rate of 0.10 µg/kg/minute, or an increase in the QTc by 65 ms[33] or to a value above 600 ms[34] during epinephrine infusions with a rate up to 0.4 µg/kg/minute. In adenosine testing, 6 mg incremental doses to a maximum of 24 mg are rapidly administered intravenously until atrioventricular block or a sinus pause of greater than 3 seconds occurs. At maximal bradycardia, a QT and QTc interval of greater than 410 and 490 ms has a sensitivity of 0.94 and 0.9 and a specificity of 0.94 and 0.85 to detect LQTS, respectively.[35] Both epinephrine and adenosine challenge are rarely performed for the primary purpose of detecting Long QT, given the utility of exercise and genetic testing.

For CPVT, a test is considered positive if bidirectional VT or polymorphic VT is induced during epinephrine infusion. This occurs in 82% of patients with CPVT.[36]

For Brugada syndrome, provocative testing is judged as positive if a type 1 Brugada ECG is detected with sodium channel blocker infusion. In patients with an SCN5A mutation, which is found in only 20% of patients with Brugada syndrome, the sensitivity of provocative testing is approximately 71%–80%.[37,38]

In elderly patients with syncope of unknown origin, there is evidence that adenosine triphosphate (ATP) hypersensitivity may guide pacemaker selection. A positive ATP is diagnosed in

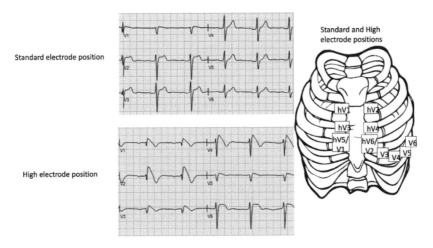

Figure 5.5 Electrocardiograms of Brugada pattern in standard and high precordial leads and electrode placement for standard and high precordial leads.

patients who have atrioventricular or sinoatrial block lasting greater than 10 seconds following a 20 mg IV bolus of ATP. In a single-blind multicenter study in 80 elderly patients (mean age 75.9±7.7 years) with syncope of unknown origin and positive ATP test, active pacing reduced recurrent syncope from 66% to 21% (hazard ratio, 0.25; 95% confidence interval, 0.12–0.56) when compared to back-up pacing.[39] Although this trial supports the use of an ATP test in this group of patients, guidelines have not endorsed it on a broad basis.

Exercise Stress Testing

Exercise stress testing (EST) is often used in the investigation of the patient with syncope, particularly if syncope has occurred during or shortly after exertion. Heart rate, blood pressure, and ECG analysis (heart rhythm, conduction, ST-T waves, and QT dynamics) during and immediately after exercise may uncover syncope attributed to coronary ischemia, tachyarrhythmias (catecholaminergic polymorphic ventricular tachycardia or ventricular fibrillation/tachycardia), exercise-induced AV block, or reflex vasodilation.

Patients with suspected ischemia should have further evaluation.

Evaluating the end of recovery (4 minutes after cessation of exercise) corrected QT interval (QTc) can help to differentiate LQTS from unaffected individuals. At this time point, a QTc cutoff value of 445 ms has a sensitivity and specificity of 92% and 88%, respectively, for distinguishing patients with LQTS from those who do not.[40] This simple cutoff and exercise testing is more accurate in females, though it performs well in both sexes.[41] Bidirectional VT or polymorphic VT is induced during exercise in 63% of patients with CPVT.[36]

Structural Heart Disease Evaluation

As the presence of structural heart disease carries a poor prognosis in the patient who has had syncope, it is essential to consider this in the initial evaluation. In patients suspected of having structural heart disease including those with symptoms, risk factors, physical findings, or a family history of structural heart disease or those with an abnormal ECG, cardiac imaging is recommended.[3] The current imaging test of choice in the evaluation of structural heart disease is echocardiography as it is non-invasive, carries no radiation exposure, and is highly accessible. Further evaluation with cardiac MRI can be considered when abnormalities are suspected but not definitive following echocardiography, or when occult cardiomyopathy is suspected.

Conclusion

A comprehensive understanding of the diagnostic tools for the investigation of syncope and how to use them is critical in the evaluation of a patient who has had syncope. By combining the information gained from the initial evaluation of history, physical examination, and ECG, the clinician can direct further testing to further risk stratify and diagnose the syncope etiology, thereby reducing anxiety and syncope-associated morbidity and mortality. Extended monitoring in multiple formats is increasingly accessible to detect or exclude a culprit arrhythmia.

REFERENCES

1. Ganzeboom KS, Mairuhu G, Reitsma JB, Linzer M, Wieling W, van Dijk N. Lifetime cumulative incidence of syncope in the general population: a study of 549 Dutch subjects aged 35–60 years. *J Cardiovasc Electrophysiol.* 2006;17:1172–1176.

2. Soteriades ES, Evans JC, Larson MG, et al. Incidence and prognosis of syncope. *N Engl J Med.* 2002;347:878–885.

3. Brignole M, Moya A, de Lange FJ, et al. and Group ESCSD. 2018 ESC guidelines for the diagnosis and management of syncope. *Eur Heart J.* 2018;39:1883–1948.

4. Kapoor WN. Syncope. *N Engl J Med.* 2000;343:1856–1862.

5. Martin GJ, Adams SL, Martin HG, Mathews J, Zull D, Scanlon PJ. Prospective evaluation of syncope. *Ann Emerg Med.* 1984;13:499–504.

6. Mitro P, Kirsch P, Valocik G, Murin P. A prospective study of the standardized diagnostic evaluation of syncope. *Europace*. 2011;13:566–571.

7. Primary Writing C, Sandhu RK, Raj SR, et al. Canadian Cardiovascular Society clinical practice update on the assessment and management of syncope. *Can J Cardiol*. 2020;36:1167–1177.

8. Shen WK, Sheldon RS, Benditt DG, et al. 2017 ACC/AHA/HRS guideline for the evaluation and management of patients with syncope: executive summary: a report of the American College of Cardiology/American Heart Association Task Force on Clinical Practice Guidelines and the Heart Rhythm Society. *J Am Coll Cardiol*. 2017;70:620–663.

9. O'Neil BJ, Hoekstra J, Pride YB, et al. Incremental benefit of 80-lead electrocardiogram body surface mapping over the 12-lead electrocardiogram in the detection of acute coronary syndromes in patients without ST-elevation myocardial infarction: Results from the Optimal Cardiovascular Diagnostic Evaluation Enabling Faster Treatment of Myocardial Infarction (OCCULT MI) trial. *Acad Emerg Med*. 2010;17:932–939.

10. Pandian PS, Mohanavelu K, Safeer KP, et al. Smart Vest: wearable multi-parameter remote physiological monitoring system. *Med Eng Phys*. 2008;30:466–477.

11. Haberman ZC, Jahn RT, Bose R, et al. Wireless smartphone ECG enables large-scale screening in diverse populations. *J Cardiovasc Electrophysiol*. 2015;26:520–526.

12. Solbiati M, Casazza G, Dipaola F, et al. Syncope recurrence and mortality: a systematic review. *Europace*. 2015;17:300–308.

13. Zimetbaum P, Goldman A. Ambulatory arrhythmia monitoring: choosing the right device. *Circulation*. 2010;122:1629–1636.

14. Krahn AD, Andrade JG, Deyell MW. Selecting appropriate diagnostic tools for evaluating the patient with syncope/collapse. *Prog Cardiovasc Dis*. 2013;55:402–409.

15. Linzer M, Yang EH, Estes NA, 3rd, Wang P, Vorperian VR, Kapoor WN. Diagnosing syncope. Part 2: Unexplained syncope. Clinical Efficacy Assessment Project of the American College of Physicians. *Ann Intern Med*. 1997;127:76–86.

16. Sarasin FP, Carballo D, Slama S, Louis-Simonet M. Usefulness of 24-h Holter monitoring in patients with unexplained syncope and a high likelihood of arrhythmias. *Int J Cardiol*. 2005;101:203–207.

17. Gibson TC, Heitzman MR. Diagnostic efficacy of 24-hour electrocardiographic monitoring for syncope. *Am J Cardiol*. 1984;53:1013–1017.

18. Croci F, Brignole M, Alboni P, et al. The application of a standardized strategy of evaluation in patients with syncope referred to three syncope units. *Europace*. 2002;4:351–355.

19. Barrett PM, Komatireddy R, Haaser S, et al. Comparison of 24-hour Holter monitoring with 14-day novel adhesive patch electrocardiographic monitoring. *Am J Med*. 2014;127:95 e11–95 e17.

20. Gula LJ, Krahn AD, Massel D, Skanes A, Yee R, Klein GJ. External loop recorders: determinants of diagnostic yield in patients with syncope. *Am Heart J*. 2004;147:644–648.

21. Sivakumaran S, Krahn AD, Klein GJ, et al. A prospective randomized comparison of loop recorders versus Holter monitors in patients with syncope or presyncope. *Am J Med*. 2003;115:1–5.

22. Krahn AD, Klein GJ, Yee R, Takle-Newhouse T, Norris C. Use of an extended monitoring strategy in patients with problematic syncope. Reveal Investigators. *Circulation*. 1999;99:406–410.

23. Seidl K, Rameken M, Breunung S, et al. Diagnostic assessment of recurrent unexplained syncope with a new subcutaneously implantable loop recorder. Reveal-Investigators. *Europace*. 2000;2:256–262.

24. Krahn AD, Klein GJ, Yee R, Skanes AC. Randomized assessment of syncope trial: conventional diagnostic testing versus a prolonged monitoring strategy. *Circulation*. 2001;104:46–51.

25. Krahn AD, Klein GJ, Yee R, Hoch JS, Skanes AC. Cost implications of testing strategy in patients with syncope: randomized assessment of syncope trial. *J Am Coll Cardiol*. 2003;42:495–501.

26. Connolly SJ, Sheldon R, Thorpe KE, et al. Pacemaker therapy for prevention of syncope in patients with recurrent severe vasovagal syncope: Second Vasovagal Pacemaker Study (VPS II): a randomized trial. *JAMA*. 2003;289:2224–2229.

27. Brignole M, Menozzi C, Moya A, et al. and International Study on Syncope of Uncertain Etiology Investigators. Pacemaker therapy in patients with neurally mediated syncope and documented asystole: Third International Study on Syncope of Uncertain Etiology (ISSUE-3): a randomized trial. *Circulation*. 2012;125:2566–2571.

28. Miyamoto K, Yokokawa M, Tanaka K, et al. Diagnostic and prognostic value of a type 1 Brugada electrocardiogram at higher (third or second) V1 to V2 recording in men with Brugada syndrome. *Am J Cardiol*. 2007;99:53–57.

29. Obeyesekere MN, Klein GJ, Modi S, et al. How to perform and interpret provocative testing for the diagnosis of Brugada syndrome, long-QT syndrome, and catecholaminergic polymorphic ventricular tachycardia. *Circ Arrhythm Electrophysiol*. 2011;4:958–964.

30. Ackerman MJ, Khositseth A, Tester DJ, Hejlik JB, Shen WK, Porter CB. Epinephrine-induced QT interval prolongation: a gene-specific paradoxical response in congenital long QT syndrome. *Mayo Clin Proc*. 2002;77:413–421.

31. Shimizu W, Noda T, Takaki H, et al. Diagnostic value of epinephrine test for genotyping LQT1, LQT2, and LQT3 forms of congenital long QT syndrome. *Heart Rhythm*. 2004;1:276–283.

32. Shimizu W, Noda T, Takaki H, et al. Epinephrine unmasks latent mutation carriers with LQT1 form of congenital long-QT syndrome. *J Am Coll Cardiol*. 2003;41:633–642.

33. Krahn AD, Gollob M, Yee R, et al. Diagnosis of unexplained cardiac arrest: role of adrenaline and procainamide infusion. *Circulation*. 2005;112:2228–2234.

34. Kaufman ES, Gorodeski EZ, Dettmer MM, Dikshteyn M. Use of autonomic maneuvers to probe phenotype/genotype discordance in congenital long QT syndrome. *Am J Cardiol*. 2005;96:1425–1430.

35. Viskin S, Rosso R, Rogowski O, et al. Provocation of sudden heart rate oscillation with adenosine exposes abnormal QT responses in patients with long QT syndrome: a bedside test for diagnosing long QT syndrome. *Eur Heart J*. 2006;27:469–475.

36. Sy RW, Gollob MH, Klein GJ, et al. Arrhythmia characterization and long-term outcomes in catecholaminergic polymorphic ventricular tachycardia. *Heart Rhythm*. 2011;8:864–871.

37. Hong K, Brugada J, Oliva A, et al. Value of electrocardiographic parameters and ajmaline test in the diagnosis of Brugada syndrome caused by SCN5A mutations. *Circulation*. 2004;110:3023–3027.

38. Meregalli PG, Ruijter JM, Hofman N, Bezzina CR, Wilde AA, Tan HL. Diagnostic value of flecainide testing in unmasking SCN5A-related Brugada syndrome. *J Cardiovasc Electrophysiol*. 2006;17:857–864.

39. Donateo P, Brignole M, Menozzi C, et al. Mechanism of syncope in patients with positive adenosine triphosphate tests. *J Am Coll Cardiol*. 2003;41:93–98.

40. Chattha IS, Sy RW, Yee R, et al. Utility of the recovery electrocardiogram after exercise: a novel indicator for the diagnosis and genotyping of long QT syndrome? *Heart Rhythm*. 2010;7:906–911.

41. Yee LA, Han HC, Davies B, et al. Sex differences and utility of treadmill testing in long-QT syndrome. *J Am Heart Assoc*. 2022;11:e025108.

6 Reflex Syncope

6A Reflex Syncope

Vasovagal Syncope

William H. Parker, Mark W. Chapleau, and Brian Olshansky

INTRODUCTION

Vasovagal syncope (VVS), also known as neurally mediated syncope or the common faint, results from paradoxical reflex disruption of effective cardiovascular regulation, resulting in transient failure to maintain homeostasis and proper blood flow to vital organs, particularly the brain. Reflex syncope, due to a specific trigger, is termed situational syncope,[1] but the overarching mechanism is related to the same vasovagal reflex. Here, we discuss the causes for and mechanisms of reflex VVS, define specific situational triggers, and consider diagnostic and therapeutic approaches to these common problems.

OVERVIEW OF VVS

Observations regarding fainting date back hundreds of years, but Sir Thomas Lewis, in 1932, characterized vasovagal syncope as a combination of vagal and vasomotor effects.[2] The incidence of clinically apparent reflex syncope in the general population is characterized by a bimodal distribution with peak incidences in teenagers and the elderly.[1] However, no evidence indicates that the vasovagal response itself is necessarily pathologic. The lifetime incidence in females can approach 50% compared to 25% in males,[3] but for most, VVS is a singular event triggered by some specific stimulus. Others have recurrent unexplained episodes that are debilitating.

A careful history is the essential first step to securing a diagnosis of reflex syncope, but further diagnostic evaluation, including electrocardiographic (ECG) monitoring[4] and tilt testing, may be required[5] even though the tilt test has problems with sensitivity and specificity[6] as it does not emulate what happens in real life. Monitoring alone does not explain the mechanism of asystolic fainting nor does it correlate the exact temporal relationship of asystole to syncope. Episodes often begin with a prodrome that can include nausea, diaphoresis, pallor, or a diminution in vision or hearing before collapse. During recovery, profound fatigue is common. A point-scoring questionnaire[7] has an 89% sensitivity and 91% specificity to diagnose VVS even though the gold standard comparison to diagnose VVS is in question.

A reproducible trigger may be present (often in older patients). Underlying acute and transient pathology may be responsible: acute myocardial infarction, aortic stenosis, hypertrophic obstructive cardiomyopathy, pulmonary hypertension, pulmonary embolus, pericardial effusion, and cardiac tamponade are potential causes. In others, daily activities (deglutition, cough, defecation, micturition, vomiting, prolonged standing, heat, noxious stimuli, and pain) can be the precipitant. For the latter group, episodes can be reproducible under similar circumstances or exist as singular events.

Although often considered pathologic, VVS can be a physiologic defense mechanism to protect the brain from ischemic injury. It is not necessarily an abnormal reflex. Much like a turtle's autonomic adjustment to maintain necessary cerebral oxygenation when diving underwater for prolonged periods[8] or a bear's vagal activation to reduce energy consumption when hibernating,[9] so too does our autonomic nervous system attempt to strike a perfect balance to meet instantaneous cardiovascular needs. Loss of consciousness with concomitant loss of muscle tone caused by VVS in humans may have specific benefits as part of the fight/flight response and may be life-saving during drowning.[8]

Cerebral perfusion requires 15%–20% of the cardiac output. Disruption of adequate cerebral blood flow for as little as 6 seconds, particularly to the claustrum, the paraventricular nucleus,[10] and the reticular activating system in the brainstem, can cause syncope. While VVS is generally an isolated low-risk event aside from the risk of injury due to falling, recurrent forms of VVS, whether it be idiopathic in younger individuals or related to the cardiovascular, neurological, or metabolic condition, require further investigation and, possibly, treatment.[11]

CLINICAL FEATURES OF VVS

When VVS affects young individuals in good health, a precursor marked by nausea, pallor, and excess diaphoresis aligned with heightened vagal activity is common.[12] Other prodromal symptoms include lightheadedness, change in perception of temperature, diaphoresis, palpitations,

DOI: 10.1201/9781003415855-7

gastrointestinal upset, visual changes, auditory manifestations, and sensory alterations. Usual triggers and preliminary symptoms provide strong indicators of an overt impending vasovagal response, but a prodrome may or may not be present or associated with a faint. Consequently, VVS may be hard to diagnose. Thus, 20%–30% of those who pass out from an undefined cause most likely have VVS. In the elderly, the history might not conform to the classical pattern observed in younger patients; there may be a specific trigger.[13]

VVS typically occurs while sitting upright or standing, especially for long periods of time. In addition to prolonged standing, VVS triggers include emotional stress, pain, or medical procedures.[4] In younger individuals, this may not be triggered by a defining event. Situational syncope in older adults may have unique triggers including deglutition, cough, etc. VVS is usually brief (seconds to minutes), yet fatigue, after recovery, might persist. Alternatively, arrhythmia-mediated syncope tends to be abrupt, lacking autonomic warning signs or post-event weariness. Seizure disorder may have a prodrome but also has a prolonged recovery.

Current European Society of Cardiology (ESC) guidelines reference a "low BP phenotype" as a subpopulation of reflex syncope.[4,14] This is better elucidated in a subsequent multicohort cross-sectional study demonstrating a different resting hemodynamic profile among patients with reflex syncope versus the general population. Namely, patients with reflex syncope have, on average, lower systolic blood pressure (BP), higher diastolic BP, lower pulse pressure, and higher heart rate (HR). These data suggest reflex syncope patients have lower stroke volume and lower venous return and rely on chronic activation of compensatory mechanisms to maintain cardiac output.[14,15]

Recurrence of reflex syncope varies based on individuals and triggers, but recurrence is common and yet often difficult to predict. In the ISSUE-3 trial, that compared the recurrence of syncope in pacemaker groups to control groups, 57% of the control group experienced a recurrence of syncope over two years.[16] Other data confirm a similar likelihood of recurrence. In patients with recurrent VVS, episodes can occur in clusters or storms of multiple syncopal events over days to weeks, followed by prolonged syncope-free periods.[17] The likely inciting initiating trigger may be excess sympathetic activation. The resulting vasovagal reflex can be a transient and self-limited phenomenon but may present in a malignant and recurrent fashion[17] which can even present as a "storm". Mechanisms driving clusters and periods of remission are uncertain.

Recurrent VVS appears to be more prevalent in certain families, with a higher likelihood of both biological parents experiencing fainting, suggesting a potential genetic component to the disease.[18] One analysis of pooled family data reported that 36%–51% of VVS patients had a family member who fainted versus 28% of controls.[19] Various studies point to genomic sites linked to VVS, but specific genes and pathways remain largely unknown. However, one multigenerational kindred candidate gene study identified three genes associated with VVS.[20] This represents an area of ongoing study.[21]

AUTONOMIC (REFLEX) CONTROL OF BLOOD PRESSURE (BP) AND HEART RATE (HR)

The autonomic nervous system regulates BP, HR, and vascular tone to maintain effective perfusion to vital organs, including during fluid shifts with postural change (Figure 6.1). Arterial baroreceptors, located in the carotid sinuses and aortic arch, and cardiopulmonary baroreceptors in the heart and great veins detect changes in arterial BP and central blood volume (e.g., left ventricular end-diastolic volume and pressure), respectively.[22,23] Afferent baroreceptor activity is transmitted to the nucleus tractus solitarius (NTS) in the medulla oblongata of the central nervous system via the glossopharyngeal (cranial nerve IX) and vagus (cranial nerve X) nerves.

When activated by increased baroreceptor activity (e.g., during increases in BP), the NTS transmits excitatory glutamatergic signals to the caudal ventrolateral medulla (CVLM), which transmits inhibitory GABAnergic signals to the rostral ventrolateral medulla (RVLM) thereby inhibiting the activity of premotor neurons that project to efferent preganglionic sympathetic neurons in the intermediolateral (IML) region of the thoracolumbar spinal cord. Decreases in central blood volume, arterial BP, and baroreceptor activity (as occur with standing) evoke the opposite reflex response, an increase in sympathetic nerve activity (SNA). From the IML, preganglionic sympathetic neurons exit the spinal cord to innervate postganglionic sympathetic neurons that project to arterial and venous blood vessels, the heart, the adrenal medulla, and other organs.

Increased SNA releases norepinephrine. This binds to cardiac β-1 adrenergic receptors to increase HR and myocardial contractility and vascular α-1 adrenergic receptors to increase vascular resistance and decrease venous compliance. Circulating norepinephrine and epinephrine released from the adrenal medulla increase HR and myocardial contractility by binding to

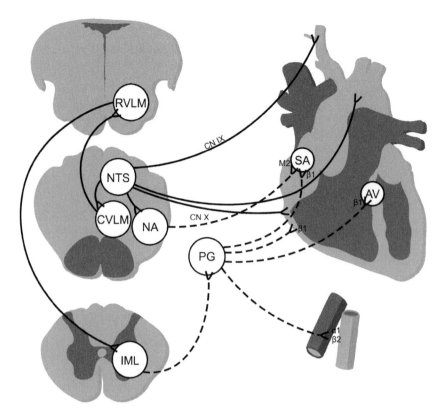

Figure 6.1 Schematic view of autonomic cardiovascular control.

cardiac β-1 adrenergic receptors and may cause vasoconstriction or vasodilation by binding to α-1 and β-2 receptors, respectively. Neuropeptide Y released from sympathetic nerves contributes to sympathetic-mediated vasoconstriction.[24] Arterial and cardiopulmonary baroreflex-mediated increases in vasopressin and renin release (activation of the renin–angiotensin system) also contribute to the vasoconstrictor response to standing.[23,25]

When activated by increased baroreceptor activity, the NTS transmits excitatory glutamatergic signals to the nucleus ambiguus and dorsal motor nucleus of the vagus, leading to increased parasympathetic nerve activity (paraSNA) to the heart, release of the neurotransmitter acetylcholine (Ach), binding of Ach to M2 muscarinic cholinergic receptors, and decreased HR.[23,25] Therefore, when central blood volume and arterial BP have decreased withstanding, the baroreflex inhibits cardiac paraSNA and increases HR.

MECHANISMS OF VVS

During vasovagal syncope, disruption in the normal homeostatic mechanisms occurs; the HR slows, and contractility can become impaired in close association with venous and arteriolar dilation. Although cerebrovascular autoregulation can compensate to a point, decreased blood flow to the reticular activating system and other integrating centers in the brain, including the thalamus[26,27] (even for 6–10 seconds), results in loss of consciousness.[28]

The arterial baroreceptor reflex normally prevents or minimizes orthostatic hypotension. Interestingly, carotid baroreflex sensitivity for control of vascular resistance is increased during 60° head-up tilt in control subjects, underscoring its importance in maintaining BP during orthostatic stress.[29] In contrast, this reflex was unchanged during head-up tilt in patients with suspected prior syncope and documented orthostatic intolerance to lower body negative pressure.[29]

The mechanisms that evoke VVS have been investigated and debated for decades. Preclinical studies have shown that severe hemorrhage and the associated decrease in central blood volume evoke paradoxical activation of mechanosensitive vagal C-fiber afferents and reflex activation of paraSNA to the heart and reflex inhibition of SNA to peripheral blood vessels.[30] Hypercontraction of an under-filled left ventricle induced by baroreflex-mediated increases in cardiac SNA and myocardial contractility is thought to cause the paradoxical mechanical activation of vagal afferents.[31] Similarly, venous pooling of blood during orthostatic stress decreases end-diastolic volume, stroke volume, cardiac output, and arterial BP followed by baroreflex-mediated increases in cardiac SNA and myocardial contractility. The role of cardiac sensory neurons in syncope has been challenged. Upright tilt-induced bradycardia, hypotension, and VVS have been demonstrated in patients after heart transplant where the heart is denervated.[32] Furthermore, measurements of left ventricular volume, stroke volume, and ejection fraction in subjects with and without VVS during upright tilt have supported[33–35] and not supported[36] the hypothesis that mechanical activation of vagal afferents triggers VVS in humans.

C-fiber vagal afferents innervating the left ventricle are also chemosensitive. Activation of C-fiber vagal afferents by metabolites, such as prostacyclin, serotonin, bradykinin, protons, and the TRPV1 agonist capsaicin, also triggers reflex inhibition of peripheral SNA, excitation of cardiac paraSNA, decreased peripheral resistance, decreased HR, and hypotension—referred to as the Bezold–Jarisch reflex.[37] Cardiac C-fiber afferents are often polymodal; metabolites produced in the heart may sensitize afferent terminals to mechanical stimulation. Interestingly, while activation of the Bezold–Jarisch reflex inhibits peripheral SNA, it exerts both inhibitory and excitatory effects on cardiac sympathetic nerve activity,[38,39] suggesting the possibility of differential effects on neuronal subtypes. Activation of the Bezold–Jarisch reflex also inhibits arterial baroreflex sensitivity via a central interaction,[40] which may contribute to orthostatic hypotension and VVS. Selective optogenetic activation of cardiac vagal afferent neurons expressing the neuropeptide Y type 2 receptor in mice evoked the classic Bezold–Jarisch reflex: bradycardia, hypotension, and decreased breathing, accompanied by syncope.[41] Ablation of these neurons abolished the reflex.[41]

VVS triggered by emotion, anxiety, or pain suggests a central mechanism mediated by brainstem interactions with higher centers committed to psychological stress and pain sensation (e.g., hypothalamus, cerebral cortex). Sensory inputs from peripheral organ systems and humoral factors may also contribute to the occurrence of VVS. Dynamic sinusoidal stimulation of the vestibulo-sympathetic reflex induces oscillations in BP and HR and subsequent vasovagal responses in rats,[42] while habituation of this reflex over days suppressed vasovagal responses.[43]

Hyperventilation induced by anxiety or emotion will decrease arterial carbon dioxide levels. The removal of the cerebral vasodilator influence of CO_2 causes cerebral vasoconstriction that can provoke syncope.[44] The proinflammatory cytokine tumor necrosis factor-alpha (TNF-α) elicits autonomic dysfunction and pathology through multiple effects on vago-vagal reflex circuits in the brainstem.[45] Epinephrine released from the adrenal medulla during orthostatic stress contributes to hypotension and syncope via β-2 adrenergic receptor-mediated vasodilation in skeletal muscle.[46–48] Multiple mechanisms can contribute to VVS.

There are various central neurological locations that lead to complex sympathetic and parasympathetic nerve processing of the afferent signals. Ironically, tonic vagal activation may inhibit the vasovagal reflex, whereas phasic or rapid parasympathetic activation occurs somewhere after the onset of the reflex to offset transient sympathetic activation. As vasodilation often proceeds changes in HR and as changes in HR start from a tachycardic response that becomes bradycardic, the process appears to involve a dynamic between the sympathetic and parasympathetic limbs, but the link between sympathoinhibition causing vasodilation peripherally and vagal activation causing bradycardia or asystole remains uncertain.

Manifestations may vary in any given individual and can include bradycardia, asystole, hypotension, a negative inotropic effect, and cerebral vasoconstriction. Furthermore, once the reflex manifests, mechanisms responsible for its resolution remain unexplored. During the vasovagal reflex, within seconds, there is a corrective response that can take a while to resolve completely but, nevertheless, prevent serious cerebrovascular repercussions even if asystolic pause and hypotension persist.

Even for those who are susceptible, the reflex is not necessarily reproducible under similar circumstances and can change over time. Why younger females and older individuals have a greater propensity to VVS is uncertain. Further, the vasovagal reflex may be life-threatening in individuals with severe underlying cardiomyopathies as it can be a final death knell causing asystole in a patient with end-stage cardiomyopathy and heart failure.[49]

Although heart responses are tightly regulated by various ganglionated plexi located in the epicardium, locations for the processing and the severity of the processing and specific ganglionated plexi remain uncertain as to their ability to generate the vasovagal reflex. The interaction between the ganglia and a global vago-sympathetic response is not well explored. Additionally, in the nucleus accumbens, nucleus tractus, and nucleus ambiguus, processing that takes place has not been well-characterized. Regulation between peripheral autonomic reflexes and the presence of loss of consciousness is only associated but, mechanistically, may not necessarily be tied tightly as central mechanisms may affect loss of consciousness or alterations in consciousness directly independent of peripheral hemodynamic alterations.[50,51]

What has been shown with tilt-table testing is that there is an early elevation in HR likely due to sympathetic activation followed by bradycardia and even asystole. This can occur concomitant to or just after there is intense sympatho-inhibition as seen by measurements of integrated sympathetic peroneal nerve traffic.[24]

HEMODYNAMIC CHANGES IN VVS

Traditionally, patients with VVS have been categorized into three subtypes depending on the predominant hemodynamic changes occurring prior to and during the syncopal event.[52] Cardioinhibitory VVS is characterized by a drop in HR, often <30 bpm, with periods of asystole and advanced AV block. A transient increase in parasympathetic activation is thought to drive this subtype. The vasodepressor subtype is characterized by a drop in systemic arterial pressure irrespective of changes in HR, with SBP often dropping below 60 mmHg at the level of the heart. A transiently decreased peripheral sympathetic tone is thought to drive this subtype. The third subtype, the most common form, is a mixed cardioinhibitory and vasodepressor response. However, for any individual with a propensity for VVS, there is no reason that one subtype is manifest. On the contrary, many individuals have one response seen on a loop recorder and a different response on a tilt-table test, but there is no reason to suspect that different responses could and do occur spontaneously.[4] Mechanisms of vasovagal syncope, even in the young, can vary such that some individuals have reduced vascular resistance versus reduced cardiac output.[53]

These subtypes of VVS, often defined by tilt-table testing, represent an oversimplified and partly factitious description of VVS. In reality, there is a high degree of inter- and intra-individual variability in tilt-table outcomes,[54] and almost all syncope patients with positive tilt testing demonstrate a combination of cardioinhibitory and vasodepressor responses.[55] Furthermore, the specific response seen on a tilt-table test does not indicate a specific action. For example, marked asystole on the tilt-table does not necessarily require ablation or pacemaker intervention.[56] Nonetheless, current ESC syncope guidelines still use these definitions to guide therapy.[4]

A modern description of VVS summarizes combined cardioinhibitory and vasodepressor responses in four phases.[55] In phase 1, there is early stability during orthostatic challenges, such as standing or tilt up. The gravity shift that accompanies standing pushes approximately 500–1,000 mL of dedicated cerebral blood volume in the thorax below the diaphragm with most of the venous pooling within the first 10 seconds of postural change.[57] HR increases may not be enough to compensate for the decrease in preload and stroke volume, the culmination of which is a drop in cardiac output by 10%–20%. Systolic blood pressure (SBP) change is variable, but baroreflex-mediated vasoconstriction causes systemic vascular resistance (SVR) and diastolic blood pressure (DBP) to increase to maintain mean arterial pressure (MAP).

Phase 2 is characterized by circulatory instability and "presyncope." A progressive increase in SVR reduces cardiac output with an eventual drop in SBP by about 20 mmHg on average. Cerebral blood volume is mildly reduced due mostly to a drop in MAP and cerebrovascular constriction to a lesser extent.[39]

Phase 3 is characterized by terminal hypotension and syncope. Reduced brainstem perfusion is rapid with a fall in SBP by about 50 mmHg on average over the final 30–60 seconds before syncope. MAP and HR decrease, with simultaneous symptoms of autonomic activation including warmth and nausea. A fall in HR occurs after a fall in MAP. The fall in MAP is attributed to decreased cardiac output (35%–48% from baseline) rather than decreased vascular tone, as SVR appears to be increased throughout phase three.

Phase 4 is the recovery phase, when the table is tilted to its horizontal starting position. In this phase, there is a rapid improvement in venous return, an increase in preload, and an increase in cardiac output. MAP recovers within 30 seconds and may temporarily elevate above the starting MAP. HR rapidly recovers to baseline.[55]

NEUROHORMONAL INVOLVEMENT IN VVS

Neurohormonal shifts occur during VVS, but the mechanistic relationship to VVS is unknown.[39] A notable early rise in circulating epinephrine occurs before syncope during tilt testing, reaching values of 6–16 times baseline,[11] whereas those who do not have VVS on tilt testing have a more marked elevation in norepinephrine. Elevated urinary epinephrine levels are present in blood donors who experienced syncope during donation compared to those who did not experience syncope with blood donation.[48] A trend toward norepinephrine elevations immediately preceding syncope is less consistent. A disproportionate rise in epinephrine over norepinephrine during tilt testing appears to predict patients who will experience VVS.[47]

Adenosine is proposed as a regulator of VVS.[58] In addition to its well-known inhibitory cardiovascular actions, adenosine has a sympathoexcitatory effect mediated via baroreflex, similar to isoproterenol, which may feed into the aforementioned autonomic cascade.[59] Theophylline has been considered a therapy for this subset of patients with syncope, but data are limited.

Additional hormone shifts studied in the context of VVS include arginine vasopressin, adrenomedullin, atrial and brain natriuretic peptides, endothelin-1, and opioids.[11,13,60,61] Nonetheless, it is currently uncertain whether these various agents collectively or individually directly impact the pathophysiology of VVS or if they primarily represent a compensatory reaction to a developing hemodynamic shift.

SYMPATHETIC AND PARASYMPATHETIC ACTIVITY IN VVS

Muscle sympathetic nerve activity (MSNA) can be recorded from the peroneal nerve using microneurography alongside hemodynamic measurements during tilt testing to directly measure beat-to-beat changes in MSNA, BP, and HR throughout the phases of VVS. Enhanced MSNA correlates well with increases in DBP due to sympathetic-mediated vasoconstriction in non-syncopal patients,[24] but the opposite occurs during VVS.

The autonomic progression of VVS occurs in stages following the transition from supine to head-up positioning on tilt testing.[24,62,63] During the first few minutes of head-up tilt, baroreflex-mediated increases in HR, MSNA, and peripheral vascular resistance maintain BP. Interestingly, these changes are accompanied by increases in the amplitude of low-frequency (LF, ~0.1 Hz) oscillations of MSNA and BP and a decrease in the amplitude of high-frequency (HF) oscillations of HR (pulse interval) in phase with breathing.[24,62,63] The decrease in HF-HR variability reflects decreased paraSNA in the heart. Continued venous pooling of blood and decreases in left ventricular stroke volume and cardiac output lead to a slow decrease in BP accompanied by decreases in the amplitude of LF-MSNA oscillations despite continued elevation in mean MSNA and LF-BP variability.[62] Subjects destined to faint demonstrate further decreases in LF-MSNA oscillations followed by sudden cessation of MSNA and marked decreases in HR and BP (presyncope) prior to syncope.[24,50,62,63] The mechanisms that cause orthostatic hypotension and rapid conversion from cardiac sympathetic to parasympathetic dominance at syncope include (1) loss of baroreceptor reflex sensitivity; (2) activation of left ventricular vagal afferent C-fibers by hypercontraction of the under-filled ventricle (as evoked by increased cardiac SNA) and/or chemical factors generated in the stressed heart; (3) sensory inputs from other organs (e.g., gut, bladder, kidney, vestibular system); and (4) central nervous system mechanisms invoked by psychological stress, emotion, or pain.

EVALUATION

The differential diagnosis for syncope is broad. Many conditions mimic syncope. On the differential are cardiac (non-autonomically mediated) syncope and orthostatic hypotension. Neurogenic orthostatic hypotension is often conflated with VVS. However, these can be differentiated based on hemodynamic response to tilt testing.[64,65] Non-syncopal episodes can also be confused for VVS, including seizures, hypoglycemia, chemical intoxication, narcolepsy, psychogenic pseudosyncope, and orthopedic falls.

Tilt testing can diagnose and assess conditions including reflex syncope, autonomic failure, delayed orthostatic hypotension, and postural orthostatic tachycardia syndrome and distinguish syncope from psychogenic pseudosyncope. While it has limited value in evaluating treatment effectiveness,[66] it can demonstrate susceptibility to reflex syncope and indicate when to initiate treatment. The specificity of tilt testing is limited in diagnosing reflex syncope, however.[67,68] While 92% of VVS patients show a positive tilt-test result, 47% of those with arrhythmic syncope also exhibit a positive tilt test.[6]

Furthermore, the introduction of pharmacological provocation (such as sublingual nitroglycerin or isoproterenol) raises the risk of inducing syncope during tilt testing, even in individuals who have never experienced a syncopal episode.[4,69] While a negative tilt-table response does not exclude a diagnosis of reflex syncope, a positive test does not necessarily indicate the cause for syncope. ESC guidelines clarify that tilt-table testing should be viewed to reveal a hypotensive tendency rather than for a definitive diagnosis of VVS.[4] A markedly positive test (marked asystole, for example) alone though is no reason to proceed with aggressive interventions.[56]

AMBULATORY VITAL SIGNS AND RHYTHM MONITORING

Key autonomic function tests include orthostatic vital signs as part of an active stand test, the Valsalva maneuver, deep breathing, and other assessments. With Valsalva, a pronounced BP drop during forced expiration, with a normal HR response, may indicate a propensity toward situational syncope and may differentiate VVS from neurogenic orthostatic hypotension. Deep breathing tests may indicate parasympathetic dysfunction, but these tests, as well as ambulatory HR and BP monitoring, have not been robust to facilitate the diagnosis of VVS. Long-term monitoring may identify HR changes consistent with VVS, but the exact temporal relationship of HR to syncope is not well defined.[70]

MANAGEMENT AND TREATMENT OF VVS

Lifestyle Interventions

Management of reflex syncope through lifestyle changes revolves around patients identifying and avoiding triggers in addition to prompt recognition of prodromal symptoms so they can rest and use counterpressure maneuvers to avoid loss of consciousness and potential physical injury. In addition, patients are generally recommended to avoid hypovolemia by consuming a set quantity of salt and volume of water daily and by wearing compression garments to maintain volume intravascularly.[13]

Physical Counterpressure Maneuvers

Counterpressure maneuvers to mitigate the risk of fainting by increasing BP and maintaining cerebral blood flow have been utilized.[71] These maneuvers include leg crossing, leg tensing, hand gripping, buttock clenching, abdominal contraction, arms tensing, calf pumping, deep breathing, and squatting. By engaging these maneuvers in time, there may be some who could abort the episode, but other data suggest that once the reflex becomes manifest, there is no way to stop it, and in fact, it may get worse as was shown in a case report.[72]

Pharmacological Interventions for VVS

Not every patient with VVS needs treatment. The goal for pharmacologic prevention of syncope in VVS is focused on increasing peripheral vascular resistance and/or increasing intravascular volume. Limited pharmacologic data have shown benefits.[73] Based on randomized clinical trials, midodrine[74,75] and fludrocortisone[76] may have modest benefits in reducing the recurrence of syncope in smaller clinical trials. While β-blockers were favored as first-line treatment, randomized controlled trials failed to demonstrate their efficacy except in those over age of 40. Consequently, the ESC guidelines advise against using β-blockers to treat reflex syncope.[4]

Likewise, because VVS can be precipitated by excess sympathetic excitation and because the sympathetic output is thought to be mediated in part by excess serotonin, selective serotonin reuptake inhibitors have been hypothesized to reduce central sympathetic nervous system activity and thus may have a role in preventing VVS. Some studies, including a randomized placebo-controlled trial, demonstrated that paroxetine,[77] but not fluoxetine,[78] was associated with a decrease in syncope recurrence in patients with VVS,[79] but this is not a widely accepted therapy.

Pacing in VVSSe Chapter 13C for a Detailed Revision

ESC recommends that for a small percentage of VVS patients older than 40 years, with cardio-inhibitory predominance and with syncope refractory to the aforementioned therapies, dual-chamber pacing should be considered.[4] Effectiveness has been studied in multiple clinical trials, which have collectively demonstrated a modest improvement in syncope recurrence in select patients receiving a pacemaker. However, this improvement was not significant when evaluating patients who are blinded to their treatment condition, with control groups receiving a pacemaker that is turned off.[80] This implies that the act of implanting a pacemaker, and not the pacing itself, may carry a large placebo effect.[81]

The SPAIN trial[82] was a double-blind, randomized crossover study of patients who had a cardioinhibitory response on the tilt-table test and recurrent episodes of syncope. Using closed-loop stimulation pacing, there was marked benefit from pacing, suggesting that patients with asystolic/cardioinhibitory recurrent vasovagal syncope may benefit from pacemaker implantation.

Cardioneuroablation (CNA)

Cardioneuroablation (CNA) to modulate the autonomic innervation of the heart is proposed as an alternative to pacing in medically refractory VVS with cardioinhibitory components. A randomized controlled clinical trial investigating CNA to treat refractory VVS demonstrated a substantial decrease in syncope recurrence, 54% in control vs. 8% in CNA, at 2-year follow-up.[83] However, this study was unblinded, and placebo may have played a strong role.[84] Additionally, patient selection and location of ablation lesions are some of the concerns.[85] Further work is eagerly anticipated and will be presented in this book in later chapters.

AREAS OF FURTHER INVESTIGATION

A small observational study investigating gut microbiota in pediatric patients with VVS found there was a correlation between the relative abundance of Ruminococcaceae in the VVS group and syncopal frequency.[86]

Various forms of meditation are shown to regulate autonomic tone. For example, meditation that developed out of certain traditions such as Vajrayana and Hindu Tantric leads to heightened sympathetic activation, while Theravada and Mahayana meditation elicit heightened parasympathetic activity.[87] No clinical trials have evaluated meditation to date. However, a small clinical trial has demonstrated a substantial reduction in syncope recurrence in VVS patients assigned to guided yoga in comparison with the control group.[88] Such a study did not and could not blind the participants to their treatment condition and thus is subject to placebo effects.

Animal models have demonstrated that vestibulo-sympathetic activation is effective in blunting syncopal episodes in VVS[89] and may thus serve as an alternative to CNA, but this has not yet been investigated in humans.

Tragus nerve stimulation has shown positive results in suppressing atrial fibrillation and alleviating post-myocardial infarction ventricular tachyarrhythmias, likely due to favorable alteration of sympatho-vagal imbalance.[90] This noninvasive intervention could be an interesting area of further study when applied to VVS.

CONCLUSION

Vasovagal (reflex) syncope is the most common cause of syncope. While many cases are benign, some are more malignant and require diligent clinical evaluation. Even if no malignant underlying pathology is identified, recurrent reflex syncope may require treatment even though no well-established treatment yet exists and is proven by carefully controlled long-term prospective studies. Because lifestyle interventions and medications alone offer only modest benefits for select patients, clinicians must also be aware of the availability and success of procedural interventions in treating refractory patients. The ideal patient for a pacemaker or CNA is one with idiopathic VVS, triggered by a specific mechanism that is understood but continues to experience syncope on a regular basis despite maximized noninvasive intervention. Tailoring therapeutic approaches to individual patient profiles and considering the nuances of various reflex subtypes are paramount to helping our patients to the greatest extent of our abilities given our current understanding of the disease.

REFERENCES

1. Colman N, Nahm K, Ganzeboom KS, et al. Epidemiology of reflex syncope. *Clin Auton Res.* 2004;14 Suppl 1:9–17.

2. Lewis T. A lecture on vasovagal syncope and the carotid sinus mechanism. *Br Med J.* 1932;1:873–876.

3. van Dijk N, Boer KR, Colman N, et al. High diagnostic yield and accuracy of history, physical examination and ECG in patients with transient loss of consciousness in FAST: the Fainting Assessment study. *J Cardiovasc Electrophysiol.* 2008;19:48–55.

4. Brignole M, Moya A, de Lange FJ, et al. 2018 ESC guidelines for the diagnosis and management of syncope. *Eur Heart J.* 2018;39:1883–1948.

5. Sutton R, Fedorowski A, Olshansky B, et al. Tilt testing remains a valuable asset. *Eur Heart J.* 2021;42:1654–1660.

6. Forleo C, Guida P, Iacoviello M, et al. Head-up tilt testing for diagnosing vasovagal syncope: a meta-analysis. *Int J Cardiol.* 2013;168:27–35.

7. Sheldon R, Rose S, Connolly S, Ritchie D, Koshman ML, Frenneaux M. Diagnostic criteria for vasovagal syncope based on a quantitative history. *Eur Heart J.* 2006;27:344–350.

8. Okuyama J, Shiozawa M, Shiode D. Heart rate and cardiac response to exercise during voluntary dives in captive sea turtles (Cheloniidae). *Biol Open.* 2020;9:bio049247.

9. Berg von Linde M, Arevström L, Fröbert O. Insights from the Den: how hibernating bears may help us understand and treat human fisease. *Clin Transl Sci.* 2015;8:601–605.

10. Zhao T, Zhu Y, Tang H, Xie R, Zhu J, Zhang JH. Consciousness: new concepts and neural networks. *Front Cell Neurosci.* 2019;13:302.

11. Benditt DG, van Dijk JG, Krishnappa D, Adkisson WO, Sakaguchi S. Neurohormones in the pathophysiology of vasovagal syncope in adults. *Front Cardiovasc Med.* 2020;7:76.

12. Linzer M, Yang EH, Estes NA, 3rd, Wang P, Vorperian VR, Kapoor WN. Diagnosing syncope. Part 1: Value of history, physical examination and electrocardiography. Clinical Efficacy Assessment Project of the American College of Physicians. *Ann Intern Med.* 1997;126:989–996.

13. Aydin MA, Salukhe TV, Wilke I, Willems S. Management and therapy of vasovagal syncope: A review. *World J Cardiol.* 2010;2:308–315.

14. Brignole M, Rivasi G, Sutton R, et al. Low-blood pressure phenotype underpins the tendency to reflex syncope. *J Hypertens.* 2021;39:1319–1325.

15. Fedorowski A, Rivasi G, Torabi P, et al. Underlying hemodynamic differences are associated with responses to tilt testing. *Sci Rep.* 2021;11:17894.

16. Brignole M, Donateo P, Tomaino M, et al. Benefit of pacemaker therapy in patients with presumed neurally mediated syncope and documented asystole is greater when tilt test is negative: an analysis from the third International Study on Syncope of Uncertain Etiology (ISSUE-3). *Circ Arrhythm Electrophysiol.* 2014;7:10–16.

17. Sahota IS, Maxey C, Pournazari P, Sheldon RS. Clusters, gaps and randomness: vasovagal syncope recurrence patterns. *JACC Clin Electrophysiol.* 2017;3:1046–1053.

18. Sheldon RS, Sandhu RK. The search for the genes of vasovagal syncope. *Front Cardiovasc Med.* 2019;6:175.

19. Mathias CJ, Deguchi K, Bleasdale-Barr K, Kimber JR. Frequency of family history in vasovagal syncope. *Lancet.* 1998;352:33–34.

20. Sheldon RS, Gerull B. Genetic markers of vasovagal syncope. *Auton Neurosci.* 2021;235:102871.

21. Aegisdottir HM, Thorolfsdottir RB, Sveinbjornsson G, et al. Genetic variants associated with syncope implicate neural and autonomic processes. *Eur Heart J.* 2023;44:1070–1080.

22. Iwase S. Structure and function. In: Hongo Y, Ga M, editor *Basic and Clinical Autonomic Nervous System.* Osaka: Iyaku Journal, 2006:1–340.

23. Wehrwein EA, Joyner MJ. Regulation of blood pressure by the arterial baroreflex and autonomic nervous system. *Handb Clin Neurol.* 2013;117:89–102.

24. Iwase S, Mano T, Kamiya A, Niimi Y, Fu Q, Suzumura A. Syncopal attack alters the burst properties of muscle sympathetic nerve activity in humans. *Auton Neurosci*. 2002;95:141–145.

25. Chapleau MW. Chapter 30: Baroreceptor reflexes. In: *Primer on the Autonomic Nervous System* (Fourth Edition). Academic Press, 2023:171–177.

26. Wu TC, Hachul DT, Darrieux F, Scanavacca MI. Carotid sinus massage in syncope evaluation: a nonspecific and dubious diagnostic method. *Arq Bras Cardiol*. 2018;111:84–91.

27. Alkire MT, Hudetz AG, Tononi G. Consciousness and anesthesia. *Science*. 2008;322:876–880.

28. Longo S, Legramante JM, Rizza S, Federici M. Vasovagal syncope: An overview of pathophysiological mechanisms. *Eur J Intern Med*. 2023;112:6–14.

29. Cooper VL, Hainsworth R. Effects of head-up tilting on baroreceptor control in subjects with different tolerances to orthostatic stress. *Clin Sci (Lond)*. 2002;103:221–226.

30. Oberg B, Thoren P. Increased activity in left ventricular receptors during hemorrhage or occlusion of caval veins in the cat. A possible cause of the vaso-vagal reaction. *Acta Physiol Scand*. 1972;85:164–173.

31. Oberg B, Thoren P. Studies on left ventricular receptors, signalling in non-medullated vagal afferents. *Acta Physiol Scand*. 1972;85:145–163.

32. Fitzpatrick AP, Banner N, Cheng A, Yacoub M, Sutton R. Vasovagal reactions may occur after orthotopic heart transplantation. *J Am Coll Cardiol*. 1993;21:1132–1137.

33. Shalev Y, Gal R, Tchou PJ, et al. Echocardiographic demonstration of decreased left ventricular dimensions and vigorous myocardial contraction during syncope induced by head-up tilt. *J Am Coll Cardiol*. 1991;18:746–751.

34. Hosaka H, Takase B, Kitamura K, et al. Assessment of left ventricular volume by an ambulatory radionuclide monitoring system during head-up tilt in patients with unexplained syncope: relation to autonomic activity assessed by heart rate variability. *J Nucl Cardiol*. 2001;8:660–668.

35. Moon J, Kim H, Kim JY, et al. Left ventricular hypercontractility immediately after tilting triggers a disregulated cardioinhibitory reaction in vasovagal syncope: echocardiographic evaluation during the head-up tilt test. *Cardiology*. 2010;117:118–123.

36. Novak V, Honos G, Schondorf R. Is the heart "empty" at syncope? *J Auton Nerv Syst*. 1996;60:83–92.

37. Mark AL. The Bezold-Jarisch reflex revisited: clinical implications of inhibitory reflexes originating in the heart. *J Am Coll Cardiol*. 1983;1:90–102.

38. Salo LM, Woods RL Anderson CR, McAllen RM. Nonuniformity in the von Bezold-Jarisch reflex. *Am J Physiol Regul Integr Comp Physiol*. 2007;293:R714–R720.

39. Larson RA, Chapleau MW. Increased cardiac sympathetic activity: Cause or compensation in vasovagal syncope? *Clin Auton Res*. 2018;28:265–266.

40. Chen HI. Interaction between the baroreceptor and Bezold-Jarisch reflexes. *Am J Physiol*. 1979;237:H655–H661.

41. Lovelace JW, Ma J, Yadav S, et al. Vagal sensory neurons mediate the Bezold-Jarisch reflex and induce syncope. *Nature*. 2023;623:387–396.

42. Yakushin SB, Martinelli GP, Raphan T, Xiang Y, Holstein GR, Cohen B. Vasovagal oscillations and vasovagal responses produced by the vestibulo-sympathetic reflex in the rat. *Front Neurol.* 2014;5:37.

43. Cohen B, Martinelli GP, Xiang Y, Raphan T, Yakushin SB. Vestibular activation habituates the vasovagal response in the rat. *Front Neurol.* 2017;8:83.

44. Norcliffe-Kaufmann LJ, Kaufmann H, Hainsworth R. Enhanced vascular responses to hypocapnia in neurally mediated syncope. *Ann Neurol.* 2008;63:288–294.

45. Hermann GE, Rogers RC. TNFalpha: a trigger of autonomic dysfunction. *Neuroscientist.* 2008;14:53–67.

46. Goldstein DS. Catecholamines and stress. *Endocr Regul.* 2003;37:69–80.

47. Goldstein DS, Holmes C, Frank SM et al. Sympathoadrenal imbalance before neurocardiogenic syncope. *Am J Cardiol.* 2003;91:53–58.

48. Chosy JJ, Graham DT. Catecholamines in vasovagal fainting. *J Psychosom Res.* 1965;9:189–194.

49. Olshansky B. For whom does the bell toll? *J Cardiovasc Electrophysiol.* 2001;12:1002–1003.

50. Iwase S, Nishimura N, Mano T. Role of sympathetic nerve activity in the process of fainting. *Front Physiol.* 2014;5:343.

51. Chen-Scarabelli C, Scarabelli TM. Neurocardiogenic syncope. *BMJ.* 2004;329:336–341.

52. Chen MY, Goldenberg IF, Milstein S et al. Cardiac electrophysiologic and hemodynamic correlates of neurally mediated syncope. *Am J Cardiol.* 1989;63:66–72.

53. Stewart JM, Pianosi P, Shaban MA et al. Postural hyperventilation as a cause of postural tachycardia syndrome: increased systemic vascular resistance and decreased cardiac output when upright in all postural tachycardia syndrome variants. *J Am Heart Assoc.* 2018;7:e008854.

54. Kaiser T, Jost WH, König J, Schimrigk K. Intra- and interindividual reproducibility of heart rate variations in the tilt-table test. *Wien Klin Wochenschr.* 2000;112:322–328.

55. Jardine DL, Wieling W, Brignole M, Lenders JWM, Sutton R, Stewart J. The pathophysiology of the vasovagal response. *Heart Rhythm.* 2018;15:921–929.

56. Carvalho MS, Reis Santos K, Carmo P et al. Prognostic value of a very prolonged asystole during head-up tilt test. *Pacing Clin Electrophysiol.* 2015;38:973–979.

57. Stewart JM, McLeod KJ, Sanyal S, Herzberg G, Montgomery LD. Relation of postural vasovagal syncope to splanchnic hypervolemia in adolescents. *Circulation.* 2004;110:2575–2581.

58. Guieu R, Degioanni C, Fromonot J et al. Adenosine, adenosine receptors and neurohumoral syncope: from molecular basis to personalized treatment. *Biomedicines.* 2022;10:1127.

59. Mittal S, Stein KM, Markowitz SM, Slotwiner DJ, Rohatgi S, Lerman BB. Induction of neurally mediated syncope with adenosine. *Circulation.* 1999;99:1318–1324.

60. Hamrefors V, Nilsson D, Melander O, Sutton R, Fedorowski A. Low adrenomedullin and endothelin-1 predict cardioinhibitory response during vasovagal reflex in adults over 40 years of age. *Circ Arrhythm Electrophysiol.* 2017;10:e005585.

61. Williford NN, Chapleau MW, Olshansky B. Neurohormones in vasovagal syncope: are they important? *J Am Heart Assoc.* 2019;8:e013129.

62. Kamiya A, Hayano J, Kawada T et al. Low-frequency oscillation of sympathetic nerve activity decreases during development of tilt-induced syncope preceding sympathetic withdrawal and bradycardia. *Am J Physiol Heart Circ Physiol.* 2005;289:H1758–H1769.

63. Schwartz CE, Lambert E, Medow MS, Stewart JM. Disruption of phase synchronization between blood pressure and muscle sympathetic nerve activity in postural vasovagal syncope. *Am J Physiol Heart Circ Physiol.* 2013;305:H1238–H1245.

64. Morillo CA, Eckberg DL, Ellenbogen KA et al. Vagal and sympathetic mechanisms in patients with orthostatic vasovagal syncope. *Circulation.* 1997;96:2509–2513.

65. Wieling W, Kaufmann H, Claydon VE et al. Diagnosis and treatment of orthostatic hypotension. *Lancet Neurol.* 2022;21:735–746.

66. Kulkarni N, Mody P, Levine BD. Abolish the tilt table test for the workup of syncope! *Circulation.* 2020;141:335–337.

67. Raddino R, Zanini G, Robba D et al. Diagnostic value of the head-up tilt test and the R-test in patients with syncope. *Heart Int.* 2006;2:171.

68. Flevari P, Leftheriotis D, Komborozos C et al. Recurrent vasovagal syncope: comparison between clomipramine and nitroglycerin as drug challenges during head-up tilt testing. *Eur Heart J.* 2009;30:2249–2253.

69. Fu Q, Verheyden B, Wieling W, Levine BD. Cardiac output and sympathetic vasoconstrictor responses during upright tilt to presyncope in healthy humans. *J Physiol.* 2012;590:1839–1848.

70. Sandesara CM, Gopinathannair R, Olshansky B. Implantable cardiac monitors: evolution through disruption. *J Innov Card Rhythm Manag.* 2017;8:2824–2834.

71. Brignole M, Croci F, Menozzi C et al. Isometric arm counter-pressure maneuvers to abort impending vasovagal syncope. *J Am Coll Cardiol.* 2002;40:2053–2059.

72. Brignole M, Maggi R, Croci F. A very prolonged asystolic vasovagal syncope is suspended but not aborted by counterpressure manoeuvre. *Europace.* 2010;12:91.

73. Vyas A, Swaminathan PD, Zimmerman MB, Olshansky B. Are treatments for vasovagal syncope effective? A meta-analysis. *Int J Cardiol.* 2013;167:1906–1911.

74. Sheldon R, Faris P, Tang A et al. Midodrine for the prevention of vasovagal syncope: a randomized clinical trial. *Ann Intern Med.* 2021;174:1349–1356.

75. Ward CR, Gray JC, Gilroy JJ, Kenny RA. Midodrine: a role in the management of neurocardiogenic syncope. *Heart.* 1998;79:45–49.

76. Sheldon R, Raj SR, Rose MS et al. Fludrocortisone for the prevention of vasovagal syncope: a randomized, placebo-controlled trial. *J Am Coll Cardiol.* 2016;68:1–9.

77. Di Girolamo E, Di Iorio C, Sabatini P, Leonzio L, Barbone C, Barsotti A. Effects of paroxetine hydrochloride, a selective serotonin reuptake inhibitor, on refractory vasovagal syncope: a randomized, double-blind, placebo-controlled study. *J Am Coll Cardiol.* 1999;33:1227–1230.

78. Theodorakis GN, Leftheriotis D, Livanis EG et al. Fluoxetine vs. propranolol in the treatment of vasovagal syncope: a prospective, randomized, placebo-controlled study. *Europace.* 2006;8:193–198.

79. Takata TS, Wasmund SL, Smith ML et al. Serotonin reuptake inhibitor (Paxil) does not prevent the vasovagal reaction associated with carotid sinus massage and/or lower body negative pressure in healthy volunteers. *Circulation.* 2002;106:1500–1504.

80. Connolly SJ, Sheldon R, Thorpe KE et al. Pacemaker therapy for prevention of syncope in patients with recurrent severe vasovagal syncope: Second Vasovagal Pacemaker Study (VPS II): a randomized trial. *JAMA.* 2003;289:2224–2229.

81. Olshansky B. Placebo and nocebo in cardiovascular health: implications for healthcare, research and the doctor-patient relationship. *J Am Coll Cardiol.* 2007;49:415–421.

82. Baron-Esquivias G, Morillo CA, Moya-Mitjans A et al. Dual-chamber pacing with closed loop stimulation in recurrent reflex vasovagal syncope: the SPAIN study. *J Am Coll Cardiol.* 2017;70:1720–1728.

83. Piotrowski R, Baran J, Sikorska A, Krynski T, Kulakowski P. Cardioneuroablation for reflex syncope: efficacy and effects on autonomic cardiac regulation – a prospective randomized trial. *JACC Clin Electrophysiol.* 2023;9:85–95.

84. Parker WH, Olshansky B. Autonomic modulation: getting it "just right". *Heart Rhythm O2.* 2023;4:414–415.

85. Brignole M, Aksu T, Calo L et al. Clinical controversy: methodology and indications of cardioneuroablation for reflex syncope. *Europace.* 2023;25.

86. Bai W, Chen S, Tang CS et al. Gut microbiota analysis and its significance in vasovagal syncope in children. *Chin Med J (Engl).* 2019;132:411–419.

87. Amihai I, Kozhevnikov M. The influence of Buddhist meditation traditions on the autonomic system and attention. *Biomed Res Int.* 2015;2015:731579.

88. Gunda S, Kanmanthareddy A, Atkins D et al. Role of yoga as an adjunctive therapy in patients with neurocardiogenic syncope: a pilot study. *J Interv Card Electrophysiol.* 2015;43:105–110.

89. Raphan T, Cohen B, Xiang Y, Yakushin SB. A model of blood pressure, heart rate and vaso-vagal responses produced by vestibulo-sympathetic activation. *Front Neurosci.* 2016;10:96.

90. Jiang Y, Po SS, Amil F, Dasari TW. Non-invasive low-level tragus stimulation in cardiovascular diseases. *Arrhythm Electrophysiol Rev.* 2020;9:40–46.

6B Reflex Syncope

Other Causes of Reflex Syncope

Piotr Kulakowski

SITUATIONAL SYNCOPE

Definition. Situational syncope is the reflex syncope associated with specific circumstances which trigger loss of consciousness.[1] The most frequent types include micturition, defecation, cough, and swallow syncope, followed by less frequent forms.[2,3] Also, some types of post-exercise syncope may be classified as situational syncope. Because in many patients there is a significant overlap between situational syncope and VVS as well as orthostatic hypotension, it is not always easy to define which type of reflex is present or predominant in a given patient. The safest way is to use the broad term "reflex syncope" which covers all these conditions.

Epidemiology. Situational syncope is less common than VVS. In one study which included 1401 patients with various forms of syncope, 252 (18%) had VVS and 55 (4%) had situational syncope.[2] In another report which encompassed 3,140 patients with presumed reflex syncope who underwent tilt testing, 354 (11%) subjects were diagnosed as having situational syncope.[3] Compared with VVS, these patients were older, were more likely to be male, had a higher prevalence of hypertension, and had a higher incidence of syncope associated with injury.[2]

Pathophysiology. Underlying mechanisms are variable and frequently not well understood. The efferent limb of the reflex and the central nervous system processing seem common to be for all types of situational syncope whereas the afferent limb is different and depends on the trigger. In addition, there is a significant overlap between VVS and situational syncope. It has been shown that approximately 50% of patients with situational syncope have features typical for VVS, demonstrated during tilt testing.[3] Moreover, syncope triggered by a "specific" trigger and classified as "situational" may be in fact VVS. For example, micturition syncope—the most frequently encountered form of situational syncope, may occur due to initiation of abnormal reflex from mechanoreceptors located in the bladder, but also due to orthostatic hypotension or VVS, especially at night after rapidly adopting the upright position and triggering further reflexes by passing urine. A simplified scheme of pathophysiological pathways operating in different forms of reflex non-VVS syncope is presented in Figure 6.1.

Prognosis. Prognosis is usually good, except in patients in whom syncope is due to the presence of a serious underlying disease like a malignant tumor or advanced organic disease.

Treatment. The first aim of therapy is to eliminate or at least reduce the trigger. Additional non-pharmacological approach and patient's education, like in VVS, are usually needed. Permanent pacing is recommended in some patients, and cardioneuroablation may be considered in selected cases. In hypotensive phenotype, medical therapy may be used.

SPECIFIC FORMS OF SITUATIONAL SYNCOPE

Micturition Syncope. This is probably the most frequent form of situational syncope, ranging from 27% to 51% of all patients.[2,3] It occurs more frequently in middle-aged males than in females. Drinking alcohol is often associated with this type of syncope.

The pathophysiology of micturition syncope is complex. The bladder contains mechanoreceptors. In some situations, sudden activation of a large number of mechanoreceptors is transmitted via afferent limb to the spinal cord and nucleus tractii solitarii which in turn increases the parasympathetic drive to the heart via vagal nerve, resulting in bradycardia or asystole. Also, paradoxical inhibition of adrenergic drive to the peripheral vessels causes vasodilatation and hypotension. Again, fainting while passing urine may also be caused by typical vasovagal reflex, and orthostatic hypotension and facilitated by performing the Valsalva maneuver, especially in older males with an enlarged prostate. The overlap between micturition syncope and VVS was shown in one study where tilting revealed vasodepressor response in 28%, cardioinhibitory in 2%, and mixed in 17% of patients with micturition syncope.[3]

Prognosis Is Good. Recurrences occur in 13% of patients.[2] Treatment consists of a typical non-pharmacological approach and patient's education. Males should be advised to pass urine while sitting and not while standing. In case of problems with passing urine due to prostatic hypertrophy, tumor, or other diseases, treatment of these conditions is mandatory.

DOI: 10.1201/9781003415855-8

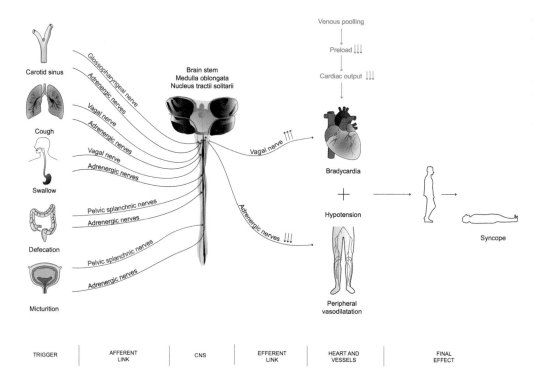

Figure 6.1 Schematic presentation of afferent and efferent pathways in situational reflex syncope and carotid sinus syndrome. The parasympathetic part is depicted by red arrows, and the sympathetic part is depicted by blue arrows.

Defecation Syncope. Defecation syncope appears to be the second most frequent form of situational syncope, accounting for 5%–29% of cases.[2–4] It tends to occur predominantly in older women. Symptoms of gastrointestinal tract dysfunction are common with chronic constipation being the most frequent complaint.

The process of bowel mobility and feces transportation is controlled by various mechanisms which include the sympathetic and parasympathetic system, intrinsic or enteric nervous system, gastrointestinal peptides, and other mechanisms.[5] Failure of any of these systems such as the loss of inhibitory sympathetic input or augmented parasympathetic drive can increase intra-bowel pressure and bowel wall tension with subsequent mechanoreceptor activation. When this information reaches the central nervous system, the efferent limb of reflex further increases vagal activity and reduces adrenergic activity, leading to bradycardia/asystole, hypotension, and syncope. In addition, the Valsalva maneuver, often performed when constipation is present, further decreases venous return and increases vagal tone, contributing to syncope.

Abnormalities of autonomic innervation of capacitance splanchnic vasculature may also play a role. These vessels have a large capacitance and even small abnormalities in their autonomic innervation may result in the sequestration of a large amount of blood, reducing venous return to the heart, decreasing stroke volume, and causing hypotension.

As with micturition syncope, subjects with defecation syncope have often abnormal tilt testing results. In one study, 23% of patients had vasodepression and 27% had a mixed type of vasovagal reaction;[3] however, this finding has not been confirmed by others.[6] This suggests that typical vasovagal reaction may also play a role in defecation syncope. It has been also reported that patients with defecation syncope suffer from autonomic failure, affecting both the sympathetic and parasympathetic parts of the autonomic nervous system.[6]

Prognosis Is Uncertain. One study showed increased mortality in these patients,[4] whereas other more recent reports documented good outcomes providing specific treatment was instituted.[2,6]

Treatment, as always, should be concentrated on specific causes of syncope in an individual patient. Proper diet, exercise, and anti-constipation drugs are of paramount value. Cessation of medications causing constipation or interfering with bowel mobility like non-selective beta-blockers is indicated.[6] Typical non-pharmacological approaches and education as in patients with VVS are often helpful. In cases with documented reflex asystole pacemaker may be effective.[6]

Swallow (Swallowing, Deglutition) Syncope. Temporal association with meal intake is characteristic of this type of situational syncope. Swallow syncope is a rather rare cause of syncope, occurring in 0.3% of all patients with syncope[7] and in 5%–6.5% of patients with situational syncope.[2,3] It occurs most commonly in adult males, whereas in the younger population female gender predominates. In many patients (up to 40%), it is associated with gastroesophageal diseases such as esophageal stricture, diverticulum or spasm, hiatus hernia, gastroesophageal reflux, esophagitis, achalasia, and esophageal carcinoma. Also, other disorders localized close to the esophagus such as lung cancer, ascending aorta aneurysm, or neck lymph node metastasis may be associated with swallow syncope.[8,9]

The most frequently postulated mechanism is the exaggerated activation of esophageal mechanoreceptors caused by swallowing solid food in the presence of esophageal abnormality. The limbs of reflex are typical—afferent limb via esophageal nerves to the medulla oblongata and nucleus tractii solitarii and efferent limb—vagal nerve increased tone leading to asystole and/or atrio-ventricular block. It has been shown that atropine prevents bradyarrhythmia. Interestingly, in this condition, atrio-ventricular block is more often seen than sinus arrest which is in slight contrast to the majority of other forms of reflex syncope (Figure 6.2).

Another speculative mechanism is the direct interaction between the esophagus and the left atrium. Because of the close relationship between the esophagus and the posterior left atrial wall, many esophageal diseases, such as inflammation, may directly affect ganglionated plexi located close to the pulmonary vein ostia. This may in turn result in bradycardia or asystole. Also, autonomic innervation of the esophagus and the heart is closely related, and changes in parasympathetic or sympathetic tone in the esophageal autonomic innervation may also affect cardiac innervation.

The prognosis obviously depends on the underlying disease. Treatment is firstly directed to elimination of the cause of esophageal disorder and consists of dilatation of esophageal stricture, surgical correction of hiatal hernia, or surgical excision of esophageal carcinoma. Also, surgical cauterization of the vagal nerve and long-term proton pump inhibitor therapy have been tried.[8,9]

Changes in dietary habits, avoiding foods triggering syncope, and swallowing slowly are recommended. Carbonated beverages have been implicated as a trigger for swallow syncope because dissolved carbon dioxide distends the gastric lumen and induces vagal reflex. Also, cold beverages, sandwiches, and sticky foods have been reported to trigger swallow syncope.[8,9]

In resistant cases, permanent pacing may be effective. Recently, several cases of successful cardioneuroablation for the treatment of swallow syncope have been described.[10,11] However, it has to be kept in mind that these procedures are reserved for patients in whom causative therapy and diet changes were ineffective.

Cough Syncope. This form of situational syncope is defined as loss of consciousness during or following a cough. A typical patient with cough syncope is a middle-aged, overweight, or muscularly built male with chronic obstructive pulmonary disease or asthma who is capable of

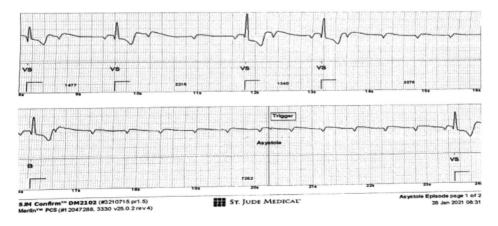

Figure 6.2 ECG recorded with implantable cardiac monitor in a patient with swallow syncope. Atrio-ventricular block with 13 non-conducted P waves is shown.

generating very high intrathoracic pressure. The incidence varies between 5% and 18%[2,3] of all patients with situational syncope.

The pathophysiology of cough syncope is complex and several mechanisms have been postulated. Firstly, it has been demonstrated that elevated intrathoracic pressure during cough is transmitted to the cerebrospinal fluid and causes an acute pressure increase in the skull, resulting in diminished brain perfusion. In addition, an acute increase of arterial, venous, and cerebrospinal fluid pressures in the skull directly compromises cerebral functions. Secondly, the increase in intrathoracic pressure diminishes venous return, cardiac filling, and subsequently cardiac output. Thirdly, increased intrathoracic pressure is transferred to the systemic circulation, causing arterial baroreflex-mediated vasodilatation. Fourthly, a neurally mediated reflex vasodepressor-bradycardia response to cough has been also proposed as a possible mechanism of cough syncope. As a result, a decrease in total peripheral resistance plays a pivotal role in the pathophysiology of cough syncope.[12,13] It has been shown that tilt testing revealed typical vasovagal reflex in 62% of patients with chronic cough.[14] Finally, chronotropic incompetence resulting in inadequate heart rhythm acceleration to combat the effects of hypotension has been described.[15]

The prognosis depends on the underlying condition. Treatment is focused on eliminating cough and its causes. Chronic cough should be treated according to guidelines. It is worth remembering that many widely used medications such as angiotensin-converting enzyme inhibitors are associated with cough and should be stopped and exchanged for a suitable alternative treatment. Also, the use of vasodilators and diuretics should be careful because these drugs may worsen hypotension. Apart from pulmonary and bronchial diseases, large pericardial effusion may also cause cough and syncope. This may occur both due to reflex as well as decreased cardiac output due to markedly reduced venous return because of the presence of pericardial effusion.[16]

Two other rare forms of situational syncope occurring while brass instrument playing or in trumpet-blowers have similar pathophysiology to cough syncope. Here, transient venous obstruction due to increased intrathoracic pressure decreases cardiac filling and output, leading to global cerebral hypoperfusion and syncope. Similar mechanisms may operate in syncope occurring during laughing, singing, sneezing, and weight-lifting.

POST-EXERCISE SYNCOPE

This type of syncope is usually due to hypotension and reflex bradycardia or asystole and is an expression of VVS. However, some of these subjects have normal tilt testing and may be classified as situational syncope. The condition is usually benign providing that cardiac causes of syncope have been excluded. Treatment consists of avoiding exaggerated physical activity and proper non-pharmacological methods. They include very intense hydration during exercise, avoiding exercising in hot environment, and proper post-exercise behavior—lying down after completion of exercise rather than keeping a standing position.

NON-CLASSICAL FORMS

These include syncopal episodes without prodromes or without apparent triggers or with atypical presentation. This group of patients is heterogeneous. The diagnosis of reflex syncope can be only suspected when other causes of syncope are excluded. Reproduction of symptoms during tilt testing reinforces the diagnosis. According to the guidelines,[1] the non-classical forms of reflex syncope include also syncope due to low adenosine plasma levels.

Another unresolved issue is the role of the brain itself in some forms of reflex syncope. The role of the central nervous system as an initial syncope trigger is unknown but probably may be responsible for these forms of reflex syncope where there is no detectable external or internal (like a pain) physical trigger. One of the examples is blood phobia which can be effectively treated using psychotherapy.[17] Also, venipuncture phobia may belong to this category of situational syncope. Intense emotional stress, consisting of anxiety, fear, and pain at the time of venipuncture, may probably lead to centrally mediated reflex syncope.[18]

Another example is sleep syncope which is usually categorized as a special form of VVS; however, it can be also classified as reflex situational syncope. Attenuation of sympathetic responses to non-baroreflex pathways has been implicated as the mechanism of sleep syncope.[19]

CAROTID SINUS SYNDROME

This type of reflex syncope occurs in subjects with carotid sinus hypersensitivity. The prevalence of carotid sinus syndrome (CSS) increases with age, reaching 40% of all causes of syncope in subjects aged >80 years[20], and is responsible for nearly 30% of unexplained syncope episodes in the elderly. It is more common in men than in women, particularly in those with concomitant chronic diseases and with neurodegenerative disorders.

The exact cause of CSS has not been fully established. Baroreceptors localized in the carotid sinus, aortic arch, and great arteries are fundamental for proper control of blood pressure and heart rate. Upon stretching due to a rise in blood pressure, baroreceptors are activated and this message is transmitted to the nucleus tractii solitarii using a glossopharyngeal nerve from the carotid sinus and vagal nerve from the aortic arch which serves as the afferent limb of the reflex. Then, parasympathetic nerves are activated and sympathetic pathways are inhibited (efferent limb) causing decrease in blood pressure and heart rate. It has been hypothesized that degenerative processes of the medullary autonomic nuclei, which sense baroreceptor's signaling, lead to an exaggerated response, causing hypotension and bradycardia.[21] Stretching or mechanical pressure over the carotid sinus overshoots signals resulting in hypotension or bradycardia or both.[22] Upregulation of the alfa-2 receptors in the brainstem and decreased arterial compliance due to atherosclerosis of the carotid arteries have also been suggested; however, the latter cause was not confirmed as the cause of CSS in more recent studies.[20,23]

CSS should be strongly suspected when there is a history of syncope associated with head-turning, shaving, or other circumstances that increase pressure over the carotid sinus (for example, tight collar). Very often there are no prodromal symptoms and loss of consciousness is sudden, frequently associated with injury which is associated with adverse prognosis in this elderly population. The final diagnosis is always based on the results of carotid sinus massage which can reproduce syncope and reveal the type of reflex—cardioinhibitory (70%), vasodepressor (10%), and mixed (20%). Details on how to perform and interpret carotid sinus massage are presented elsewhere. Of note, in all patients with positive results of carotid sinus massage other autonomic tests should be also performed because there is a significant overlap between CSS, orthostatic hypotension, and VVS.

The prognosis is usually good and depends on the underlying disease and concomitant disorders. Because CSS predominantly occurs in the elderly, comorbidities and injuries associated with syncope are frequent and worsen the outcome. In rare cases when head or neck tumors are responsible for CSS, the prognosis may be poor.

Treatment depends on the type of reflex elucidated by carotid sinus massage and is described in detail in this book elsewhere. In brief, in the asystolic form of CSS permanent pacing has an established role and class IIa recommendation in the ESC syncope guidelines[1] and class I recommendation in the ECS 2021 pacing guidelines.[24] It is especially effective in those patients with CSS who have no other forms of reflex syncope, especially vasodepressor reaction, documented by negative tilt testing results. When vasodepressor reflex is documented, pacing may be ineffective, and pharmacological treatment with midodrine or fludrocortisone, together with proper fluid intake and avoiding triggers, may be tried. However, there is not much evidence that these agents are effective in CSS and in fact are frequently contraindicated because patients with CSS have very often concomitant hypertension. Also, frequent side effects of midodrine like urinary retention in males limit wider usage. Other therapeutic options include surgical adventitial tripping of carotid sinus which was reported many years ago to be extremely effective;[25] however, it did not gain further support. Another new option, especially for the cardioinhibitory type of CSS, is cardioneuroablation.[26]

REFERENCES

1. Brignole M, Moya A, de Lange FJ, et al. 2018 ESC guidelines for the diagnosis and management of syncope. *Eur Heart J*. 2018;39:1883–1948.

2. Wenzke KE, Walsh KE, Kalscheur M, et al. Clinical characteristics and outcome of patients with situational syncope compared to patients with vasovagal syncope. *Pacing Clin Electrophysiol*. 2017;40:591–595.

3. Zou R, Wang S, Lin P, et al. The clinical characteristics of situational syncope in children and adults undergoing head-up tilt testing. *Am J Emerg Med*. 2020;38:1419–1423.

4. Kapoor WN, Peterson J, Karpf M. Defecation syncope. A symptom with multiple etiologies. *Arch Intern Med*. 1986;146:2377–2379.

5. Grubb BP. Defaecation syncope: new light on an old problem. *Europace*. 2004;6:189–191.

6. Allan L, Johns E, Doshi M, Anne Kenny R, Newton JL. Abnormalities of sympathetic and parasympathetic autonomic function in subjects with defaecation syncope. *Europace*. 2004;6:192–198.

7. Mathias CJ, Deguchi K, Schatz I. Observations on recurrent syncope and presyncope in 641 patients. *Lancet*. 2001;357:348–353.

8. Uraguchi K, Kariya S, Makihara S, et al. Dangerous noodle: a case of swallowing syncope and a review of 122 cases from the literature. *J Arrhythm*. 2018;35:145–148.

9. Siew KSW, Tan MP, Hilmi IN, Loch A. Swallow syncope: a case report and review of literature. *BMC Cardiovasc Disord*. 2019;19:191.

10. Stiavnicky P, Wichterle D, Hrosova M, Kautzner J. Cardioneuroablation for the treatment of recurrent swallow syncope. *Europace*. 2020;22: 1741.

11. Miranda-Arboleda AF, Burak C, Abdollah H, Baranchuk A, Aksu T, Enriquez A. Cardioneuroablation for swallowing-induced syncope: to pace or to ablate, that is the question. *HeartRhythm Case Rep*. 2023;9:283–286.

12. Dicpinigaitis PV, Lim L, Farmakidis C. Cough syncope. *Respir Med*. 2014;108:244–251.

13. Krediet CT, Wieling W. Edward P. Sharpey-Schafer was right: evidence for systemic vasodilatation as a mechanism of hypotension in cough syncope. *Europace*. 2008;10:486–488.

14. Mereu R, Taraborrelli P, Sau A, et al. Diagnostic role of head-up tilt test in patients with cough syncope. *Europace*. 2016;18:1273–1279.

15. Dickinson O, Akdemir B, Puppala VK, et al. Blunted chronotropic response to hypotension in cough syncope. *JACC Clin Electrophysiol*. 2016;2:818–824.

16. Evans J, Ullah S. Pericardial effusion presenting as cough syncope. *Acute Med*. 2020;19:106–109.

17. Van Dijk N, Velzeboer SC, Destrée-Vonk A, Linzer M, Wieling W. Psychological treatment of malignant vasovagal syncope due to bloodphobia. *Pacing Clin Electrophysiol*. 2001;24:122–124.

18. Win NN, Kohase H, Miyamoto T, Umino M. Decreased bispectral index as an indicator of syncope before hypotension and bradycardia in two patients with needle phobia. *Br J Anaesthesia*. 2003;91:749–752.

19. Jardine DL, Davis J, Frampton CM, Wieling W. Sleep syncope: a prospective cohort study. *Clin Auton Res*. 2022;32:19–27.

20. Amin V, Pavri BB. Carotid sinus syndrome. *Cardiol Rev*. 2015;23:130–134.

21. Miller VM, Kenny RA, Slade JY, Oakley AE, Kalaria RN. Medullary autonomic pathology in carotid sinus hypersensitivity. *Neuropathol Appl Neurobiol*. 2008;34:403–411.

22. Sutton R. Carotid sinus syndrome: progress in understanding and management. *Glob Cardiol Sci Pract*. 2014;18;1–8.

23. Parry SW, Baptist M, Gilroy JJ, Steen N, Kenny RA. Central alpha2 adrenoceptors and the pathogenesis of carotid sinus hypersensitivity. *Heart*. 2004;90:935–936.

24. Gilkson M, Nielsen JC, Kronberg MB, et al. 2021 ESC guidelines on cardiac pacing and cardiac resynchronization therapy. *Eur Heart J*. 2021;00:1–94

25. Toorop RJ, Scheltinga MR, Huige MC, Moll FL. Clinical results of carotid denervation by adventitial stripping in carotid sinus syndrome. *Eur J Vasc Endovasc Surg.* 2010;39:146–152.

26. Francia P, Viveros D, Falasconi G, et al. Cardioneuroablation for carotid sinus syndrome: a case series. *Heart Rhythm.* 2023;20:640–641.

7 Adenosine-Sensitive Syncope

Diagnosis and Management

Régis Guieu, Michele Brignole, and Jean Claude Deharo

INTRODUCTION

Adenosine-sensitive syncope has been identified as a subtype of unexplained syncope.

Over the last few years, it has become clear that there is a link between adenosine and unexplained syncope and adenosine, whether from an endogenous or exogenous source.

The aim of this chapter is to clarify the possible roles of adenosine and its receptors, particularly when administered exogenously, in the screening of syncope.

ADENOSINE AND ATP METABOLISM

Adenosine is a nucleoside synthesized in a lot of tissues, especially in endothelial and muscle cells, and that mainly comes from the dephosphorylation of ATP, while a short proportion comes from the methionine cycle (Figure 7.1). Adenosine is naturally released in the extracellular spaces via an equilibrative nucleoside transporter ($ENT_{1,2}$) present at the surface of most cells, while a concentrative sodium-dependent transport exists in monocytes. The half-life of adenosine in the blood is short around 30s due to the quick uptake by red blood cells via the ENT_1 on one hand and to the deamination of adenosine-by-adenosine deaminase (ADA) both at the intracellular

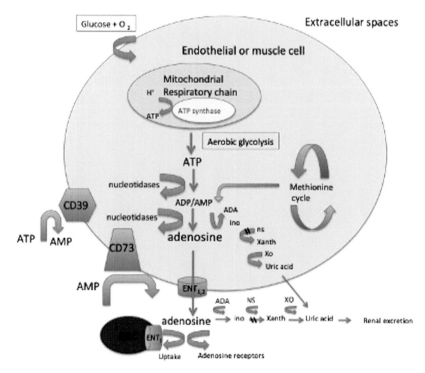

Figure 7.1 Schematic representation of adenosine metabolism. *At the intracellular level, adenosine comes mainly from the dephosphorylation of ATP, which itself synthesizes at the mitochondrial level mainly through the aerobic glycolysis pathway using the proton pump. ATP is dephosphorylated into ADP and AMP via intracellular nucleotidases. Part of adenosine is deaminated into inosine by the adenosine deaminase (ADA), and its degradation joins the uric acid metabolism through the xanthine oxidase (XO) pathway. Part of adenosine is released from the cell via an equilibrative nucleoside transporter 1 or 2 (ENT1,2) depending on cell subtype. At the extracellular level, adenyl nucleotides (ATP, AMP) are hydrolyzed via CD39 and CD73 ectonucleotidases. Adenosine is quickly uptake by red blood cells (RBC, via ENT1), while a part joints the uric acid metabolism in the same manner as for intracellular procedure.*

DOI: 10.1201/9781003415855-9

and extracellular levels (see Figure 7.1). The half-life of ATP in the blood is also short due to the active ectonucleotidases notably CD39 (see Figure 7.1). Thus, the turnover of ATP is very high since humans synthesize and hydrolyze the equivalent of their own weight every 24 hours. The main source of ATP is glycolysis, while other macromolecules like proteins or lipids degradation leads also to ATP formation. ATP is synthesized mainly via the aerobic glycolysis pathway through the respiratory chain in the mitochondria (see Figure 7.1). Part of adenosine or ATP that has not been dephosphorylated by ectonucleotidases, deaminated by adenosine deaminase, or uptaken by red blood cells or other tissues, acts on purinergic receptors.

ADENOSINE AND ADP/ATP RECEPTORS

Purinergic receptors are divided into P1 (adenosine) or P2 (ATP or ADP) receptors. Adenosine strongly impacts the cardiovascular system via its four membrane receptors named A_1 R, A_{2A} R, A_{2B} R, and A_3 R. Activation of A_1 R or A_3 R leads to cAMP production inhibition, while the activation of A_2 Rs leads to cAMP production. While in physiological conditions extracellular adenosine concentration remains low (0.4–0.8 µM),[1,2] this concentration increases strongly in pathophysiological conditions such as hypoxia, ischemia, inflammation, or tissue stress.[3] The main effects of adenosine on the cardiovascular system are summarized in Figure 7.2. Note that in the context of syncope, the A_3 R is likely poorly concerned.

Activation of A_1 R leads to the activation of an inward potassium channel (IK_{ado}), leading to K^+ outward flux and synaptic membrane hyperpolarization. This direct effect (cAMP-independent) mostly concerns the sinus node (SN), and the atrioventricular node (AVN) leads to negative chronotropic and dromotropic effects (see Figure 7.2). The indirect effects occur through the inhibition of cAMP production and lead to the inhibition of cAMP-dependent neurotransmitter release notably catecholamines.

Thus, the consequences of the activation of A_1R are similar to those found during Ach muscarinic M1 receptor (vagal stimulation) activation. While vagal stimulation can participate in unexplained syncope, this notion could introduce some confusion because activation of A_1 R mimics vagal activation. Therefore, we would like to emphasize that there is no rationale supporting the use of cardioneuroablation in low adenosine syncope. Indeed, low adenosine syncope shares cardioinhibition with cardioinhibitory reflex syncope but the mechanism is mediated by A1R activation instead of muscarinic receptor activation. Denervation of vagal endings by cardioneuroablation, which appears to be effective in some forms of reflex syncope with severe cardioinhibition,[4] may not be effective in low adenosine syncope.

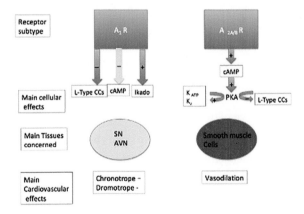

Figure 7.2 Schematic representation of the transduction pathways concerning adenosine receptors. *Activation of A_1 receptors (A_1R) leads to inward potassium channel activation (IKAdo, direct effects), voltage-gated calcium channel inhibition (L-type calcium channels (CCs)), and cAMP production inhibition (indirect effects). The main tissue targets are the sinus node (SN) and atrioventricular node (AVN) leading to negative chronotropic and dromotropic effects. Activation of A_{2A} adenosine receptors (A_{2A} R) leads to cAMP production and thus to protein kinase A (AMP-dependent kinase, PKA). The activation of PKA leads to activation of potassium channels, (Kv) and ATP-sensitive potassium channels (K_{ATP}) through their phosphorylation. Conversely, the phosphorylation of L-type CCs by PKA leads to their inhibition. The resulting effects are strong vasodilation through the smooth muscle cell relaxation of artery walls.*

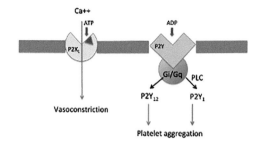

Figure 7.3 Schematic representation of P2 receptor activation. *ATP through P2X ion channel receptor subtypes favors calcium influx through smooth muscle cells that contribute to vasoconstriction. Via P2Y subtype, which are G protein membrane receptors (Gi or Gq), activation by adenosine diphosphate (ADP) leads to platelet aggregation via a signal transduction cascade depending on receptor subtype. PLC, phospholipase C.*

Among adenosine receptors, A_1R exhibits a higher affinity with a K_D around 0.8 μM for the high-affinity A_1R subtype.[5]

While A_{2A}Rs are also implicated in the control of heart rhythm, the main effects concern vaso-dilation of arteries. These effects occur mainly through cAMP production (indirect effects) via a protein kinase (PKA) pathway and activation of K_{ATP} and K_V channels (see Figure 7.2).[6] The affinity of adenosine for A_{2A} R ranges around 1.8 μM,[7] while the affinity of A_{2B} receptors for adenosine is very high[8] and thus probably poorly concerned by the syncope mechanism.

ATP acts through P2X and P2Y subtypes. P2X is subdivided into seven subtypes (P2X 1 to 7) and is ion channel receptor, while P2Y subtypes belong to the G-coupled receptor family (P2Y 1 to 14). mRNAs for P2X1, P2X4, and $P2Y_1$, $P2Y_2$, $P2Y_4$, $P2Y_6$, $P2Y_{12}$, and $P2Y_{14}$ receptors are expressed in human SA node, with $P2Y_{14}$ receptors showing the highest level.[9] ATP has negative chronotropic and dromo-tropic effects. Adenosine and ATP, via P1 receptors, suppress the pacemaker activity of the SA node. While activation of the PX1 receptor subtype modulates Ca^{++} influx (see Figure 7.3), the activation of P2Y subtypes is especially involved in platelet aggregation.[9]

Adenosine, via A_1 receptors, or ATP inhibits AV nodal conduction and suppresses the pacemaker activity of the SA node. ATP, but not adenosine, triggers a vagal reflex, which mediates, in part, the transient negative chronotropic and dromotropic effects on the sinus node and atrioventricular node, respectively.[9] In an animal model, ATP increases SA conduction time in isolated blood-perfused atrium, increases sinus cycle length in the heart in vivo, and induces negative chronotropic and dromotropic effects that were antagonized by aminophylline.[10] In humans, intravenous ATP admin-istration produces AV block via P1 receptor mediation. These two results suggest that not only ATP but also its degradation product adenosine may act predominantly. ATP also induces NO release from endothelial cells that probably involves Ca^{2+}-activated Cl^- channels, via the PKA pathway.[9]

Finally, ATP as a co-transmitter, seems to play a major role in the pressor during sino-carotid reflex and in sensory-motor nerve regulation during vascular axon reflex activity.[9]

ADENOSINE AND ATP IN THE DIAGNOSIS OF UNEXPLAINED SYNCOPE

There is a lot of evidence that adenosine and its receptors are implicated in the pathophysiology of unexplained syncope (for review, see Refs. [11,12]). In an animal model of vasovagal syncope (VVS), the use of aminophylline, a non-specific adenosine receptor antagonist, inhibits bradycar-dia.[13] In humans, high adenosine plasma level and high A_{2A} adenosine receptor expression have been reported in patients with VVS.[14,15] Theophylline, a non-specific adenosine receptor antagonist, has been shown in a small series of patients to be effective in the treatment of syncope, particu-larly in those with low plasma adenosine concentration and no prodromes.[16,17] Furthermore, the use of adenosine administration as a provocative agent, remains a matter of debate and current guidelines do not provide any clear recommendation.[18,19] However, it seems that the ATP test (or adenosine test) and HUT did not explore the same population of patients, and those with a positive ATP test do not show the same symptoms as those with a positive HUT. Indeed, bradycar-dia is the most frequent finding in patients with positive ATP/adenosine test,[20] while vasoplegia is more frequent in patients with positive HUT.[14] The absence of prodromal symptoms is particularly common in patients with a positive ATP test.

In a study including 175 patients with unexplained syncope and who underwent both ATP test and HUT, among the entire patient population, 64% had a positive HUT while only 15% displayed a positive ATP test.[21] Furthermore, patients with positive ATP tests were older compared with those with positive HUT.[21] In a study of 46 patients with unexplained syncope, 39% had positive HUT, 23% had positive ATP test, 17% had negative tests, and only 19% exhibited both HUT- and ATP-positive tests.[15] It has also been reported that patients with positive ATP test have lower adenosine plasma level and lower A_{2A} R expression.[15] Interestingly, those with positive ATP test and negative HUT have a very low plasma adenosine concentration, while those with positive HUT have higher plasma adenosine concentration. Intermediate values of adenosine were found in patients with both positive tests.[15,22] Thus, it was concluded that the concentration of plasma adenosine could predict the positivity of the ATP test, with low APL being associated with a high probability of a positive ATP test.[15] While there is an overlap between the population with positive HUT and positive ATP/adenosine test, it seems that these tests explore different populations of patients.

In these conditions, how can we explain the fact that in a proportion of patients the HUT test is negative while the ATP test is positive and conversely that in some patients with positive HUT, the ATP test is negative? One possible explanation could be as follows: In patients with a positive ATP test, the basal plasma adenosine concentration is often low or very low (mostly under the K_D values for high-affinity A_1 R), the lower the plasma adenosine concentration, the higher the probability of ATP test positivity.[15] Conversely, in the VVS group, basal adenosine plasma concentration is high.[14,15] During the HUT adenosine plasma concentration rises as a result of relative hypoxemia linked to the influx of blood to the lower body. This increase is sufficient to activate low-affinity A_1 receptors and/or A_{2A} receptors and can induce vasoplegia and/or bradycardia, depending on the subtype of the activated receptor. On the other hand, in patients with very low basal concentrations, HUT does not allow adenosine levels to rise sufficiently, whereas abrupt iv administration of adenosine or ATP does, leading to activation mainly of A_1 R. Conversely, in VVS patients with positive HUT, the basal adenosine plasma level is very high. In this context, the administration of ATP or adenosine intravenously does not change the response. However, this last hypothesis needs further investigation.

Note that an increase in plasma adenosine concentration may sometimes occur as a collateral effect of some treatments. For example, ticagrelor used as an antiplatelet agent, may be accompanied by a rapid rise in adenosine concentration[23] that may induce AVB.[24-26]

ADENOSINE TEST, SICK SINUS SYNDROME, OR CAROTID SINUS SYNDROME (CSS)

Brignole et al.[18] explored the effects of ATP on the heart rhythm in patients affected by unexplained syncope or sick sinus syndrome or both syndromes and in healthy subjects. During ATP infusion, the sinus cycle lengthened to >2 seconds in 4% (among 76) of patients with unexplained syncope, in 23% patients with sick sinus syndrome, and in 42% patients with both neurally mediated and sick sinus syndromes. AVB occurred in nearly half of the controls, in 38% of patients with unexplained syncope, in 18% of patients with sick sinus syndrome, and finally in 42% of patients with both neurally mediated syncope and sick sinus syndrome. It was concluded that ATP administration exerts different effects on patients with unexplained syncope and patients with sick sinus syndrome and that the effect of ATP on atrioventricular conduction is greater than that on sinus node and is of similar magnitude in patients and controls; thus, the clinical meaning of ATP induced atrioventricular block remains uncertain.

Adenosine is well known to excite carotid chemoreceptors in animals,[27,28] and adenosine is thought to facilitate the baroreflex leading to a decrease in heart rate and blood pressure.[29,30]

ARE ATP OR ADENOSINE ADMINISTRATION THE SAME TESTS?

The mechanism of the action of ATP on the sinus node or the atrioventricular node remains unclear.

This is due to the rapid dephosphorylation of ATP by leucocyte ectonucleotidase CD39; thus, when administered ATP intravenously, it is likely that only a weak concentration of ATP reaches the target tissue, notably SN and AVN. It has been argued that ATP induced negative chronotropic and dromotropic effects via P1 activation.[9] However, the main target of ATP remains P2 receptors.[31]

Thus, it is likely that following ATP administration, only ATP breakdown products including mostly adenosine act at the sinus and atrioventricular nodes.

Note that since the molecular weight of ATP is almost twice that of adenosine (507 mg/mole vs. 267 g/mole), 10 mg of adenosine corresponds to approximately 20 mg of ATP.

Conclusion

While the ATP test has been used for many years to pinpoint the origin of syncope, the study of the adenosinergic profile seems to be a more useful aid for diagnostic orientation and above all for the management of syncope.

REFERENCES

1. Guieu R, Paganelli F, Sampieri F, Bechis G, Levy S, Rochat H. The use of HPLC to evaluate the variations of blood coronary adenosine levels during percutaneous transluminal angioplasty. *Clin Chim Acta*. 1994;230(1):63–68. https://doi.org/10.1016/0009-8981(94)90089-2.

2. Brignole M, Groppelli A, Brambilla R, et al. Plasma adenosine and neurally mediated syncope: ready for clinical use. *Europace*. 2020;22(6):847–853. https://doi.org/10.1093/europace/euaa070.

3. Gaubert M, Marlinge M, Kerbaul F, et al. Adenosine plasma level and A2A receptor expression in patients with cardiogenic shock. *Crit Care Med*. 2018;46(9):e874–e880. https://doi.org/10.1097/CCM.0000000000003252.

4. Aksu T, Golcuk E, Yalin K, Guler TE, Erden I. Simplified cardioneuroablation in the treatment of reflex syncope, functional AV block, and sinus node dysfunction. *Pacing Clin Electrophysiol*. 2016;39(1):42–53. https://doi.org/10.1111/pace.12756.

5. Cohen FR, Lazareno S, Birdsall NJ. The affinity of adenosine for the high- and low-affinity states of the human adenosine A1 receptor. *Eur J Pharmacol*. 1996;309(1):111–114. https://doi.org/10.1016/0014-2999(96)00415-3.

6. Kleppisch T, Nelson MT. Adenosine activates ATP-sensitive potassium channels in arterial myocytes via A2 receptors and cAMP-dependent protein kinase. *Proc Natl Acad Sci U S A*. 1995;92(26):12441–12445. https://doi.org/10.1073/pnas.92.26.12441.

7. Shryock JC, Snowdy S, Baraldi PG, et al. A2A-adenosine receptor reserve for coronary vasodilation. *Circulation*. 1998;98(7):711–718. https://doi.org/10.1161/01.cir.98.7.711.

8. Beukers MW, den Dulk H, van Tilburg EW, Brouwer J, Ijzerman AP. Why are A(2B) receptors low-affinity adenosine receptors? Mutation of Asn273 to Tyr increases affinity of human A(2B) receptor for 2-(1-hexynyl)adenosine. *Mol Pharmacol*. 2000; 58(6):1349–1356. https://doi.org/10.1124/mol.58.6.1349.

9. Burnstock G. Purinergic signaling in the cardiovascular system. *Circ Res*. 2017;120(1):207–228. https://doi.org/10.1161/CIRCRESAHA.116.309726.

10. Chorro FJ, Pardo JD, Sanchis J, et al. Estudio experimental de los efectos del ATP sobre el automatismo sinusal y la conducción en el nodo auriculoventricular [Experimental study of the effects of ATP on sinus automatism and atrioventricular node conduction]. *Rev Esp Cardiol*. 1989;42(5):329–336.

11. Deharo JC, Brignole M, Guieu R. Adenosine and neurohumoral syncope. *Minerva Med*. 2022;113(2):243–250. https://doi.org/10.23736/S0026-4806.21.07537-6.

12. Guieu R, Fromonot J, Mottola G, et al. Adenosinergic system and neuroendocrine syncope: what is the link? *Cells*. 2023;12(16):2027. https://doi.org/10.3390/cells12162027.

13. Waxman MB, Asta JA. Role of adenosine receptors in the paradoxic bradycardia response of rats to inferior vena cava occlusion during an infusion of isoproterenol. *Circulation*. 1998;98(12):1228–1235.

14. Saadjian AY, Lévy S, Franceschi F, Zouher I, Paganelli F, Guieu RP. Role of endogenous adenosine as a modulator of syncope induced during tilt testing. *Circulation*. 2002;106(5):569–574. https://doi.org/10.1161/01.cir.0000023924.66889.4c.

15. Deharo JC, Mechulan A, Giorgi R, et al. Adenosine plasma level and A2A adenosine receptor expression: correlation with laboratory tests in patients with neurally mediated syncope. *Heart*. 2012;98(11):855–859. https://doi.org/10.1136/heartjnl-2011-301411.

16. Brignole M, Iori M, Solari D, et al. Efficacy of theophylline in patients with syncope without prodromes with normal heart and normal ECG. *Int J Cardiol*. 2019;289:70–73. https://doi.org/10.1016/j.ijcard.2019.03.043.

17. Brignole M, Iori M, Strano S, et al. Theophylline in patients with syncope without prodrome, normal heart, and normal electrocardiogram: a propensity-score matched study verified by implantable cardiac monitor. *Europace*. 2022;24(7):1164–1170. https://doi.org/10.1093/europace/euab300.

18. Brignole M, Menozzi C, Alboni P, et al. The effect of exogenous adenosine in patients with neurally-mediated syncope and sick sinus syndrome. *Pacing Clin Electrophysiol*. 1994;17(11 Pt 2):2211–2216. https://doi.org/10.1111/j.1540-8159.1994.tb03828.x.

19. Shen WK, Hammill SC, Munger TM, et al. Adenosine: potential modulator for vasovagal syncope. *J Am Coll Cardiol*. 1996;28(1):146–154. https://doi.org/10.1016/0735-1097(96)00100-3.

20. Donateo P, Brignole M, Menozzi C, et al. Mechanism of syncope in patients with positive adenosine triphosphate tests. *J Am Coll Cardiol*. 2003;41(1):93–98. https://doi.org/10.1016/s0735-1097(02)02621-9.

21. Brignole M, Gaggioli G, Menozzi C, et al. Clinical features of adenosine sensitive syncope and tilt induced vasovagal syncope. *Heart*. 2000;83(1):24–28. https://doi.org/10.1136/heart.83.1.24.

22. Franceschi F, By Y, Peyrouse E, et al. A2A adenosine receptor function in patients with vasovagal syncope. *Europace*. 2013;15(9):1328–1332. https://doi.org/10.1093/europace/eut066.

23. Bonello L, Laine M, Kipson N, et al. Ticagrelor increases adenosine plasma concentration in patients with an acute coronary syndrome. *J Am Coll Cardiol*. 2014;63(9):872–877. https://doi.org/10.1016/j.jacc.2013.09.067.

24. Unlu M, Demirkol S, Yildirim AO, Balta Ş, Öztürk C, Iyisoy A. Atrioventricular block associated with ticagrelor therapy may require permanent pacemaker. *Int J Cardiol*. 2016;202:946–947. https://doi.org/10.1016/j.ijcard.2015.08.067.

25. De Maria E, Borghi A, Modonesi L, Cappelli S. Ticagrelor therapy and atrioventricular block: Do we need to worry? *World J Clin Cases*. 2017;5(5):178–182. https://doi.org/10.12998/wjcc.v5.i5.178.

26. Li X, Xue Y, Wu H. A case of atrioventricular block potentially associated with right coronary artery lesion and ticagrelor therapy mediated by the increasing adenosine plasma concentration. *Case Rep Vasc Med*. 2018;2018:9385017. https://doi.org/10.1155/2018/9385017.

27. McQueen DS, Ribeiro JA. Effect of adenosine on carotid chemoreceptor activity in the cat. *Br J Pharmacol*. 1981;74(1):129–136. https://doi.org/10.1111/j.1476-5381.1981.tb09964.x.

28. Chen S, Fan ZZ, He RR. [Adenosine facilitates carotid baroreflex in rats]. *Sheng Li Xue Bao*. 1998;50(3):296–302. Chinese.

29. Su X, Zhang WY, Ho SY. Effect of adenosine on carotid chemoreceptor activity in the rabbit. *Sheng Li Xue Bao.* 1991;43(3):291–295. Chinese.

30. Parry SW, Nath S, Bourke JP, Bexton RS, Kenny RA. Adenosine test in the diagnosis of unexplained syncope: marker of conducting tissue disease or neurally mediated syncope? *Eur Heart J.* 2006;27(12):1396–1400. https://doi.org/10.1093/eurheartj/ehi844.

31. Linden JM. *Basic Neurochemistry: Molecular, Cellular and Medical Aspects*, 6th edition. In: Siegel GJ, Agranoff BW, Albers RW, et al., editors. Philadelphia, PA: Lippincott-Raven, 1999.

8 Disorders of Orthostatic Intolerance

Orthostatic Hypotension and Postural Orthostatic Tachycardia Syndrome

Jacquie R. Baker and Satish R. Raj

GENERAL INTRODUCTION

Hemodynamic adjustments to physiological stressors are critical for adequate organ and tissue perfusion. Autonomic nervous system control of the cardiovascular system and local adjustments of the microvasculature ensure blood supply to vital organs such as the heart and brain is effectively regulated. If these systems become impaired, then the body can no longer adjust to gravitational stressors, resulting in hemodynamic instability and chronic intolerance to upright posture.

OH is a common form of orthostatic intolerance that becomes increasingly prevalent with increasing age and age-related diseases (e.g., Parkinson's disease, diabetes).[1] OH is characterized by excessive reductions in blood pressure on standing.[2] POTS is another chronic form of orthostatic intolerance that predominantly affects females of child-bearing age.[3] POTS is characterized by excessive orthostatic tachycardia in the absence of orthostatic hypotension and chronic (>3 month) symptoms.[2,3] Patients with chronic forms of orthostatic intolerance often experience daily, debilitating symptoms (e.g., light-headedness, brain fog, syncope, shortness of breath), which are exacerbated during upright position and relieved by recumbency.

In this chapter, we (1) review two common disorders of orthostatic intolerance, namely OH and POTS; (2) discuss current management options to help guide patient care; and (3) introduce novel therapeutic approaches.

PHYSIOLOGY OF STANDING

Upon standing, there is an instantaneous shift of 500–1,000 mL of blood to the capacitance vessels in the lower extremities and splanchnic circulation,[4] which leads to a reduction in cardiac venous return and reduced filling pressure. Consequently, cardiac output and stroke volume are reduced, which leads to small reductions in systolic blood pressure (~5 mmHg). In healthy individuals, unloading of high-pressure arterial baroreceptors leads to a reflexive increase in sympathetic nerve activity to increase cardiac contractility, heart rate, and systemic vascular resistance. In disorders of chronic orthostatic intolerance, this healthy reflex response to gravitation stress can become impaired, resulting in abnormal hemodynamic responses to upright posture, as seen in OH and POTS.

ORTHOSTATIC HYPOTENSION

OH is a debilitating autonomic nervous system disorder characterized by significant hemodynamic instability, crippling symptoms, and a reduced quality of life.[2,5] OH occurs due to the failure of the autonomic nervous system to reflexively control sympathetic nervous system activity in the vasculature, resulting in impaired vascular resistance. Classic OH is defined as a sustained drop in systolic (≥20 mmHg) or diastolic (≥10 mmHg) blood pressure within 3 minutes of active standing or during a ≥60° head-up tilt test.[2]

Common Clinical Features

Symptoms

Patients with OH may be symptomatic or asymptomatic.[6,7] Commonly reported symptoms include light-headedness, fatigue with standing, blurry vision, and shoulder and neck pain ("coat hanger pain"). Other less specific symptoms include generalized weakness, shortness of breath, chest pain, and headache. While the specific symptoms can vary, they should occur in the upright position and resolve with recumbence. Other factors supportive of OH include symptoms that are worse with high ambient temperatures, hot showers and baths, exertion, following large meals, and early in the morning. For patients who are not frequently symptomatic, syncope becomes a common comorbid condition, resulting in high rates of OH-related hospitalizations.[8] Additionally, ~50% of patients with OH related to baroreflex failure (i.e., nOH) also have concomitant supine hypertension (systolic ≥150 mmHg or diastolic ≥90 mmHg),[9] with a slightly greater prevalence in females (63% vs. 52%).[10] Although supine hypertension is a common side effect of most anti-hypotensive (or pressor) agents, multiple studies have reported evidence of supine hypertension even in untreated patients, suggesting it is part of the pathophysiology of autonomic failure.[11,12]

DOI: 10.1201/9781003415855-10

When supine hypertension is present, a systolic drop ≥30 mmHg or a diastolic drop ≥15 mmHg is required for a diagnosis of OH, as the magnitude of the blood pressure drop is dependent on the baseline blood pressure.[9]

Common Causes

The prevalence of OH increases with age. The association between OH and aging is complex, but it is likely in part due to normal age-associated decreases in baroreceptor sensitivity and blood pressure regulatory mechanisms.[13,14] Other common causes of OH include endocrine issues, hypovolemia, and medication side effects. Neurogenic OH (nOH) is a subtype of OH characterized by disruption of central and/or peripheral pathways within the baroreflex, leading to insufficient norepinephrine release from sympathetic neurons and a subsequent inability to constrict the peripheral vasculature. nOH is a feature of several neurodegenerative α-synucleinopathies and peripheral neuropathies.[2]

Synucleinopathies

α-Synucleinopathies are a collection of neurodegenerative disorders characterized by the deposition and aggregation of misfolded α-synuclein, leading to neuronal degeneration and death. The clinical phenotype depends on the anatomical location of α-synuclein aggregates within the nervous system but can involve autonomic, motor, and/or cognitive features. *Multiple system atrophy (MSA)*: MSA (formerly referred to as Shy-Drager syndrome) is a sporadic and fatal, adult-onset, neurodegenerative disorder characterized by parkinsonian features or cerebellar ataxia, and progressive autonomic failure.[15] The prevalence of MSA ranges from 4 to 5 cases/100,000 persons, increasing to 7.8 cases/100,000 in individuals >40 years of age.[15,16] Glial cytoplasmic inclusions containing aggregates of misfolded α-synuclein are a biological hallmark of MSA.[15] *Parkinson's disease (PD)*: While PD is primarily regarded as a movement disorder, nOH is a common non-motor feature. Lewy bodies and Lewy neurites are the pathological hallmarks of PD, with α-synuclein aggregates present in the neurons of the brainstem, intermediolateral cell column, and peripheral autonomic nervous system. *Dementia with Lewy bodies (DLB)*: DLB accounts for 5% of all dementia cases in older adults[17] and is the second most common neurodegenerative dementia after Alzheimer's disease. DLB is characterized by autonomic dysfunction, cognitive decline, and hallucinations.[1] *Pure autonomic failure (PAF)*: Previously called Bradbury-Eggleston syndrome, PAF is a rare neurodegenerative disorder with no known environmental or genetic cause.[18] PAF may be a forme fruste of one of the aforementioned disorders. In a longitudinal study, over 30% of patients with PAF "phenoconverted" into either MSA, PD, or DLB.[1]

Peripheral Neuropathies

Diabetic autonomic neuropathies secondary to long-standing and/or poorly controlled diabetes mellitus are the most common autonomic neuropathies in the developed world. In addition to diabetes, other causes of small or unmyelinated fiber autonomic neuropathies that can lead to nOH include amyloidosis, hereditary neuropathies, immune-mediated autonomic neuropathies, and neuropathies associated with toxins and infectious diseases.[19,20] For an in-depth review of autonomic neuropathies, readers are encouraged to review these articles.[19,20]

Epidemiology

In community-dwelling adults, the prevalence of OH strongly correlates with age,[21,22] ranging from 5% to 7% in adults years 45–65,[23,24] increasing to 10%–18% in adults ≥60 years,[21] and 30% in adults ≥75 years.[8,25] OH is also prevalent in diabetes, with an estimated pooled prevalence of 24% (95% CI: 19%–28%),[26] and is a key feature of the neurodegenerative α-synucleinopathies. In MSA, OH is evident in 54% of patients within 3 minutes of standing and 72% of patients after 10 minutes.[27] In PD, a systematic review of 25 studies (n=5,070) reported OH rates ranging from 9.6% to 64.9% with an estimated pooled prevalence of 30.1% (95% CI: 22.9%–38.4%).[28] OH is also present in 30%–50% of patients with DLB[1] and all patients with PAF.[18]

POSTURAL ORTHOSTATIC TACHYCARDIA SYNDROME

POTS is a debilitating and chronic form of orthostatic intolerance characterized by excessive orthostatic tachycardia (≥30 bpm) in the absence of orthostatic hypotension (≥20/10 mmHg)[2,3,29] and chronic (≥3 month) symptoms. POTS is an under-recognized and often misdiagnosed condition[30] that significantly negatively impacts patient quality of life and day-to-day functioning of patients to a similar extent as heart failure.[31]

Common Clinical Features

In addition to excessive orthostatic tachycardia, patients can also experience a combination of cardiac (e.g., rapid heart palpitations, light-headedness, chest pain/discomfort, and difficulty breathing) and non-cardiac (e.g., mental clouding [i.e., "brain fog"], headaches, nausea, shakiness, blurred vision, sleep disturbances, exercise intolerance, and fatigue) symptoms.[3,30] Even routine activities of daily living can significantly exacerbate symptoms, leading to increased fatigue and reduced functional capacity. Although many patients experience symptoms of pre-syncope, only ~30% of patients with POTS faint.[3]

Common Causes

POTS represents the final common clinical presentation of various pathophysiological pathways, which may include selective lower limb sympathetic denervation, central hyperadrenergic states, norepinephrine transporter deficiencies, hypovolemia with impaired blood volume regulation, and mast cell activation.[3] POTS is also associated with several comorbidities including irritable bowel syndrome, myalgic encephalomyelitis or chronic fatigue syndrome (ME/CFS), Ehlers–Danlos syndrome,[30] and Long-COVID.[32] When taking a medical history, it is important to inquire about significant events that occurred before the onset of these symptoms, including viral infections, illness, pregnancy, or major surgical procedures, as symptoms can often manifest after such events.

Epidemiology

The prevalence of POTS in the general population is unknown, but it is estimated to be up to 1%. In the United States, POTS was estimated to affect 3,000,000 individuals before COVID-19, but these numbers are likely higher now as there has been an emergence of studies reporting new-onset POTS in patients with Long-COVID.[32] While POTS can affect individuals of any sex at any age, >90% of individuals are young, pre-menopausal females.[30]

TREATMENT OPTIONS FOR ORTHOSTATIC INTOLERANCE

Treatment decisions should be based on the individual cardiovascular profile, with the primary goals being to mitigate symptoms, avoid falls, and maintain quality of life. Initial steps should include a review of current medications and withdrawal of drugs that exacerbate hemodynamic instability (e.g., diuretics, daytime nitrates, α_1-blockers, tricyclic antidepressants). Patients should also be educated on factors that can aggravate symptoms (i.e., hot showers/baths, high ambient temperatures, post-prandial hypotension). Prior to pharmacological intervention, the following non-pharmacological strategies can be implemented as a first pass to help mitigate symptoms in both OH and POTS (Table 8.1).

Table 8.1: Summary of Non-Pharmacological Interventions

Non-Pharmacological Intervention	Implementation	Purpose
Counter-maneuvers[1,39]	Muscle tensing maneuvers (e.g., leg-crossing, thigh and buttocks tensing, [half-] squatting)	Prevent venous pooling Increase cardiac venous return
Physical activity[1,3,39]	Primarily recumbent aerobic exercise Lower limb resistance training	Reduce orthostatic tachycardia Increase blood volume, stroke volume, and left ventricular mass
Fluid hydration[1,3,39]	2–3 L/day of water-equivalents in nOH >3 L/day of water-equivalents in POTS	Increase blood volume Provide increase in blood pressure
Adequate sodium intake[1,3,39]	2–6 g/day for patients with nOH 10 g of sodium/day for patients with hypovolemic POTS	Increase intravascular volume
Compression garments[1,3,39]	Abdominal binders and waist-high compression garments	Reduce venous pooling Increase cardiac venous return
[a]Head-up sleeping[1,9]	Raise head of the bed 6–9 inches (15–30 cm)	Helps shift fluid to the lower body and reduce central blood volume Reduce renal hyper-perfusion Reduce pressure diuresis and natriuresis

[a] For supine hypertension often seen in patients with nOH.

Non-Pharmacological Interventions
Counter Maneuvers and Physical Activity

Simple physical counter-maneuvers can be incorporated into activities of daily living to improve orthostatic tolerance. Muscle tensing maneuvers such as leg-crossing, thigh and buttocks tensing, and (half-) squatting prevent venous pooling and increase cardiac venous return and cardiac output,[33] resulting in improved standing hemodynamics for patients.[34,35] Additionally, all patients should be encouraged to incorporate/maintain physical activity and exercise. To avoid symptoms of orthostatic intolerance, patients should be educated to start with supine or recumbent exercises, moving progressively toward upright exercises as tolerated.

Increase Plasma Volume

Increasing dietary sodium intake and maintaining adequate hydration help maintain plasma volume and improve orthostatic tolerance. Consensus guidelines recommend that patients with OH drink 2 L of water/day and ingest 2–6 g of sodium/day.[1] Moreover, rapid ingestion (within 3–4 minutes) of 500 mL of water produces marked, acute pressor effects (33–37 mmHg) for patients with OH that are sustained for about 1 hour.[36–38] In POTS, patients are encouraged to drink >3 L of water/day and to ingest ~10 g of sodium/day.[39] Of note, the long-term risks of high-sodium diets (e.g., edema, increased blood pressure) have not been well studied.

Compression Garments

Compression garments are often recommended for patients with orthostatic intolerance. In the upright position, patients can experience considerable venous pooling within the splanchnic circulation,[40,41] which exacerbates upright hemodynamic instability. Abdominal/waist-high compression minimizes blood pooling, which in turn has been shown to reduce orthostatic blood pressure drops in OH,[42] reduce tachycardia in POTS,[43] and reduce symptoms in both groups.[42,43]

Head-Up Sleeping (for Supine Hypertension)

Sleeping with the head of the bed raised 6–9 inches (15–30 cm) helps shift fluid to the lower body and reduce central blood volume, resulting in reduced nocturnal renal perfusion and reduced nocturnal pressure diuresis and natriuresis.[9] Additionally, by activating the renin–angiotensin–aldosterone system, head-up sleeping reduces sodium and water excretion leading to improved fluid retention[44] and orthostatic tolerance.[45] For patients with severe supine hypertension (systolic >160 mmHg), additional short-acting anti-hypertensive agents (e.g., nitroglycerine patches, clonidine, angiotensin-converting enzyme inhibitors, calcium channel blockers) can be considered for use overnight.

Current Pharmacological Interventions for Both OH and POTS
Midodrine

Midodrine is an FDA-approved α_1-agonist prodrug that promotes vaso- and venoconstriction, which helps increase cardiac venous return, stroke volume, and subsequently blood pressure (Figure 8.1).[46–48] Midodrine is often prescribed every 4 hours. Due to its relatively short duration

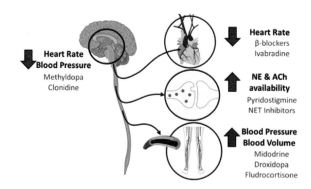

Figure 8.1 Current pharmacological interventions for disorders of orthostatic intolerance. Summary of pharmacological therapies for disorders of orthostatic intolerance and their physiological effects. NE, norepinephrine; Ach, acetylcholine; NET, norepinephrine transporters.

of onset (30–45 minutes) and short half-life, midodrine can be titrated to day-to-day activities and symptoms. Importantly, midodrine has an FDA black-box warning, the highest safety-related warning, due to its risk for supine hypertension.[46,48,49] As such, midodrine should not be taken within 4 hours of bedtime, and patients should be instructed not to lie down for 4 hours after taking the midodrine.

Fludrocortisone

Fludrocortisone is an FDA-approved drug commonly used off-label for disorders of orthostatic intolerance. Fludrocortisone is a synthetic mineralocorticoid that expands intravascular blood volume by increasing renal sodium and water reabsorption (Figure 8.1). Fludrocortisone also renders α-adrenoreceptors more sensitive to circulating catecholamines and can therefore be combined with drugs like droxidopa or midodrine to augment their effectiveness in managing orthostatic intolerance.[50,51] Typically prescribed at doses ranging from 0.1 to 0.3 mg daily, fludrocortisone should be taken regularly, usually in the morning as opposed to on an "as needed" basis, due to its long-lasting effects and the potential for exacerbating supine hypertension.[9,50] The onset of action occurs over three to seven days, with increased vascular resistance contributing to its long-term effectiveness. Higher doses of fludrocortisone may elevate the risk of adverse effects, including supine hypertension, hypokalemia, and edema,[44] and potentially lead to hypothalamic–pituitary axis suppression. Patients should be educated to maintain adequate salt and fluid consumption to increase effectiveness.

Pyridostigmine

Pyridostigmine is another FDA-approved drug often used off-label for disorders of orthostatic intolerance.[52] Pyridostigmine is a peripheral acetylcholinesterase inhibitor that enhances synaptic acetylcholine levels in both the autonomic ganglia and peripheral muscarinic parasympathetic receptors (Figure 8.1). Typical doses range from 30 to 60 mg three times daily. For patients with OH and concomitant supine hypertension, pyridostigmine is postulated to promote enhanced cholinergic transmission more when patients are upright (when there is more physiological acetylcholine release) than while they are supine (with less physiological acetylcholine release), thereby causing less supine hypertension.[53] Pyridostigmine has also shown promise in patients with POTS, with roughly 50% of patients reporting symptom improvement.[54,55] Side effects related to cholinergic stimulation (e.g., abdominal cramps, enhanced bowel motility, excessive sweating, and urinary incontinence) are common reasons for discontinuation and should be considered when prescribing this medication. Conversely, these effects may be salutary in patients who are prone to constipation.

Current Pharmacological Interventions for nOH
Droxidopa

Droxidopa is an FDA-approved prodrug of norepinephrine that undergoes conversion to norepinephrine in both the central and peripheral nervous systems. The primary mechanism behind droxidopa's efficacy lies in replenishing neural norepinephrine levels to improve standing blood pressure (Figure 8.1). Droxidopa is typically prescribed two to three times daily in doses ranging from 100 to 600 mg. Droxidopa increases circulating plasma catecholamine levels, reaching peak levels around 6 hours with sustained effects for up to 46 hours after treatment.[56] Overall, droxidopa has demonstrated its safety and effectiveness in the short-term management of nOH symptoms. Side effects can include headache, nausea, fatigue, and supine hypertension.[9]

General Comments About Pharmacological Interventions for nOH

Importantly, nearly all anti-hypotensive agents can cause or exacerbate supine hypertension, which can then worsen renal and cardiovascular outcomes. Shorter-acting pressor agents (e.g., midodrine, droxidopa) are preferred over longer-acting medications (e.g., fludrocortisone) since they can be used just during the daytime. Additionally, regular monitoring with adjustments to daytime medications and/or the use of short-acting antihypertensives at night are sometimes required.

Novel Pharmacological Interventions for nOH
Norepinephrine Transporter Inhibitors (Atomoxetine/Ampreloxetine)

Atomoxetine, a norepinephrine transporter (NET) blocker, increases synaptic norepinephrine availability by impeding its reuptake and clearance (Figure 8.1).[57] In patients with intact peripheral noradrenergic function (i.e., MSA), an acute 18 mg dose of atomoxetine elevated seated systolic blood pressure by ~50 mmHg and plasma norepinephrine levels by 26% compared to placebo.[58] In subsequent studies, atomoxetine exhibited equal or superior pressor responses upon standing compared to midodrine and alleviated clinical symptoms compared to placebo.[59,60] The efficacy of atomoxetine in patients with intact peripheral sympathetic fibers is likely due to "augmented" residual sympathetic tone, which is unopposed because of the loss of baroreflex restraint. By taking advantage of residual sympathetic tone, pharmacological inhibition of the NET represents a promising approach. Importantly, long-term data on the use of NET inhibitors for nOH are currently lacking. *Ampreloxetine*, a novel selective long-acting NET inhibitor, is under evaluation as a once-daily oral treatment for symptomatic nOH in autonomic synucleinopathies. In phase 2 clinical trial (NCT02705755), escalating doses (1–20 mg over five days) led to peak plasma ampreloxetine concentrations 6–9 hours post-administration. The optimal doses ranged from 5 to 10 mg, resulting in a ~15.7 mmHg increase in seated blood pressure 4 hours after ampreloxetine, compared to a 14 mmHg drop with placebo.[61] During a 20-week open-label treatment, steady-state plasma ampreloxetine concentrations were reached within two weeks, leading to stable levels over 24 hours (median dose: 10 mg daily). Plasma norepinephrine increased by 71%, while the norepinephrine metabolite (i.e., dihydroxyphenylglycine) decreased by 22%,[62] indicating reduced neuronal reuptake and metabolism of norepinephrine in postganglionic sympathetic neurons. Ampreloxetine not only significantly improved symptoms and increased standing systolic blood pressure, but its impact on supine blood pressure was also minimal. Overall, ampreloxetine was well-tolerated and improved orthostatic blood pressure and symptoms. A phase-3 multi-centered clinical trial of ampreloxetine for nOH in MSA is currently underway (NCT05696717).

Neurostimulators

Implantable devices, including epidural electrical stimulation, offer a novel non-pharmacological approach to improving standing blood pressure in patients with nOH. In a case report of a patient with MSA, electrical stimulation delivered over the thoracic spinal cord increased seated systolic blood pressure by 20 mmHg, a pressor response that increased linearly with the stimulation amplitude.[63] The initial evaluation of the acute efficacy showed that the magnitude of the drop in blood pressure with upright posture was similar with and without neurostimulation, but the drop occurred more gradually (over 10 minutes) when neurostimulation was used. Following three months of rehabilitation, the patient was able to complete the entire 10-minute tilt test, reported almost no syncope when upright, and showed improved ambulation. While the efficacy and potential complications of long-term use remain uncertain, implantable neurostimulators are becoming more sophisticated and may eventually become part of clinical care.

Current Pharmacological Interventions for POTS
Beta-Blockers

Beta (β)-adrenergic blockers are frequently used to reduce tachycardia in patients with POTS (Figure 8.1), although patients may report excessive fatigue or intolerance with these medications.[3] The decision to prescribe β-blockers requires careful consideration, as it could be counterproductive if excessive tachycardia is compensatory for other physiological deficits, such as low stroke volume, but beneficial if tachycardia is an "over-compensatory" response.[3] Research, primarily focused on the non-selective β-adrenergic receptor antagonist propranolol, has shown that low doses (10–20 mg orally, four times per day) are better tolerated than higher doses[64] and are highly effective at reducing standing heart rate, alleviating symptoms, and improving exercise capacity in POTS patients.[3,39]

Sympatholytics (Clonidine/Methyldopa)

Central sympatholytic medications, such as clonidine and methyldopa, offer valuable treatment options for individuals with POTS with hyperadrenergic features (Figure 8.1).[3,39] *Clonidine*, an α_2-adrenergic receptor agonist, exerts its effects centrally by reducing sympathetic nerve traffic. Clonidine can be administered in doses of 0.1–0.2 mg PO twice daily or via a long-acting transdermal patch.[3] *Methyldopa* (125–250 mg PO at bedtime, sometimes an additional morning dose) is converted into α-methyl-norepinephrine, which, like clonidine, can act on central α_2 receptors, reducing central sympathetic nervous system activity. Unfortunately, both drugs can exacerbate fatigue and symptoms of cognitive impairment, so they need to be used carefully. These medications can be valuable options for patients with high sympathetic nervous system activity who have not responded adequately to other treatments.[3,39]

Novel Pharmacological Interventions for POTS
Ivabradine

Ivabradine is a newer drug that selectively blocks I_f channels on the sinoatrial node, which in turn selectively reduces heart rate with potentially less effects on blood pressure or sympathetic nerve activity (Figure 8.1).[65,66] A recent systematic review identified 13 studies ($n=132$) exploring the safety and efficacy of ivabradine in POTS.[67] Overall, ivabradine lowered the heart rate and provided symptomatic relief without affecting blood pressure. In a recent randomized, double-blinded, placebo-controlled crossover trial, ivabradine reduced heart rate and significantly improved quality of life.[68] Across these studies, initial oral doses ranged from 2.5 to 7 mg, 1–2×/day. The most common side effects reported included visual phosphenes, nausea, headaches, and fatigue (Table 8.2).

CONCLUSIONS

Disorders of chronic orthostatic intolerance represent an important health problem that remains poorly understood. POTS, one of the most common forms of orthostatic intolerance, is a disabling

Table 8.2: Summary of Pharmacological Interventions

Pharmacological Drug	Dose	Drug Class	Side Effects	Use in POTS	Use in OH
Mechanism: Reduce sinus tachycardia					
Propranolol	PO 10–20 mg QID	Non-selective β-blocker	Fatigue, exercise intolerance, rarely weight gain	X	
Methyldopa (hyperadrenergic POTS)	PO 125–250 mg BID	Central sympatholytic	Sedation, dry mouth, orthostatic hypotension, mental clouding	X	
Clonidine (hyperadrenergic POTS)	PO 0.1–0.2 mg BID	Central sympatholytic	Sedation, dry mouth, orthostatic hypotension, mental clouding	X	
Mechanism: Expand Intravascular Volume					
Fludrocortisone	PO 0.1–0.3 mg QID	Mineralocorticoid	Migraine headache, heart failure, edema, hypokalemia	X	X
Mechanism: Vasoconstriction					
Midodrine	PO 2.5–15 mg q4H x3	α_1-adrenergic agonist	Supine hypertension (avoid dosing within 4 hours of lying down), piloerection, scalp itch, urinary retention, headache	X	X
Pyridostigmine	PO 30–60 mg TID	Peripheral acetylcholinesterase inhibitor	Nausea, vomiting, diarrhea, reduced heart rate (very good for constipation)	X	X
Droxidopa	PO 100–600 mg TID	Prodrug of norepinephrine	Supine hypertension, avoid lying down 5 hours following dose		X
Novel Therapeutic Interventions					
Ivabradine	PO 2.5–7.5 mg BID	"Funny channel" blocker	Light-headedness, fatigue, teratogenic	X	
Atomoxetine	PO 18 mg BID	Norepinephrine reuptake inhibitor	Nausea, vomiting, loss of appetite, fatigue, dry mouth		X
Ampreloxetine	PO 5–10 mg QID	Norepinephrine reuptake inhibitor	Headache, hypertension		X
Neurostimulator	N/A	Electrical activity delivered to thoracic spinal cord	Potential complications associated with surgery and anesthesia Lower back pain		X

BID, twice daily; mg, milligram; OH, orthostatic hypotension; PO, by mouth; POTS, postural orthostatic tachycardia syndrome; q4H x3, every 4 hours three times daily; QD, once daily; QID, four times daily; SC, subcutaneous; TID, three times daily.

and chronic condition that predominantly (>90%) affects young females (13–50 years). OH is another highly prevalent form of chronic orthostatic intolerance that becomes increasingly prevalent with increasing age. Through a combination of non-pharmacological and pharmacological approaches, it is possible to improve both the symptoms of orthostatic intolerance and the overall quality of life for some patients. There is still a critical need to understand the mechanisms underlying orthostatic intolerance and to develop new strategies to optimize care, treatment, and health outcomes for patients with chronic forms of orthostatic intolerance.

REFERENCES

1. Freeman R, Abuzinadah AR, Gibbons C, Jones P, Miglis MG, Sinn DI. Orthostatic hypotension: JACC state-of-the-art review. *J Am Coll Cardiol*. 2018;72(11):1294–1309. https://doi.org/10.1016/j.jacc.2018.05.079

2. Freeman R, Wieling W, Axelrod FB, et al. Consensus statement on the definition of orthostatic hypotension, neurally mediated syncope and the postural tachycardia syndrome. *Clin Auton Res*. 2011;21(2):69–72.

3. Raj SR. Postural tachycardia syndrome (POTS). *Circulation*. 2013;127(23):2336–2342.

4. Smith JJ, Porth CM, Erickson M. Hemodynamic response to the upright posture. *J Clin Pharmacol*. 1994;34(5):375–386. https://doi.org/10.1002/j.1552-4604.1994.tb04977.x

5. Farrell MC, Shibao CA. Morbidity and mortality in orthostatic hypotension. *Auton Neurosci*. 2020;229:102717. https://doi.org/10.1016/j.autneu.2020.102717

6. Freeman R, Illigens BMW, Lapusca R, et al. Orthostatic hypotension symptom recognition is impaired in patients with orthostatic hypotension. *Hypertension*. 2020;75:1325–1332. https://doi.org/10.1161/HYPERTENSIONAHA.119.13619

7. Isik AT, Kocyigit SE, Smith L, Aydin AE, Soysal P. A comparison of the prevalence of orthostatic hypotension between older patients with Alzheimer's disease, Lewy body dementia, and without dementia. *Exp Gerontol*. 2019;124:110628. https://doi.org/10.1016/j.exger.2019.06.001

8. Shibao C, Grijalva CG, Raj SR, Biaggioni I, Griffin MR. Orthostatic hypotension-related hospitalizations in the United States. *Am J Med*. 2007;120(11):975–980. https://doi.org/10.1016/j.amjmed.2007.05.009

9. Baker J, Kimpinski K. Management of supine hypertension complicating neurogenic orthostatic hypotension. *CNS Drugs*. 2017;8:653–663.

10. Shannon J, Jordan J, Costa F, Robertson R, Biaggioni I. The hypertension of autonomic failure and its treatment. *Hypertension*. 1997;30(5):1062–1067.

11. Goldstein DS, Pechnik S, Holmes C, Eldadah B, Sharabi Y. Association between supine hypertension and orthostatic hypotension in autonomic failure. *Hypertension*. 2003;42(2):136–142. https://doi.org/10.1161/01.HYP.0000081216.11623.C3

12. Biaggioni I, Robertson RM. Hypertension in orthostatic hypotension and autonomic dysfunction. *Cardiol Clin*. 2002;20(2):291–301. https://doi.org/10.1016/S0733-8651(01)00005-4

13. Davy KP, Seals DR, Tanaka H. Augmented cardiopulmonary and integrative sympathetic baroreflexes but attenuated peripheral vasoconstriction with age. *Hypertension*. 1998;32(2):298–304. https://doi.org/10.1161/01.HYP.32.2.298

14. Gribbin B, Pickering TG, Sleight P, Peto R. Effect of age and high blood pressure on baroreflex sensitivity in man. *Circ Res*. 1971;29(4):424–431. https://doi.org/10.1161/01.RES.29.4.424

15. Fanciulli A, Wenning GK. Multiple-system atrophy. *N Engl J Med.* 2015;372:249–263. https://doi.org/10.1056/NEJMra1311488

16. Vanacore N, Bonifati V, Fabbrini G, et al. Epidemiology of multiple system atrophy. *Neurol Sci.* 2001;22(1):97–99. https://doi.org/10.1007/s100720170064

17. Hogan DB, Fiest KM, Roberts JI, et al. The prevalence and incidence of dementia with lewy bodies: A systematic review. *Can J Neurol Sci.* 2016;43(S1):S83–S95. https://doi.org/10.1017/cjn.2016.2

18. Coon EA, Singer W, Low PA. Pure autonomic failure. *Mayo Clin Proc.* 2019;94(10):2087–2098. https://doi.org/10.1053/j.gastro.2016.08.014.CagY

19. Freeman R. Autonomic peripheral neuropathy. *Neurol Clin.* 2007;25(1):277–301. https://doi.org/10.1016/j.ncl.2007.01.001

20. Dineen J, Freeman R. Autonomic neuropathy. *Semin Neurol.* 2015;35:458–468. https://doi.org/10.1001/archinte.143.8.1635

21. Rutan G, Hermanson B, Bild D, Kittner S, LaBaw F, Tell G. Orthostatic hypotension in older adults: The cardiovascular health study. *Hypertension.* 1992;19(6):508–519. https://doi.org/10.1007/978-3-030-62493-4

22. Masaki K, Schatz I, Burchfiel C, et al. Orthostatic hypotension predicts mortality in elderly men: The Honolulu Heart Program. *Circulation.* 1998;98:2290–2295. https://doi.org/10.1007/978-3-642-95642-3_32

23. Finucane C, O'Connell MDL, Fan CW, et al. Age-related normative changes in phasic orthostatic blood pressure in a large population study: Findings from the Irish longitudinal study on ageing (TILDA). *Circulation.* 2014;130(20):1780–1789. https://doi.org/10.1161/CIRCULATIONAHA.114.009831

24. Juraschek SP, Daya N, Appel LJ, et al. Orthostatic hypotension in middle-age and risk of falls. *Am J Hypertens.* 2017;30(2):188–195. https://doi.org/10.1093/ajh/hpw108

25. Tilvis RS, Hakala S, Valvanne J, Erkinjuntti T. Postural hypotension and dizziness in a general aged population: A four-year follow-up of the Helsinki aging study. *J Am Geriatr Soc.* 1996;44(7):809–814.

26. Zhou Y, Ke SJ, Qiu XP, Liu LB. Prevalence, risk factors, and prognosis of orthostatic hypotension in diabetic patients. *Med (United States).* 2017;96(36):1–11. https://doi.org/10.1097/MD.0000000000008004

27. Pavy-Le Traon A, Piedvache A, Perez-Lloret S, et al. New insights into orthostatic hypotension in multiple system atrophy: A European multicentre cohort study. *J Neurol Neurosurg Psychiatry.* 2016;87(5):554–561. https://doi.org/10.1136/jnnp-2014-309999

28. Velseboer DC, De Haan RJ, Wieling W, Goldstein DS, De Bie RMA. Prevalence of orthostatic hypotension in Parkinson's disease: A systematic review and meta-analysis. *Parkinsonism Relat Disord.* 2011;17(10):724–729.

29. Raj SR, Guzman JC, Harvey P, et al. Canadian Cardiovascular Society position statement on postural orthostatic tachycardia syndrome (POTS) and related disorders of chronic orthostatic intolerance. *Can J Cardiol.* 2020;36:357–372. https://doi.org/10.1016/j.cjca.2019.12.024

30. Shaw BH, Stiles LE, Bourne K, et al. The face of postural tachycardia syndrome – insights from a large cross-sectional online community-based survey. *J Intern Med.* 2019;286(4):438–448. https://doi.org/10.1111/joim.12895

31. Benrud-Larson L, Dewar M, Sandroni P, Rummans T, Haythornthwaite J, Low P. Quality of life in patients with postural tachycardia syndrome. *Mayo Clin Proc.* 2002;77(6):531–537. https://doi.org/10.4065/77.6.531

32. Hira R, Baker JR, Siddiqui T, et al. Objective hemodynamic cardiovascular autonomic abnormalities in post-acute sequelae of COVID-19. *Can J Cardiol.* 2023;39(6):767–775. https://doi.org/10.1016/j.cjca.2022.12.002

33. Van Lieshout JJ, Pott F, Madsen PL, Van Goudoever J, Secher NH. Muscle tensing during standing: Effects on cerebral tissue oxygenation and cerebral artery blood velocity. *Stroke.* 2001;32(7):1546–1551. https://doi.org/10.1161/01.STR.32.7.1546

34. Harms MPM, Wieling W, Colier WNJM, Lenders JWM, Secher NH, Van Lieshout JJ. Central and cerebrovascular effects of leg crossing in humans with sympathetic failure. *Clin Sci.* 2010;118(9):573–581. https://doi.org/10.1042/CS20090038

35. Wieling W, van Dijk N, Thijs RD, de Lange FJ, Krediet CTP, Halliwill JR. Physical countermeasures to increase orthostatic tolerance. *J Intern Med.* 2015;277(1):69–82. https://doi.org/10.1111/joim.12249

36. Jordan J, Shannon JR, Shannon JR, et al. A potent pressor response elicited by drinking water. *Lancet.* 1999;353(9154):723.

37. Jordan J, Shannon JR, Black BK, et al. The pressor response to water drinking in humans: A sympathetic reflex? *Circulation.* 2000;101(5):504–509.

38. Oyewunmi O, Lei L, Laurin J, Morillo C, Sheldon R, Raj S. Hemodynamic effects of the osmopressor response: A systematic review and meta-analysis. *J Am Heart Assoc.* 2023;12(21):1–12. https://doi.org/10.1161/JAHA.122.029645

39. Mar P, Raj S. Postural orthostatic tachycardia syndrome: Mechanisms and new therapies. *Annu Rev Med.* 2020;71:235–248. https://doi.org/10.14503/THIJ-19-7060

40. Stewart JM, Medow MS, Glover J, Montgomery LD. Persistent splanchnic hyperemia during upright tilt in postural tachycardia syndrome. *Am J Physiol Hear Circ Physiol.* 2006;290(2):H665–H673. https://doi.org/10.1152/ajpheart.00784.2005.Persistent

41. Denq JC, Opfer-Gehrking TL, Giuliani M, Felten J, Converti VA, Low PA. Efficacy of compression of different capacitance beds in the amelioration of orthostatic hypotension. *Clin Auton Res.* 1997;7(6):321–326. https://doi.org/10.1007/BF02267725

42. Podoleanu C, Maggi R, Brignole M, et al. Lower limb and abdominal compression bandages prevent progressive orthostatic hypotension in elderly persons a randomized single-blind controlled study. *J Am Coll Cardiol.* 2006;48(7):1425–1432. https://doi.org/10.1016/j.jacc.2006.06.052

43. Bourne KM, Sheldon RS, Hall J, et al. Compression garment reduces orthostatic tachycardia and symptoms in patients with postural orthostatic tachycardia syndrome. *J Am Coll Cardiol.* 2021;77(3):285–296. https://doi.org/10.1016/j.jacc.2020.11.040

44. van Lieshout JJ, ten Harkel AD, Wieling W. Fludrocortisone and sleeping in the head-up position limit the postural decrease in cardiac output in autonomic failure. *Clin Auton Res.* 2000;10(1):35–42.

45. Cooper VL, Hainsworth R. Head-up sleeping improves orthostatic tolerance in patients with syncope. *Clin Auton Res.* 2008;18(6):318–324. https://doi.org/10.1007/s10286-008-0494-8

46. Low PA. Efficacy of Midodrine vs Placebo in neurogenic orthostatic hypotension. *JAMA*. 1997;277(13):1046. https://doi.org/10.1001/jama.1997.03540370036033

47. Shibao C, Okamoto L, Biaggioni I. Pharmacotherapy of autonomic failure. *Pharmacol Ther*. 2012;134(3):279–286. https://dx.doi.org/10.1016/j.pharmthera.2011.05.009

48. Parsaik AK, Singh B, Altayar O, et al. Midodrine for orthostatic hypotension: A systematic review and meta-analysis of clinical trials. *J Gen Intern Med*. 2013;28(11):1496–1503. https://doi.org/10.1007/s11606-013-2520-3

49. Low PA, Gilden JL, Freeman R, Sheng KN, McElligott MA. Efficacy of midodrine vs placebo in neurogenic orthostatic hypotension. A randomized, double-blind multicenter study. Midodrine Study Group. *JAMA*. 1997;277(13):1046–1051.

50. Chobanian AV, Volicer L, Tifft CP, Gavras H, Liang CS, Faxon D. Mineralocorticoid-induced hypertension in patients with orthostatic hypotension. *N Engl J Med*. 1979;301(2):68–73.

51. Davies B, Bannister R, Sever P, Wilcox C. The pressor actions of noradrenaline and angiotension II in chronic autonomic failure treated with indomethacin. *Br J Clin Pharmacol*. 1979;8:253–260. https://doi.org/10.1111/j.1365-2125.1980.tb01748.x

52. Singer W, Opfer-Gehrking TL, Nickander KK, Hines SM, Low PA. Acetylcholinesterase inhibition in patients with orthostatic intolerance. *J Clin Neurophysiol*. 2006;23(5):476–481.

53. Singer W, Sandroni P, Opfer-Gehrking TL, et al. Pyridostigmine treatment trial in neurogenic orthostatic hypotension. *Arch Neurol*. 2006;63(4):513–518.

54. Kanjwal K, Karabin B, Sheikh M, et al. Pyridostigmine in the treatment of postural orthostatic tachycardia: A single-center experience. *PACE – Pacing Clin Electrophysiol*. 2011;34(6):750–755. https://doi.org/10.1111/j.1540-8159.2011.03047.x

55. Raj SR, Black BK, Biaggioni I, Harris PA, Robertson D. Acetylcholinesterase inhibition improves tachycardia in postural tachycardia syndrome. *Circulation*. 2005;111(21):2734–2740. https://doi.org/10.1161/CIRCULATIONAHA.104.497594

56. Kaufmann H, Saadia D, Voustianiouk A, et al. Norepinephrine precursor therapy in neurogenic orthostatic hypotension. *Circulation*. 2003;108(6):724–728.

57. Sauer JM, Ring BJ, Witcher JW. Clinical pharmacokinetics of atomoxetine. *Clin Pharmacokinet*. 2005;44(6):571–590. https://doi.org/10.2165/00003088-200544060-00002

58. Shibao C, Raj SR, Gamboa A, et al. Norepinephrine transporter blockade with atomoxetine induces hypertension in patients with impaired autonomic function. *Hypertension*. 2007;50(1):47–53. https://doi.org/10.1161/HYPERTENSIONAHA.107.089961

59. Ramirez C, Okamoto L, Arnold A, et al. Efficacy of atomoxetine versus midodrine for the treatment of orthostatic hypotension in autonomic failure. *Hypertension*. 2014;64(6):1235–1240. https://doi.org/10.1161/HYPERTENSIONAHA.114.04225.EFFICACY

60. Byun JI, Kim DY, Moon J, et al. Efficacy of atomoxetine versus midodrine for neurogenic orthostatic hypotension. *Ann Clin Transl Neurol*. 2020;7(1):112–120. https://doi.org/10.1002/acn3.50968

61. Kaufmann H, Vickery R, Wang W, et al. Safety and efficacy of ampreloxetine in symptomatic neurogenic orthostatic hypotension: A phase 2 trial. *Clin Auton Res*. 2021;31(6):699–711. https://doi.org/10.1007/s10286-021-00827-0

62. Lo A, Norcliffe-Kaufmann L, Vickery R, Bourdet D, Kanodia J. Pharmacokinetics and pharmacodynamics of ampreloxetine, a novel, selective norepinephrine reuptake inhibitor, in symptomatic neurogenic orthostatic hypotension. *Clin Auton Res.* 2021;31(3):395–403. https://doi.org/10.1007/s10286-021-00800-x

63. Squair JW, Berney M, Castro Jimenez M, et al. Implanted system for orthostatic hypotension in multiple-system atrophy. *N Engl J Med.* 2022;386(14):1339–1344. https://doi.org/10.1056/nejmoa2112809

64. Raj S, Black B, Biaggioni I, et al. Propranolol decreases tachycardia and improves symptoms in the postural tachycardia syndrome (POTS): Less is more. *Circulation.* 2009;120(9):725–734. https://doi.org/10.1161/CIRCULATIONAHA.108.846501.Propranolol

65. Ewan V, Norton M, Newton JL. Symptom improvement in postural orthostatic tachycardia syndrome with the sinus node blocker ivabradine. *Europace.* 2007;9(12):1202. https://doi.org/10.1093/europace/eum235

66. McDonald C, Frith J, Newton JL. Single centre experience of ivabradine in postural orthostatic tachycardia syndrome. *Europace.* 2011;13(3):427–430. https://doi.org/10.1093/europace/euq390

67. Gee ME, Watkins AK, Brown JN, Young EJA. Ivabradine for the treatment of postural orthostatic tachycardia syndrome: A systematic review. *Am J Cardiovasc Drugs.* 2018;18(3):195–204. https://doi.org/10.1007/s40256-017-0252-1

68. Taub PRP, Zadourian A, Lo HCH, Ormiston CKC, Golshan S, Hsu JCJ. Randomized trial of ivabradine in patients with hyperadrenergic postural orthostatic tachycardia syndrome. *J Am Coll Cardiol.* 2021;77(7):861–871. https://doi.org/10.1016/j.jacc.2020.12.029

9 Cardiac Syncope

Angel Moya-Mitjans and Jaume Francisco-Pascual

INTRODUCTION

The term *cardiac syncope* refers to those episodes where the cause of the cerebral hypoperfusion is directly related to a cardiac disorder.[1] It is the second most frequent cause of syncope and the most threatening while it presents the worst prognosis, and it can be a harbinger of sudden cardiac death (SCD).[2]

This prognostic implication is mostly associated with the underlying cause of syncope rather than syncope itself. Patients with cardiac syncope have been reported to have an overall mortality rate of approximately 50% within 5 years, with a 30% incidence of death in the first year.[1,2] Additionally, in patients with syncope of unknown origin, the mere presence of structural heart disease (SHD) or conduction abnormalities is linked to a fivefold increased risk of death. On the other hand, a structurally normal heart with a normal electrocardiogram (ECG) is usually associated with a benign etiology for syncope and a favorable prognosis.[1,3]

Identifying patients with cardiac syncope or those at high risk of life-threatening causes is crucial to performing thorough investigations and specific treatments, while also allowing for reasonable reassurance and avoiding unnecessary tests in most patients who will have benign causes of syncope.

CLASSIFICATION AND MAIN CAUSES

Cardiac syncope can be classified according to the physiopathological cause (Figure 9.1), but also depending on the underlying SHD.

Arrhythmias are the most common cause of cardiac syncope. Both bradyarrhythmia and tachyarrhythmia can lead to a sudden decrease in cardiac output, resulting in syncope.[3] Furthermore, an abrupt change in heart rate, as occurs in most arrhythmias, can also lead to a drop in blood pressure due to impaired vasomotor function, especially in an upright position.

Non-arrhythmic causes of cardiac syncope are usually related to SHD that obstruct the outflow and/or inflow of blood. Severe aortic stenosis (AS), hypertrophic cardiomyopathy (HCM), mitral stenosis, or atrial myxoma are some examples. Cardiopulmonary disorders, such as severe pulmonary hypertension or pulmonary thromboembolism, as well as pathologies of the great

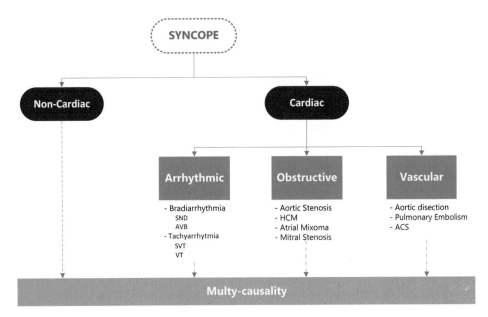

Figure 9.1 Main causes of cardiac syncope. SND, sinus node dysfunction; AVB, atrioventricular block; SVT, supraventricular tachycardia; VT, ventricular tachycardia; HCM, hypertrophic cardiomyopathy; ACS, acute coronary syndrome.

DOI: 10.1201/9781003415855-11

vessels like aortic dissection, can also cause syncope. Furthermore, myocardial ischemia and acute ischemic syndromes may also precipitate syncope through multiple mechanisms.[1]

Most heart diseases that cause outflow tract obstruction can also be associated with arrhythmias or reflex syncope. The mere presence of SHD associated with obstruction does not imply that syncope is due to this mechanism, and in many cases, it will be necessary to rule out other possible causes, especially arrhythmic ones.[1,4]

Additionally, in patients with SHD, the possibility of multi-causality cause of syncope is increased. Different contributing factors such as polypharmacy or some degree of autonomic dysfunction are commonly present in elderly patients with SHD or arrhythmias.[5]

The most important causes as well as underlying conditions related to cardiac syncope are:

- **Bradyarrhythmias**: Bradycardia resulting from sinus pauses or high-grade atrioventricular block (AVB) is the most common cause. These conditions may arise from a broad spectrum of underlying disorders, such as age-related fibrosis of the conduction system, coronary artery disease, or other cardiomyopathies. Primary genetic disorders are rare. Additionally, drugs and metabolic or hormonal imbalances may contribute to their occurrence; however, in such cases, bradyarrhythmia is typically reversible.

- **Ventricular Tachycardia**: Syncope due to ventricular tachycardia (VT) most commonly occurs in the setting of SHD, particularly in ischemic heart disease. Additionally, polymorphic ventricular tachycardia may be associated with channelopathies like Brugada syndrome, catecholaminergic polymorphic ventricular tachycardia, idiopathic ventricular fibrillation, and long QT (LQT) and short QT syndromes. Severe hydroelectrolytic imbalances can also cause polymorphic VT. It should be noted that ventricular fibrillation (VF) rarely causes syncope, as it is infrequently self-terminated.

- **Supraventricular Tachycardia:** Only on rare occasions, supraventricular tachycardia (SVTs) cause syncope. Typically, they occur during the onset of the episode when the vasomotor tone is compromised. In some cases, an SVT may trigger a vasovagal reflex. In patients with compromised ventricular inflow or outflow, the hemodynamic repercussions of an SVT can be more pronounced.

- **Conduction Disturbances**: In patients with bundle branch block (BBB), whereas AVB is the most common cause of syncope, accounting for up to 50% of patients in some series,[6] other causes may also be present.[6]

- **Ischemic Heart Disease**: During the *acute phase*, the dispersion of repolarization due to ongoing ischemia may result in polymorphic VT and VF. Monomorphic VT is less common. Additionally, AVB due to ischemia or hyper-vagotonia may also be present. In the *chronic setting*, a frequent mechanism is a ventricular arrhythmia due to macro-reentry in well-established ventricular scars.[3] The risk of ventricular arrhythmias is much higher among those patients with low ventricular ejection fraction.[7]

- Even though VT should be ruled out, it is not the most common cause of syncope. Some other factors like polypharmacy or conduction disturbances commonly present in these patients can contribute to syncope.[5,8] It is worth noting that if an EPS is negative, reflex and orthostatic hypotension (OH) syncope are the most plausible etiologies.[9,10]

- **Hypertrophic Cardiomyopathy:** Patients with HCM can present several factors that potentially may cause syncope, such as left ventricular outflow tract obstruction, conduction system disorders, sustained VT, abnormal vascular reflexes, or enhanced susceptibility to hypovolemia. Arrhythmic syncope is one of the most concerning causes that must be ruled out in this population. Moreover, syncope of unknown origin has been associated with a higher risk of SCD.[11]

- **Other Cardiomyopathies:** The risk of cardiac syncope depends on the subtype of cardiomyopathies, the degree of myocardial dysfunction, and, most notably, the presence of myocardial scar. Fibrosis and scar are strongly linked not only to a higher risk of VT and sudden cardiac death (SCD) but also to conduction disturbances.[8,12] Importantly, specific genetic variations are also associated with a higher risk of arrhythmias.[7]

- **Aortic Stenosis:** Syncope is more frequent in severe AS, but it can also occur in patients with moderate AS when experiencing other hemodynamic disturbances. In a recent study conducted by our group on a cohort of patients with severe AS and syncope of unknown origin, we observed that in only 17.5% of patients, the obstruction caused by AS was the primary cause of syncope.[4] Conduction system disease and reflex syncope were frequent causes of syncope in this population. Pharmacologic hypotension and atrial arrhythmias were also frequently observed.

- **Channelopathies**: Syncope in these patients might be due to non-sustained polymorphic VT or VF. However, benign causes are also frequent, which makes the evaluation of these populations especially challenging. In most channelopathies, the presence of syncope of unknown origin is considered a risk factor for presenting SCD and must be considered when the indication of an implantable cardiac defibrillator (ICD) is evaluated.[7] Arrhythmic syncope in patients with catecholaminergic polymorphic ventricular tachycardia is normally related to exercise or emotional stress. Patients with LQT syndrome may also present exertional syncope (especially in type 1 LQT) or during emotional stress (typical of type 2 LQT). Arrhythmic syncope in Brugada syndrome is rare.[13]

SYNCOPE DIAGNOSTIC APPROACH AND WORK-UP

Once a syncope diagnosis has been established, special attention should be paid to determining the underlying cause, especially cardiac causes. Risk stratification is crucial for identifying patients at high risk of cardiac syncope who will benefit from more in-depth investigations. Risk stratification is mostly based on clinical history and the ECG (Figure 9.2). Table 9.1 summarizes the most relevant high-risk features that may suggest cardiac syncope.

Additionally, to a detailed clinical history and physical examination, several other tests may be useful for evaluating patients with T-LOC. The diagnostic yield of these explorations depends not only on the specific test itself but also on the subgroup of patients being evaluated and the timing of the assessment. For this reason, it is important to systematically perform these tests in a specific order according to the patients' characteristics.

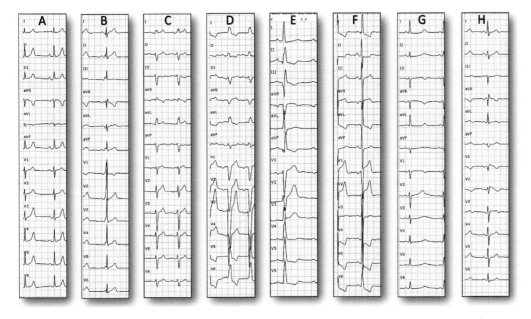

Figure 9.2 Examples of pathological ECG that should lead to suspicion of an arrhythmic origin of the syncope. Suspected supraventricular tachycardia: A: Bayes syndrome (biphasic p wave in inferior leads compatible with interatrial block, which is related to atrial arrhythmias); B: preexcitation syndrome. Suspected AV block: C: long PR interval and left anterior fascicular hemiblock. D: Left bundle branch block. Suspected VT: E: inferior necrosis (Q waves); F: hypertrophic cardiomyopathy. Suspected polymorphic VT: G: long QT syndrome; H: Brugada syndrome.

Table 9.1: High-Risk Features Suggesting Cardiac Syncope

Past Medical History

Previous myocardial infarction

Previous cardiovascular condition (i.e., IHD, Brugada syndrome, HCM, long QT syndrome)

Syncopal Event

Syncope during exertion or in supine position

Syncope associated with chest pain, palpitations, breathlessness, or abdominal pain

Physical Examination

Signs of heart failure

Cardiac murmur suggesting specific condition (i.e., aortic stenosis)

Signs of shock

Electrocardiogram

Conduction disturbance (AV block, bundle branch block)

Pathological Q waves

Long QT and short QT interval

Malignant early repolarization pattern

Preexcitation syndrome

Negative T waves

IHD, ischemic heart disease; HCM, hypertrophic cardiomyopathy; AV, atrioventricular.

Figure 9.3 provides a comprehensive step-by-step approach that can be useful for most syncope patients with a high-risk profile.

In patients with severe SHD or genetic disease and with criteria for ICD implantation according to specific guidelines, an ICD must be implanted irrespective of the completion of the diagnostic work-up for the etiology of syncope. Additionally, the underlying heart disease should be evaluated by the heart team and managed appropriately.

We propose a three-step diagnostic protocol.

Step 1 involves an initial assessment, usually performed in the emergency department (ED) including clinical history, physical examination, assessment for OH, and carotid sinus massage (for patients older than 40 years). General bloodwork, 12-lead ECG, 12–24-hour telemetry monitoring, and an echocardiogram are recommended. When no definite or highly probable diagnosis is reached, syncope is considered unexplained, and the patient should be admitted, or for intermediate-risk patients, an early outpatient evaluation in a clinical syncope unit is an alternative.[1,14] Additional cardiac tests may be carried out at the discretion of the physician based on the suspected diagnosis.

Step 2 involves hospital admission with continuous ECG monitoring or an early evaluation in a syncope unit. An electrophysiological study (EPS) should be considered if the following criteria are met: (1) presence of conduction disorder on ECG, (2) evidence of myocardial scar, and (3) history of palpitations preceding syncope. If these criteria are not met, an EPS is not indicated.

The diagnostic yield of EPS for syncope is typically low, especially in patients without SHD and a normal ECG.[1] However, the EPS still plays a significant role in high-risk patients, particularly those with myocardial scar or conduction disturbances.[1,6,8,15] In addition to providing specific diagnoses, the EPS is likely an effective tool for identifying low-risk patients. Several studies in different patient subgroups have demonstrated a low risk of arrhythmias following a negative EPS. However, its negative predictive value is suboptimal (around 70%),[1,3,6,15] and in most cases, further evaluation is still warranted.

Step 3 involves the insertion of an implantable cardiac monitor (ICM) with subsequent clinical monitoring.

The implantation of an ICM allows for additional diagnostic yield, and it is safe, as it has been shown in several studies. In our opinion, in patients with arrhythmic risk, the implantation of an ICM should be considered as the final step. However, some studies have used early ICM implantation as a first-line diagnostic approach. This approach may be less safe in high-risk patients. The potential to register the arrhythmic cause of a SCD raises concerns when monitoring high-risk

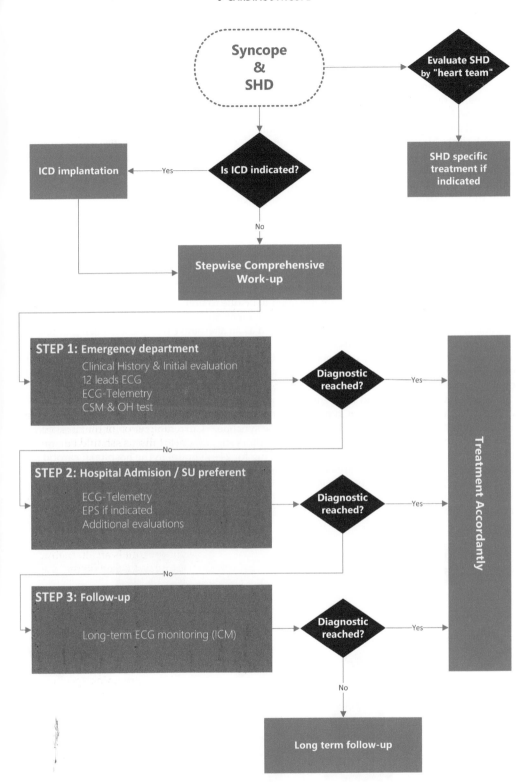

Figure 9.3 Stepwise diagnostic approach. SHD, structural heart disease; ICD, implantable cardiac defibrillator; ECG, electrocardiogram; CSM, carotid sinus massage; OH, orthostatic hypotension; EPS, electrophysiological study; ICM, implantable cardiac monitor.

patients. It is likely that the most severe patients at a higher risk of arrhythmic events leading to SCD would be identified in Steps 1 and 2.[8-10]

Other types of ECG monitoring systems, such as external loop recorders or ECG patches, may serve as alternatives to the ICM in selected patients with very frequent syncopal episodes. It's important to remember that the diagnostic yield of ECG monitoring systems primarily depends on the frequency of the symptoms and the duration of the recording. Therefore, short-term monitoring systems, like 24 hours, offer a very limited diagnostic yield as a routine exploration.[3] However, in-hospital monitoring with telemetry or continuous Holter is highly recommended in patients with high-risk clinical features, especially if the monitoring is applied immediately after syncope.[1,16,17]

Finally, it is worth mentioning that the tilt test has a limited role in the evaluation of high-risk patients and should not be routinely performed. It is useful for detecting an individual's susceptibility to a vasovagal response. However, in the context of high-risk patients, it has low specificity for the diagnosis of reflex syncope, while a significant proportion of patients with arrhythmic syncope may have a positive tilt test.[1]

TREATMENT

Syncope Secondary to Arrhythmias

Syncope Secondary to Bradycardia

In this section, we exclude the treatment of cardioinhibitory reflex syncope.

When syncope has been clearly demonstrated to be due to bradycardia, either sinus bradycardia or advanced or paroxysmal AVB, treatment is permanent cardiac pacing[1] (Figure 9.4).

Recently, cardioneuroablation (CNA) has emerged as an alternative treatment to pacing in some patients with cardioinhibitory reflex syncope.[18] While in patients with cardioinhibitory reflex syncope, many observational series[19] and one controlled trial[20] have been published suggesting its efficacy, in patients with primary sinus node dysfunction, intrinsic AVB, or AVB in the presence of bundle branch conduction system disease, currently there are no data supporting that CNA can be useful.[19]

In patients with syncope and BBB, with preserved left ventricular ejection fraction, although AVB may be the cause of syncope in many of them, other mechanisms, such as reflex, ventricular, or supraventricular tachycardia or OH, may cause syncope.[21] Currently, two different possible strategies are proposed in these patients. Some authors suggest performing a stratified diagnostic study consisting of electrocardiographic monitoring for 24–48 hours in the hospital,[17] carotid sinus massage, EPS, and, if these tests are negative, insertion of an ICM.[1,21-25] If any of these tests provide the diagnosis, patients should be treated accordingly. Other authors advocate implanting a pacemaker in all patients with syncope and BBB.[1,26,27] There is not enough evidence to recommend one or the other alternative, and at this time, the final decision must be individualized.[1]

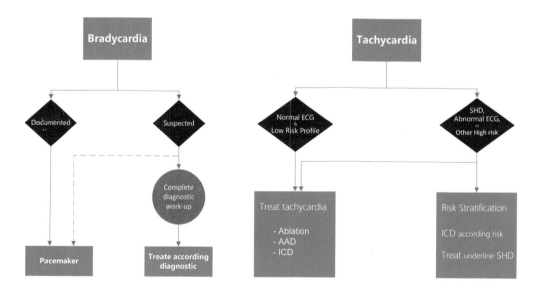

Figure 9.4 Treatment. AAD, antiarrhythmic drugs; ICD, implantable cardiac defibrillator; SHD, structural heart disease.

In patients with syncope, BBB, and left ventricular ejection fraction less than 35%, an ICD is indicated.[1] In patients with mid-range LVEF, the indication of an ICD must be individualized.[7,8] Furthermore, if they have some specific underlying SHD, it must be treated accordingly (see below).

Syncope Secondary to Tachycardias

Supraventricular Tachycardia

Syncope may be due to the presence of episodes of SVT: atrioventricular node reentry tachycardia, atrioventricular reentrant tachycardia due to an apparent or concealed accessory pathway, atrial tachycardia, or atrial flutter.

In these cases, the first therapeutic option is to treat the mechanism of tachycardia, almost always with catheter ablation. If ablation is not possible or not effective, in the absence of SHD, antiarrhythmic drugs can be considered.[1]

Some patients present with syncope in the context of episodes of paroxysmal atrial fibrillation (AF). In these patients, syncope may occur at the beginning of the episode, due, as in other episodes of tachycardia, to inadequate initial vasoconstriction at the beginning of the episode or to the presence of an asystolic pause at the end of the episode before sinus rhythm is restored (tachycardia–bradycardia syndrome). Although a few years ago, the implantation of a pacemaker was recommended in some of these patients, both to avoid prolonged pauses and to allow treatment with antiarrhythmic drugs to prevent recurrences of rapid episodes of AF, AF ablation is currently recommended as a first-line treatment.[1] A pacemaker should only be considered if ablation is not feasible or effective.

Ventricular Tachycardia

Most patients with syncope secondary to VT have some underlying cardiac abnormality, either a channelopathy, acquired cardiomyopathy, or congenital heart disease. There are very few patients with syncopal VT and without any evidence of SHD.

In any case, if VT is the cause of syncope, it should be treated, preferably with ablation, with or without additional drug therapy or implantation of an ICD (Figure 9.4).

In patients with SHD, ablation is usually less effective than in patients without SHD, because the substrate for arrhythmias is in general less localized and the disease is progressive.

In patients with cardiac abnormalities, either channelopathy or structural, in addition to treating the mechanism of syncope, a comprehensive risk stratification, taking into consideration the underlying cardiac disorder, must be performed to decide if additional measures are needed, such as implantation of an ICD to prevent the recurrence of malignant ventricular arrhythmias and SCD.[1,7] The current ESC guidelines provide detailed recommendations about the indication of ICD.[1,7] In general, the presence of syncope in patients with electrical or SHD is an additional risk for SCD, and usually, those patients are more likely candidates for ICD implantation.

In recent years, in patients with Brugada syndrome, epicardial ablation at the area of the right ventricular outflow tract, where abnormal electrograms are found, has shown to be useful in reducing the number of VF episodes and consequently decreasing the number of ICD discharges; however, it should not be considered as an alternative to ICD implantation.[28]

Syncope Secondary to Structural Heart Disease

In some patients, syncope is the clinical manifestation of acute cardiovascular disease, such as acute myocardial infarction, pulmonary thromboembolism, or acute pulmonary dissection. In those patients, syncope should not be specifically treated, and treatment must be addressed to the underlying acute cardiovascular process.[1,4]

In other patients, such as those with AS, or HCM, syncope can be due to different mechanisms, such as obstruction, reflex, AVB, SVT, or VT.[4] In those patients, a comprehensive diagnostic approach must be performed. If the mechanism of syncope is diagnosed, it must be specifically treated, in addition to treating the underlying SHD.

REFERENCES

1. Brignole M, Moya A, De Lange FJ, et al. 2018 ESC guidelines for the diagnosis and management of syncope. *Eur Heart J*. 2018;39(21):1883–1948. https://doi.org/10.1093/eurheartj/ehy037.

2. Soteriades ES, Evans JC, Larson MG, et al. Incidence and prognosis of syncope. *N Engl J Med*. 2002;347(12):878–885. https://doi.org/10.1056/NEJMoa012407.

3. Francisco Pascual J, Jordan Marchite P, Rodríguez Silva J, Rivas Gándara N. Arrhythmic syncope: from diagnosis to management. *World J Cardiol*. 2023;15(4):119–141. https://doi.org/10.4330/wjc.v15.i4.119.

4. Francisco-Pascual J, Rodenas E, Belahnech Y, et al. Syncope in patients with severe aortic stenosis: more than just an obstruction issue. *Can J Cardiol*. n.d.;37(2):284–291. https://doi.org/10.1016/j.cjca.2020.04.047.

5. De Ruiter SC, Wold JFH, Germans T, Ruiter JH, Jansen RWMM. Multiple causes of syncope in the elderly: diagnostic outcomes of a Dutch multidisciplinary syncope pathway. *Europace*. 2018;20(5):867–872. https://doi.org/10.1093/europace/eux099.

6. Moya A, García-Civera R, Croci F, et al. Diagnosis, management, and outcomes of patients with syncope and bundle branch block. *Eur Heart J*. 2011;32(12):1535–1541. https://doi.org/10.1093/eurheartj/ehr071.

7. Zeppenfeld K, Tfelt-Hansen J, de Riva M, et al. 2022 ESC guidelines for the management of patients with ventricular arrhythmias and the prevention of sudden cardiac death. *Eur Heart J*. 2022;43(40):3997–4126. https://doi.org/10.1093/EURHEARTJ/EHAC262.

8. Francisco-Pascual J, Rodenas E, Rivas-Gándara N, et al. Etiology and prognosis of patients with unexplained syncope and mid-range left ventricular dysfunction. *Heart Rhythm*. 2020. https://doi.org/10.1016/j.hrthm.2020.12.009.

9. Menozzi C, Brignole M, Garcia-Civera R, et al. Mechanism of syncope in patients with heart disease and negative electrophysiologic test. *Circulation*. 2002;105(23):2741–2745. https://doi.org/10.1161/01.CIR.0000018125.31973.87.

10. Shenthar J, Prabhu MA, Banavalikar B, Benditt DG, Padmanabhan D. Etiology and outcomes of syncope in patients with structural heart disease and negative electrophysiology study. *JACC Clin Electrophysiol*. 2019:871. https://doi.org/10.1016/j.jacep.2019.01.021.

11. Mascia G, Crotti L, Groppelli A, et al. Syncope in hypertrophic cardiomyopathy (part I): an updated systematic review and meta-analysis. *Int J Cardiol*. 2022;357:88–94. https://doi.org/10.1016/J.IJCARD.2022.03.028.

12. Di Marco A, Anguera I, Schmitt M, et al. Late gadolinium enhancement and the risk for ventricular arrhythmias or sudden death in dilated cardiomyopathy: systematic review and meta-analysis. *JACC Heart Fail*. 2017. https://doi.org/10.1016/j.jchf.2016.09.017.

13. Hernandez-Ojeda J, Arbelo E, Jorda P, et al. The role of clinical assessment and electrophysiology study in Brugada syndrome patients with syncope. *Am Heart J*. 2020;220:213–223. https://doi.org/10.1016/J.AHJ.2019.10.016.

14. Numeroso F, Mossini G, Giovanelli M, Lippi G, Cervellin G. Short-term Prognosis and Current Management of Syncopal Patients at Intermediate Risk: Results from the IRiS (Intermediate-Risk Syncope) Study. *Acad Emerg Med*. 2016 Aug;23(8):941–8. doi: 10.1111/acem.13013. Epub 2016 Aug 1.PMID: 27178670.

15. Francisco-Pascual J, Rivas-Gándara N, Maymi-Ballesteros M, et al. Arrhythmic risk in single or recurrent episodes of unexplained syncope with complete bundle branch block. *Revista Española de Cardiología (English Edition)* 2022. https://doi.org/10.1016/J.REC.2022.11.009.

16. Thiruganasambandamoorthy V, Rowe BH, Sivilotti MLA, et al. Duration of electrocardiographic monitoring of emergency department patients with syncope. *Circulation*. 2019;139(11):1396–1406. https://doi.org/10.1161/CIRCULATIONAHA.118.036088.

17. Benezet-Mazuecos J, Ibanez B, Rubio JM, et al. Utility of in-hospital cardiac remote telemetry in patients with unexplained syncope. *Europace*. 2007;9(12):1196–1201. https://doi.org/10.1093/europace/eum239.

18. Brignole M, Aksu T, Calò L, et al. Clinical controversy: methodology and indications of cardioneuroablation for reflex syncope. *Europace*. 2023;25(5). https://doi.org/10.1093/europace/euad033.

19. Vandenberk B, Lei LY, Ballantyne B, et al. Cardioneuroablation for vasovagal syncope: a systematic review and meta-analysis. *Heart Rhythm*. 2022;19(11):1804–1812. https://doi.org/10.1016/j.hrthm.2022.06.017.

20. Piotrowski R, Baran J, Sikorska A, Krynski T, Kulakowski P. Cardioneuroablation for reflex syncope: efficacy and effects on autonomic cardiac regulation – a prospective randomized trial. *JACC Clin Electrophysiol*. 2023;9(1):85–95. https://doi.org/10.1016/j.jacep.2022.08.011.

21. Moya A, García-Civera R, Croci F, et al. Diagnosis, management, and outcomes of patients with syncope and bundle branch block. *Eur Heart J*. 2011;32(12):1535–1541. https://doi.org/10.1093/eurheartj/ehr071.

22. Glikson M, Nielsen JC, Kronborg MB, et al. 2021 ESC guidelines on cardiac pacing and cardiac resynchronization therapy. *Eur Heart J*. 2021:3427–3520. https://doi.org/10.1093/eurheartj/ehab364.

23. Roca-Luque I, Francisco-Pascual J, Oristrell G, et al. Syncope, conduction disturbance, and negative electrophysiological test: predictive factors and risk score to predict pacemaker implantation during follow-up. *Heart Rhythm*. 2019;16(6). https://doi.org/10.1016/j.hrthm.2018.12.015.

24. Roca-Luque I, Oristrell G, Francisco-Pasqual J, et al. Predictors of positive electrophysiological study in patients with syncope and bundle branch block: PR interval and type of conduction disturbance. *Clin Cardiol*. 2018. https://doi.org/10.1002/clc.23079.

25. Roca-Luque I, Francisco-Pasqual J, Oristrell G, et al. Flecainide versus procainamide in electrophysiological study in patients with syncope and wide QRS duration. *JACC Clin Electrophysiol*. 2019;5(2). https://doi.org/10.1016/j.jacep.2018.09.015.

26. Ammirati F, Colivicchi F, Santini M. Permanent cardiac pacing versus medical treatment for the prevention of recurrent vasovagal syncope a multicenter, randomized, controlled trial. Circulation. 2001; 104(1):52-7. doi: 10.1161/hc2601.091708.

27. Sheldon R, Talajic M, Tang A, et al. Randomized pragmatic trial of pacemaker versus implantable cardiac monitor in syncope and bifascicular block. *Clin Electrophysiol*. 2022;8(2):239–248. https://doi.org/10.1016/J.JACEP.2021.10.003.

28. Krahn AD, Behr ER, Hamilton R, Probst V, Laksman Z, Han HC. Brugada syndrome. *JACC Clin Electrophysiol*. 2022:386–405. https://doi.org/10.1016/j.jacep.2021.12.001.

10 Syncope in Children

Khalil Kanjwal, Wasim Rashid, and Blair P. Grubb

INTRODUCTION

Syncope is not a disease but a symptom of various disease processes and has been derived from the Greek word 'synkoptein," which means "to cut short." This disorder is characterized by transient, spontaneously self-terminating loss of consciousness with brief duration and complete recovery.[1] This situation is usually alarming for the families of patients. The mechanism of syncope is transient global brain hypoperfusion to levels below those tolerated by cerebrovascular autoregulation. Regardless of the underlying etiology, multiple studies confirm that syncope decreases one's quality of life to a degree similar to other chronic illnesses. In one study of pediatric patients with syncope, PedsQL total scores were lower than in patients with diabetes and similar to those in patients with asthma, end-stage renal disease, and obesity.[2] Attention to and management of pediatric syncope can decrease patient and family anxiety as well as improve quality of life.

EPIDEMIOLOGY

Syncope is common at all ages. Approximately 40% of all people experience at least one syncope in their life. It has been reported that approximately 15% of children experience at least 1 episode of syncope before their 18th birthday. The proportion of syncope among children and adolescents is 25%, with a predominance between the ages of eight and 18 years, and it is the reason for 0.9% of consultations in emergency departments. Syncope accounts for approximately 126/100,000 children coming to medical attention in one population-based study; 1 of every 2000 emergency department visits is due to syncope. Syncope has been reported as more common in girls, and the peak of 3,700 patients aged between three months and 21 years with syncope showed that the neurally mediated etiology is the most common (52.2%), followed by postural orthostatic tachycardia syndrome (POTS) (13.1%). The cardiac cause was responsible for 4% of the cases of syncope and in 18.3% the cause was not identified.[3-6]

DIAGNOSTIC APPROACH AND TERMINOLOGY

Syncope is a heterogeneous syndrome with complex underlying mechanisms, hence, the spectrum of patients presenting with syncope is broad. A diagnosis is often not made, due to a limited overview of possible causes and inappropriate evaluation. Diagnostic failure is explicable since syncope and its mimics may be due to cardiological, neurological, medical, or psychiatric disorders. Diagnosis is made even more difficult, firstly by inconsistent definitions that incorrectly include concussion, epilepsy, metabolic disorders, stroke, transient ischemic attacks, and other conditions such as syncope in adults and children. Secondly, some classifications ignore helpful features such as the duration of unconsciousness. A recent systematic review revealed so many definitions and classification problems that the authors called for more diagnostic consistency.[7-9]

The diagnosis of syncope begins with history taking, and an accurate diagnosis can be established through correct history taking and interpretation. In this regard, ESC definitions were formulated for pragmatic diagnostic utility starting with clues to recognize the apparent loss of consciousness (LOC) through history taking requiring three obligatory features:

1. Loss of motor control: this always comprises a tendency to fall but also has variable features: tone is flaccid or stiff, eyes are open or closed, limbs and neck may be flexed or extended, myoclonic jerks are present or absent

2. Loss of response to touch/speech

3. Amnesia for the period of LOC

The presence of all three features guarantees that patients appear unconscious but do not prove gross cortical dysfunction as in syncope or generalized seizure, thus retaining functional causes.

The next step defines the major category "transient loss of consciousness" (TLOC) as LOC of brief duration with spontaneous recovery.[1,8] Including eyewitness overestimation, a pragmatic maximum duration for TLOC is 5 minutes. Separating TLOC from other causes of LOC dramatically reduces the number of causes, mainly by excluding long-lasting LOC.[10] Diagnosing syncope

DOI: 10.1201/9781003415855-12

requires a hierarchical procedure assessing the sequence of LOC, TLOC, syncope, and type of syncope (Figures 10.1 and 10.2) to achieve the most specific diagnosis the data permit.

Syncope partially overlaps with "orthostatic intolerance." The term orthostatic intolerance or OI simply means developing symptoms upon standing up or sometimes even sitting up from supine. Symptoms may include dizziness, palpitation, blurred vision, muffled hearing, nausea, or even syncope. OI by itself is not a diagnosis and merely expresses a condition that warrants further investigation. OI can also be divided based on its acuity. Acute and subacute OI are conditions when symptoms last less than one week and less than three months, respectively. In chronic OI, symptoms persist for more than three months. POTS falls into the category of chronic OI. In postural orthostatic tachycardia syndrome (POTS), syncope appears no more common than in the general population and is commonly VVS.[11,12]

The clinical history and physical examination performed with proficiency allow for differentiating the cause of syncope in up to 60% of cases. A diagnosis using initial examination differs between expert (~85%) and nonexpert (60%–70%) physicians owing to history taking as a main factor.[13] In evaluation, the main aim is to decide whether loss of consciousness is related to real syncope or not. Also, it is very important to exclude cardiovascular causes due to the high mortality and high incidence of sudden death.

---

1. Is there an apparent loss of consciousness (LOC)?
  a. LOC requires non-responsiveness, abnormal motor control with falling, and amnesia
   All three aspects must be present
  b. Counter-examples not meeting all three criteria
   a. Sleep-responsive
   b. Narcolepsy/cataplexy—no amnesia
   c. Absence/focal seizures with altered awareness—no loss of postural tone
2. Is LOC transient and resolving spontaneously?
  a. Transient loss of consciousness (TLOC): LOC of short duration with spontaneous complete recovery
  b. Counter-examples of longer-lasting or non-transient LOC
   a. Coma
   b. Intoxications
   c. Metabolic (e.g. hypoglycaemia)
  c. Counter-examples with recovery due to resuscitation
   a. Promptly resuscitated sudden cardiac death
   b. Promptly resuscitated from a potentially lethal drug overdose
3. Which type of TLOC?
  a. Traumatic brain injury (concussion)
  b. Syncope = TLOC + global cerebral hypoperfusion
  c. Tonic–clonic seizures
  d. Psychogenic/functional TLOC
  e. Other causes
4. If it is syncope, which type of syncope is it?
  a. Reflex syncope
  b. Syncope due to OH
  c. Cardiac syncope

Figure 10.1 Herarchical procedure assessing the sequence of LOC, TLOC, syncope, and type of syncope LOC (Loss of Consciousness), TLOC (Transient Loss of Consciousness).

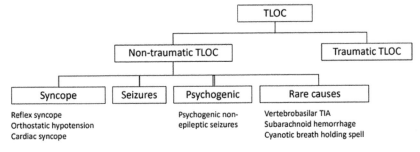

Figure 10.2 Stepwise approach to the patient presenting with TLOC.

HISTORY TAKING

In children and adolescents presenting with loss of consciousness questions regarding the patient's medical and family history as well as the history surrounding the event should be elicited. Defining the circumstances under which the child fainted and thoroughly understanding the patient's past medical and family history may uncover important clues as to the etiology of the event. When asking questions about family history, it is important to ask specific questions about cardiac family history. A family history of cardiomyopathy, arrhythmia (including congenital long QT syndrome, and Brugada syndrome), placement of a pacemaker or defibrillator, sudden cardiac death, or death from an unknown cause may suggest a cardiac cause for syncope. A complete neurological family history is also important and should include detailed inquiry regarding family members with seizures, including type, age of onset, type and duration of treatments required, epilepsy-associated deaths, or multigenerational seizure syndromes (juvenile myoclonic epilepsy, childhood absence epilepsy, channelopathies, etc.) Inquiry regarding family history of migraine, neurovascular disease (stroke, arterial dissection, vascular malformations), sleep disorders, vestibular disorders, or neurocutaneous disorders may also be helpful depending on clinical suspicion.[14-16]

Event History

It is essential to ask questions about the loss of consciousness event or events. Typically, patients with syncope can recall triggers or symptoms preceding the event. Specific triggers to ask about include positional changes, intercurrent illness, an emotional or painful stimulus, or a hot environment. These symptoms are typical for benign NMS. Chest pain or palpitations immediately before syncope and syncope that occurs without warning or during exercise are red flags for more serious cardiac etiologies and should result in restrictions from exercise and referral to a pediatric cardiologist. Positional triggers can be an important neurological warning sign, but unlike position changes associated with NMS (prolonged standing, quick change to a more upright position), the neurological concern would be heightened by position changes that provide a mechanism for CSF flow obstruction, such as bending forward at the waist with head lowered. Some stiffening or jerking of extremities or eyes following syncope is not unusual, but prolonged low-frequency, high-amplitude, clearly rhythmic bilateral jerking may increase concern for seizure particularly if accompanied by fecal or urinary incontinence or lateral tongue biting. However, it is important to note that urinary incontinence in isolation may occur with non-seizure events such as syncope and that depending on the direction of the fall, lip or tongue injuries may also be sustained in syncope. One of the most critical features distinguishing seizures from convulsive syncope is a post-ictal state of confusion lasting many minutes to hours. There can be a prolonged state of tiredness following vasovagal syncope, but this is not typically accompanied by confusion. Any focal neurological sign should raise concern for seizure and prompt consideration of further testing. Focal signs could conceivably precede an event of loss of consciousness such as definitive head or eye deviation before collapse. Focal signs such as weakness of the face or extremity might also follow a syncopal event. It is also important to elicit a psychological history, especially in patients presenting with frequently recurring loss of consciousness. Mental stressors can increase the incidence or frequency of syncope. Anxiety and depression have been identified as comorbidities with NMS. Multiple syncopal events throughout the day without any triggers or presyncope should raise concern for a psychological origin. In addition, further psychological assessment should be completed in a patient who has syncope while seated or prone.[17]

PHYSICAL EXAMINATION

A complete physical examination, including appropriate cardiac and neurological examination, should be performed. Heart rate and rhythm should be noted, specifically identifying any heart rhythm irregularities. Auscultation should be performed to listen for any new or loud murmurs or gallops. Palpation of the precordium will help identify a left or right ventricular heave.

Obtaining orthostatic vital signs may also help confirm the diagnosis. With the patient in the supine position, blood pressure and heart rate are recorded. The patient is then asked to stand for 3 minutes, and the measurements are repeated. A drop in systolic blood pressure of greater than 20 mmHg or a rise in heart rate of more than 30 beats per minute when standing is consistent with the diagnosis of neurally mediated hypotension that may result in NMS.[18]

It is imperative to review all organ systems for any clues of autonomic dysfunction. The same diligence should be applied when examining POTS patients. Pallor, jitteriness, sweaty palms, mydriasis, and sinus tachycardia suggest a particular form of POTS termed hyperadrenergic POTS. On the other side, significant hyperemia in the legs or even in the hands is suspicious of the neuropathic form of POTS. The presence of hives may indicate concomitant mast cell activation syndrome. Lax joints point to joint hypermobility in general or Ehlers–Danlos syndrome in particular.[19]

ADDITIONAL CARDIAC EVALUATION

Each patient presenting with loss of consciousness should have at least one 12-lead **electrocardiography**, a good screening tool in pediatrics for underlying cardiac abnormalities. Typically, a cardiac examination and electrocardiography with normal findings and a history consistent with NMS are sufficient to rule out a serious cardiac cause.[20]

An **echocardiogram** may be ordered if abnormalities are noted on the EKG or cardiovascular examination.

Long-term ECG monitoring either as (a) Holter (24 hours or three days)—will be useful for daily syncopal events, with normal/unclear presenting ECG, or as (b) external loop recorder (3–30 days)—for a less frequent event and implantable loop recorder (ILR) (up to three years)—for infrequent events only in patients with high suspicion of arrhythmic cause.

Video recording has allowed physicians to see real episodes and, when combined with physical monitoring, including continuous ECG and EEG, may help provide improved diagnostic yield.

Rarely, in cases where the mechanism of syncope is believed to be NMS but symptoms are atypical, a **tilt-table test** may be ordered. In the tilt-table test, the child or adolescent is placed on a table and tilted to 70 degrees while being monitored by electrocardiography and an automated blood pressure monitor. This test creates an artificial orthostatic stress that often provokes a drop in heart rate and/or blood pressure, which can be suggestive of a diagnosis of NMS. Tilt-table testing (TTT) has been considered complementary to clinical examination since its inception in 1986.[21] The test is typically carried out after 2–4 hours fasting that involves ≥20 minutes supine phase (post-venous cannulation) followed by ≥20 minutes of tilt (60–80 degrees) (passive phase) with or without the use of a provocative agent (nitroglycerine, isoproterenol, or clomipramine) for 5–20 minutes (active phase) if the first phase of the test is negative. TTT is considered to be positive only if there is syncope during the testing.[22] The positivity rate of TTT depends upon the indication for the test and provocative agent used—highest for vasovagal or emotional syncope with clomipramine (>90%), around 50% for atypical syncope (without classical features of vasovagal syncope) with nitroglycerine, and lowest ≤30% for unexplained syncope. The sensitivity and specificity of TTT with the use of isoproterenol or sublingual nitrate have been reported to be similar (sensitivity: 61–69%; specificity: 92–94%).[23–25]

Recently, there have been contrasting publications regarding the usefulness of TTT. One of these has advocated the abolishment of the test in view of no additional diagnostic benefit, high false positivity rates, use of active standing test instead of TTT in patients with OH or postural orthostatic tachycardia syndrome, and no mortality benefit.[26] The other has highlighted the benefits of TTT as an ancillary test in the evaluation of suspected syncope and reiterated that it should be used as a part of the diagnostic workup, not as a standalone to draw any conclusions.[27] Tilt testing should now be considered a means of exposing a hypotensive tendency rather than being diagnostic of VVS. According to the Consensus statement of the European Federation of Autonomic Societies, TT must be considered under the following conditions[28,29]:

- when the clinical history, physical examination, and ECG did not allow a definitive diagnosis of vasovagal syncope and POTS or for clarification of patients or family members or legal issues to differentiate syncope from seizure

- to differentiate vasovagal syncope from psychogenic causes for diagnosis of delayed OH, which occurs with more than 3 minutes of standing to guide patients

- [30]to avoid episodes of reflex syncope.

An **exercise test** and echocardiogram are also important tests in patients who experience syncope during exercise. Additional cardiac tests in this population have a high cost and low diagnostic yield.[31]

Finally, there is some evidence that individuals with neurally mediated hypotension have a higher prevalence than the general population of low iron storage and serum ferritin; this is the case even in the presence of a normal blood count or only mild anemia. Given this association, obtaining a complete blood count as well as iron and ferritin levels can be helpful in identifying patients with NMS without a classic clinical history.[32]

ADDITIONAL NEUROLOGICAL EVALUATION

Although a complete neurological examination can be performed, in most cases, detailed cranial nerve examination, funduscopic examination to rule out signs of increased intracranial pressure, and testing of the vestibular system are sufficient to confirm the diagnostic impressions created after obtaining a detailed history and to exclude serious intracranial pathology. Additional neurological testing including head and brain imaging and electroencephalogram is not necessary, unless there is history or examination evidence for underlying neurological pathology.[33]

PEDIATRIC APPLICATION OF SYNCOPE DIAGNOSTIC SCORES BASED ON HISTORICAL FEATURES

Syncope diagnostic scores based on historical features designed or applied to the pediatric population are summarized below:

1. **Differentiating between seizures and syncope**

   To the best of our knowledge, a diagnostic score based on a quantitative history taking to differentiate between seizures and syncope in children has not yet been established. The most frequently used diagnostic score for differentiating between syncope and seizure in adults is the Calgary Syncope Seizure Score (CSSS) from the Calgary Syncope Symptom Study, which was investigated by Sheldon et al.[34] The Modified Calgary score derived from the Calgary score for adults was developed for children. This score consists of seven diagnostic questions related to medical history with scores for positive answers to each question. The score ranges from –14 to +6. A score <–3 suggests cardiac syncope. The sensitivity and specificity of scores below –2.5 are 96.3% and 72.7%, respectively, for differentiating cardiac syncope from POTS.[29]

2. **Differentiating cardiogenic from other syncope types**

   Although no quantitative diagnostic score is available for children, a score from the Evaluation of Guidelines in Syncope Study (EGSYS), which was designed to differentiate between cardiac and non-cardiac causes of syncope in adult patients, has been reported.[35] Környei et al. applied this score to children with channelopathy. Among 48 affected children, 13 presented with syncope. Seven of eight children (87%) with witnessed syncope events had a score of ≥3.64. The striking finding of this study was that half of the patients presenting with syncope were initially misdiagnosed as having epilepsy and were followed up for 2–14 years for "therapy-resistant" or "atypical" epilepsy. This study underscores the need for caution in diagnosing recurrent syncope-like events.[36] The multivariable EGSYS score seems to identify syncope of arrhythmic origin, even in children who were previously misdiagnosed with epilepsy.

3. **Differentiating between psychogenic pseudosyncope and VVS**

   A recent systematic review reported that psychogenic pseudosyncope is rarer than cardiac syncope, with an average of 1.7% of all TLOC cases.[5] Zhang et al. analyzed the clinical features of 150 children with VVS and 26 with pseudosyncope and established a scoring model that could differentiate between the two groups. This study evaluated clinical symptoms and ECG data and vital signs. They showed that QT dispersion (QTd), syncope duration, and upright posture at inducement were independent factors for differentiating VVS from pseudosyncope. A total score of ≥3 predicted the likelihood of pseudosyncope versus VVS. This scoring system showed a sensitivity of 91% and a specificity of 76.9%.[37]

   Li et al. analyzed 183 children with VVS and 50 with pseudosyncope. They assigned the following four independent variables: no upright posture, LOC duration ≥9 minutes, daily frequency of attacks ≥2, and body mass index ≥20.5 kg/m^2. When a total score ≥5 points was used as the cutoff value for the initial differentiation between VVS and pseudosyncope, the sensitivity and specificity for the diagnosis of pseudosyncope were 92.0% and 90.7%, respectively.[38] However, further validation of these scoring systems is required.

SYNCOPE CLASSIFICATION

The three major syncope groups are reflex, orthostatic hypotension, and cardiac as per the European Practice Guidelines.

REFLEX SYNCOPE/NEURALLY MEDIATED SYNCOPE

Reflex syncope is defined as syncope due to a reflex that causes vasodilatation and/or bradycardia. A normal reflex for hypotension increases peripheral resistance and cardiac output by mediating an increase in sympathetic tone and the withdrawal of parasympathetic outflow. However, an inappropriate reflex may be triggered under certain conditions, including an increase in the parasympathetic tone and the inhibition of sympathetic outflow. This results in sudden hypotension and bradycardia, ultimately reducing cerebral perfusion. Consequently, reflex syncope occurs when a reflex temporarily responds inappropriately. Stimulation of the medullary vasodepressor region of the brain stem might be related to the mechanisms of bradycardia and/or vasodilatation in reflex syncope. This brain region can be stimulated by various receptors, including cardiac C fibers, cardiopulmonary baroreceptors, cranial nerves, cerebral cortex, gastrointestinal, and genitourinary mechanoreceptors. Therefore, they can occur in various situations in which such receptors are stimulated.[39,40] Neurally mediated syncope is synonymous with reflex syncope because the reflex arc is composed of afferent, central, and efferent pathways of the autonomic nervous system. The function of each reflex arc component is typically normal during reflex syncope. The term "neurocardiogenic syncope" is also frequently used to describe reflex syncope; however, the term is misleading, because this syncope is not caused by a cardiac condition, and the neural reflex does not involve the heart.

Vasovagal syncope (VVS) is the most common form of syncope in the pediatric and adult populations. VVS is defined as a relatively sudden change in autonomic nervous system activity leading to a fall in blood pressure, heart rate, and cerebral perfusion. The syncope begins with prodromes like dizziness, nausea, pallor, diaphoresis, yawning, sighing, visual and auditory disturbances. Following a period of unconsciousness, patients wake with a feeling of weakness, continued dizziness, and confusion. Some patients experience tonic movements that are usually symmetric. In one study, 66% of patients during the head-up tilt-table test showed seizure-like activities.[41] While brief symmetric myoclonic activities are common during syncope, true seizures may occur even with vasovagal syncope. True seizures coincide with profound bradycardia and/or long sinus pauses.

Vasovagal syncope may have the VAsovagal Syncope International Study (VASIS) classification modified,[42] according to the tilt-table response patterns.

- Type 1 mixed: there is a drop in blood pressure (BP) and heart rate (HR). BP falls before HR falls. The ventricular rate does not fall to 10 seconds.

- Type 2A, or cardioinhibitory without asystole: there is a drop in HR, with a ventricular rate of 10 seconds.

- Type 2B, cardioinhibition with asystole: there is asystole >3 seconds duration. BP decrease occurs simultaneously or before HR fall coincides with or precedes BP fall.

- Type 3 vasodepressor: there is a decrease in BP below 80 mmHg, but HR does not fall >10%, from its peak.

Management of VVS in Children

Management of vasovagal syncope begins with the reassurance of the patient that this type of fainting is not lethal and is different from highly publicized cases of sudden cardiac arrest in public arenas. Despite the limited literature on evidence of nonpharmacological and pharmacological management of NMS in the pediatric population, the initial guidelines are class I recommendations. These initial guidelines to prevent the recurrence of vasovagal syncope include clarification of its reflex mechanism, identification of precipitating factors, water (2 L/day) and salt intake, and physical counterpressure maneuvers.[43] The physical counterpressure maneuvers should be performed during the onset of prodromes in order to avoid syncope. Examples of these maneuvers are the movements of sitting, lying down, squatting, crossing legs, grasping hands and tensing them, pressing buttocks against each other, and raising the lower limbs. Another isometric exercise such as squeezing an object of 6 cm in diameter in the dominant hand may also be oriented as the child's age. Since these maneuvers depend on the duration of the prodromes, they are class IIa of recommendation, according to some guidelines, and are considered the first-line approach in patients with prodromal symptoms.[29,44]

A recent meta-analysis of five randomized controlled trials in the pediatric population (average age from 11 to 13 years) with 233 in the intervention group and 175 in the control group demonstrated the efficacy of water and salt intake in preventing vasovagal syncope. The dose per day of supplemental water was 500 mL and that of salt was 5.125 or 14.75 g. However, between a third and a half of the children had unsatisfactory results.[45]

Orthostatic training can be effective in motivated young people, and the lower acceleration index can be a predictor of its effectiveness in children.[46,47]

Pharmacological treatment with fludrocortisone and midodrine is class IIb recommendation if there is a failure of the initial steps.[48] In the multicenter randomized, placebo-controlled, double-blind, Prevention of Syncope Trial 2 (POST 2) study, there was a reduction in syncope recurrence after two weeks of fludrocortisone dose stabilization.[49] This efficacy in reducing the recurrence of syncope episodes was also observed in a retrospective observational study with 67 young people aged between 10 and 20 years, which compared the group of 28 patients using 0.1 mg once a day of fludrocortisone with the non-medication group.[50]

Midodrine has been recommended for the pediatric population. This alpha-agonist vasopressor was safe and effective for reducing the recurrence of vasovagal syncope in children at a dose of 2.5 mg twice a day, as included in a randomized study with 26 patients.[51,52]

There is a prospective, multicenter, randomized study (Prevention of Syncope Trial 5) in progress to verify whether beta-blocker therapy, such as metoprolol, would be effective in vasovagal syncope in patients over 40 years. Notwithstanding, there is still no evidence from randomized, placebo-controlled trials for the use of beta-blockers in children and adolescents with recurrent vasovagal syncope.

Other pharmacological treatment options are emerging, but in young and adult subjects with vasovagal syncope, reboxetine, sibutramine, and atomoxetine, which act as inhibitors of the norepinephrine transporter and therefore prevent hypotension, may be promising drugs for the treatment of vasovagal syncope.[53]

Syncope guidelines in the pediatric population also include pacemaker therapy and cardioneuroablation. A study of 11 children with cardioinhibitory syncope refractory to conventional treatment, with a median age of 2.7 years, demonstrated abolition of syncope in 10 children with ventricle pacing and sensing (VVI mode) with hysteresis.[54] However, regarding the pacemaker, there is evidence of a reduction in the risk of reflex syncope due to asystole in patients aged at least 40 years, especially with closed-loop system dual chamber pacing.[55] According to the Expert Consensus Statement on the indications of cardiovascular implantable electronic devices in pediatric patients,[56] the indication for pacemaker implantation can be considered if there is an association between significant bradycardia or asystole and clinical syncope on more than one occasion in children or adolescents refractory to other conservative treatment options. This approach can improve the quality of life in selected pediatric patients.

Catheter ablation to attenuate vagal activity on the sinus and AV node has evolved as one of the treatment modalities in a subgroup of patients not responsive to other treatments.[57,58] This technique of treatment of bradyarrhythmia is termed CNA. In this technique, ganglionated plexi (GPs) are targeted systematically—left-sided plexi first, aorto-superior vena cava (Ao-SVC) GP (for tackling atrial vagal innervations), posteromedial left GP (in case of AV block as the presenting feature), and an additional right-sided ablation if left-sided ablation was not sufficient. 138 has been performed to attenuate vagal activity in adult patients with vasovagal syncope.[59] However, there are no data on this procedure in relation to the pediatric population. This has recently been compared with conventional management without the use of CNA in the propensity-matched patient subset (recurrent syncope with VASIS-type 2B response or >3 seconds asystole), which showed that CNA caused a significant reduction in syncope recurrence (four-year syncope free rate—CNA: 0.86 vs conventional therapy: 0.50).[60] Also, the same group has recently shown that CNA reduces QTc through neuromodulation which is not noted in the patients treated with pacemaker implantation for reflex syncope.[61]

ORTHOSTATIC HYPOTENSION

Typical or classic orthostatic hypotension (OH) is defined as a sustained, ≥20 mmHg reduction of systolic blood pressure or ≥10 mmHg reduction of diastolic blood pressure within 3 minutes after standing. In some patients, the sustained blood pressure drop starts after 3 minutes from standing or head-up tilt test. This form of orthostatic hypotension is called delayed orthostatic hypotension. Classic orthostatic hypotension and delayed orthostatic hypotension are generally seen in the adult population. On the other side, initial OH is seen commonly in children and adults. Initial OH (iOH) is defined as a decline of systolic blood pressure of greater than 40 mmHg or a decline of diastolic blood pressure of greater than 20 mmHg within 15 seconds of standing. In children, iOH can present clinically as significant dizziness upon standing which resolved quickly.

At times, iOH can lead to syncope. In one study, iOH was the second most common cause of syncope. iOH is believed to be due to excessive venous pooling, inappropriate low systemic vascular resistance, or low muscle tone. iOH carries a good prognosis[62] and can be managed with lifestyle modification (rising slowly), hydration, and chronic regular exercise. At times, employing an alpha-agonist like midodrine may become necessary for a short period of time.[62–64]

For patients with OH syncope, fluid and salt intakes are recommended and, in the case of neurogenic OH, midodrine can be used. Measures such as discontinuation of vasodilators, raising the headboard above 10, and approach to dysautonomia should be taken if they are involved with OH.[65]

POTS

POTS has evolved from its first description. Although not comprehensive and inclusive, the current definition of POTS calls for a sustained heart rate increase of at least 30 bpm (40 bpm increase in individuals <19 years) or a heart rate increase above 120 bpm (or 140 bpm in children) in an upright position without hypotension. In an upright position, patients develop any or all symptoms including dizziness, palpitations, headache, pallor, nausea, and at times vasovagal syncope. These postural symptoms resolve or improve upon recumbency. Often, patients complain of non-postural symptoms like sleep disturbance, headache, cognitive clouding, a slew of gastrointestinal symptoms, voiding problems, and chronic fatigue.[62,66,67]

The onset of POTS may be precipitous and insidious. Some patients may recall the date when their first symptoms began. Others cannot pinpoint a date but point to a gradual increase in their symptoms. Not infrequently in children, patients suffer for years of chronic headache or constipation, before the orthostatic symptoms appear.

POTS has been divided, based on the clinical presentation, into subtypes, although there is no complete agreement on what should be included as a separate subtype. Most experts agree on the following subtypes: Neuropathic, hyperadrenergic, and hypovolemic. Some may add deconditioning as a subtype. Hyperadrenergic POTS is recognized in patients with significant orthostatic tachycardia and hypertension, elevated orthostatic norepinephrine above 600 pg/mL, and overshoot in phase IV of Valsalva. In a small population, a mutation in NET (norepinephrine transporter) has been shown as the etiology of hyperadrenergic POTS.[68]

Management of POTS requires a multipronged approach that includes nonpharmacological therapy, pharmacological therapy, and exercise. Addressing hypovolemia is crucial. To that effect, increased water intake, approximately 2–3 L, in addition to 5–10 g of salt per day can alleviate symptom burden a great deal. Wearing compression stockings and in more severe cases abdominal binders can prevent significant venous pooling. Many medications have been used over the years, but most experts agree that beta-blockers can be of great help. In addition, fludrocortisone, midodrine, and pyridostigmine are used frequently. In adults, clonidine, an alpha-2 agonist, and carbidopa, a false neurotransmitter, are used to blunt the sympathetic activity. Most recently, ivabradine, an HCN-4 channel blocker, has been used in adults with POTS with symptomatic improvement in 60% of patients.[69–71]

CARDIAC SYNCOPE

Although a cardiac cause of syncope is rare in children, it has a higher mortality and higher incidence of sudden death. There are certain red flags in history and investigations that point toward a cardiac cause of syncope. Supine syncope is a cardiac danger sign because it suggests a circulatory standstill: in most reflex syncope and OH, the circulation does not stop altogether, so lying or sitting alleviates complaints. When these do not help, a circulatory standstill implying cardiac syncope is more likely. VVS evoked by needles may well occur in patients already lying down and is then usually due to asystole causing a circulatory standstill, but not a dangerous one. Also, note that epileptic seizures and functional TLOC may occur while lying. Syncope during exercise is also a danger sign, although this can also occur in VVS. Syncope just after exercise also carries risks: while occurring often in VVS (and cOH), it also occurs in arhythmic syncope. Exercise stress testing is essential. Always ask for unexpected deaths in family members as these suggest inherited cardiomyopathy or arrhythmia. An ECG is essential, as many cases of cardiac syncope occur in existing although undetected structural heart disease. Most ECG abnormalities are relevant, although evidence of ischemia is rare in pediatrics (anomalous coronary artery). Echocardiography is necessary if the history suggests cardiac syncope, even with normal ECG.[7]

ARRHYTHMIA

Syncope from primary arrhythmia is typically due to an abnormally high heart rate ("tachyarrhythmia"), rarely due to low HR ("bradyarrhythmia"). Diagnosis can be made by extended external or internal ECG loop recording (ILR).[72] When myocardial function is normal, HR must be extremely high for syncope to occur, although standing increases the chance, by decreasing venous return. Most pediatric supraventricular tachycardias (SVT) and many ventricular tachycardias (VT) are tolerated with mild symptoms and palpitations. In contrast, very rapid VT, as seen with many channelopathies, causes syncope if lasting more than 3–5 seconds. There are typically no prodromes, so LOC occurs without warning. If a tachyarrhythmia with syncope reverts spontaneously to sinus rhythm, consciousness is rapidly regained. When episodes last <30 seconds, the patient appears normal immediately and asks, "What happened?" without recall of onset; this suggests an arrhythmic cause. If LOC due to arrhythmia is ended by resuscitation, this should be termed "aborted sudden cardiac death," not syncope, as underlying causes differ. Arrhythmic syncope in children and adolescents is often due to genetic causes. The resting ECG may contain clues, such as prolonged/abnormal QT interval. Inherited arrhythmic syncope may have specific triggers, e.g., startle such as by loud noise or cold water on the face (long QT syndrome), sudden onset syncope during fever (Brugada syndrome), and syncope during exercise/excitement (catecholaminergic polymorphic VT or arrhythmogenic right ventricular cardiomyopathy).[7]

Long QT Syndrome

Patients with long QT syndrome usually present with syncope associated with emotions or exercise and have a structurally normal heart. They are prone to develop a polymorphic ventricular tachycardia torsade's de pointes, which can lead to hemodynamic compromise and subsequent syncope. They may also suffer abrupt-onset syncope in response to a fright or awakening by a loud noise, such as an alarm clock. Usually, patients may exhibit symptoms during the second decade of life. Beta-blocker therapy may reduce mortality (from 70% in untreated patients) to 7%. Some patients may be candidates for ICD implantation. Sympathetic ganglionectomy has been reserved for severe refractory cases.[73]

Brugada Syndrome

Brugada syndrome is a hereditary disorder resulting from a mutation in a subunit of sodium channel protein involving the SC5NA gene. It manifests as an incomplete right bundle branch block and ST elevation in leads V1 to V3. Patients with Brugada syndrome are at risk of syncope and sudden cardiac death from polymorphic ventricular tachycardia. Many patients with Brugada syndrome have a normal ECG and manifest typical Brugada pattern only after a drug challenge either with ajmaline or procainamide. In an earlier published study on a population of children affected by Brugada syndrome, fever was found to be the most important precipitating factor for any arrhythmic event and the risk of fatal arrhythmias was significantly higher in previously symptomatic patients and in those demonstrating a spontaneous type I ECG (60% vs 7%). These patients should receive ICD if they have a cardiac arrest or have documented ventricular tachycardia even without cardiac arrest or a spontaneous type I ECG with syncope.[74]

Catecholaminergic Polymorphic Ventricular Tachycardia

Catecholaminergic polymorphic ventricular tachycardia is another rare inherited arrhythmic disorder affecting up to 1/10,000 people. It is an autosomal dominant disorder resulting from a mutation in the ryanodine receptor 2 (RYR2) gene. Less commonly, autosomal recessive variant has been seen resulting from the CASQ2 gene. Patients with CPVT suffer from disruption of the calcium handling within cardiac myocytes, which leads to ventricular tachycardia especially following exercise and emotional stress. They may present with bidirectional ventricular tachycardia as well. Beta-blockers are the only proven therapy in these patients, and ICDs have been used especially in patients with recurrent cardiac arrests on beta-blockers.[75]

Arrhythmias may also result from repaired or palliated structural heart disease. Sinus node dysfunction has been reported to occur after atrial repair surgeries. If severe enough, these patients may suffer symptomatic bradycardia and syncope. Similarly, AV block in pediatric patients is either congenital (seen in maternal lupus), which may not require pacing, or acquired from infections, such as diphtheria, endocarditis, Lyme disease, and Rocky Mountain spotted fever. Ventricular tachycardia, although rare, has been reported to occur in patients with corrected tetralogy of Fallot. Usually, these arrhythmias originate close to the ventricular path, especially in the septum and outflow tract.[40]

Supraventricular tachycardia, like in adults, rarely presents as syncope in children. The most common causes of supraventricular tachycardia, including AV reciprocating tachycardia and AV reentrant tachycardia, have clinical presentations similar to those seen in adults.

STRUCTURAL HEART DISEASE

Structural disease can cause syncope if cardiac output becomes insufficient to meet metabolic demands. Echocardiography is required. In children, causes include aortic stenosis, coarctation of the aorta, anomalous coronary arteries, tetralogy of Fallot, and transposition of great arteries. Many congenital heart diseases especially those with a ventricular surgical scar can trigger arrhythmia, and residual heart disease can trigger cardiac syncope. Conditions presenting more commonly in adolescence are primary pulmonary hypertension and hypertrophic or dilated cardiomyopathy.

Hypertrophic Cardiomyopathy

Hypertrophic cardiomyopathy (HCM) affects approximately 0.2% of the general population. Although a significant number of patients suffer a spontaneous mutation, it has also been reported that both autosomal dominant and recessive variants also exist. HCM is characterized usually by asymmetric septal hypertrophy, which produces a dynamic left ventricular outflow tract obstruction. Symptoms usually include dyspnea, fatigue, palpitations, near syncope, or syncope (either from abnormal blood pressure responses during exercise or from serious ventricular tachyarrhythmias). Although syncope occurs in up to 20% of patients in general, it is less common in the pediatric population. When present, however, syncope carries a more ominous prognosis in children. Early onset of disease in infancy carries a worse prognosis, and a majority (85%) of the infants die by age of one year. The aim of therapy is to provide symptomatic relief and decrease the risk of sudden cardiac death from ventricular tachycardia. Negative inotropes, such as b-blockers, calcium channel blockers, and disopyramide, may provide symptomatic relief. Surgical myotomy and myomectomy may help relieve symptoms but carry an operative mortality of almost 2%. Implantable cardioverter defibrillators (ICDs) are now commonly used in patients with recurrent syncope, ventricular arrhythmia, or a family history of sudden cardiac death.[76,77]

Aortic Stenosis

Aortic valve stenosis causes a fixed obstruction to blood flow. Congenital aortic stenosis accounts for approximately 5% of congenital cardiac anomalies in children. The bicuspid aortic valve is more common and is seen in up to 2% of the general population. In pediatric patients, more severe cases of aortic stenosis are seen in patients suffering from unicommissural aortic valves. Approximately 25% of these patients have other cardiac anomalies, such as aortic coarctation. As the disease progresses and the stenosis becomes severe, these patients may develop syncope from the reduction in cardiac output and cerebral perfusion. These patients are also at an increased risk of sudden cardiac death from ischemia, which results from both increased demand and decreased supply from hypotension. Therapy is aimed at either balloon valvuloplasty or surgical correction.[77,78]

Primary Pulmonary Hypertension

Primary pulmonary hypertension is a diagnosis of exclusion. It is defined as mean pulmonary artery pressure of greater than 25 mmHg at rest and greater than 30 mmHg during exercise. It affects approximately 1/1,000,000–2/1,000,000 in Western countries and has more female predominance, which may be seen even in early childhood as well. Up to 50% of the children with pulmonary hypertension suffer syncope. Syncope may result from both arrhythmias and obstruction to blood flow. Vasodilators, including calcium channel blockers and prostaglandins, are used to alleviate symptoms. Most of these patients are also treated with anticoagulation.[79]

Other Structural Cardiac Causes of Syncope in Children

Primary myocardial dysfunction Cardiomyopathies are rarely seen in children and syncope seen in these patients may be due to ischemia, arrhythmias, or some inflammatory process. Neuromuscular dystrophies, such as Duchenne, Becker, and Emery–Dreifuss muscular dystrophies, may present as myocardial dysfunction as well as bradyarrhythmias from AV block.

Myocarditis resulting in ventricular tachycardia may also present as syncope in children and unrecognized myocarditis may be an important cause of sudden unexplained death in children.

Myocardial ischemia is rarely seen in children and usually results from anomalous left main coronary artery arising from a pulmonary trunk or to the interarterial course of the left coronary artery between the aorta and pulmonary artery making it vulnerable to compression. These patients usually have exercise-related syncope because the blood flow to both aorta and pulmonary artery increases during exercise making the left coronary artery more vulnerable to compression.[40]

Another rare condition, seen in children of Asian descent under the age of five years, is Kawasaki disease. Syncope may occur especially during acute myocarditis from ventricular arrhythmias.[80] Arrhythmogenic right ventricular dysplasia can result in ventricular tachycardia and syncope. It should be suspected in children with exercise-induced syncope and left bundle branch pattern of ventricular tachycardia. Usually, this disorder becomes manifest in the 3rd–4th decades of life and, rarely, rarely early. Cardiac MRI shows classic involvement of the right ventricle. Many of these patients may need ICDs.[81]

Other causes of syncope include patients with Eisenmenger syndrome, tetralogy of Fallot, pulmonary stenosis, and right ventricular outflow tract obstruction.

OTHER TLOC FORMS

"Reflex anoxic seizures" and "breathholding spells"

Both terms refer to TLOC in infants/toddlers. The word "seizure" in reflex anoxic seizures may suggest epilepsy, but the spells are in fact cardioinhibitory VVS with asystole, evoked by unpleasant or surprising stimuli. To avoid confusion, ESC Guidelines recommend "VVS in infants." A typical episode comprises a trigger, a fall, no cry, a child lying still, eyes open and upwards, stiffening with rigid extension, and a few jerks. Pallid and cyanotic types of breath-holding spells describe facial color during an attack. Both start at ~10 months of age. Pallid breath-holding is synonymous with "reflex anoxic seizures," i.e., VVS in infants, so "breath-holding" is a misnomer for these events. In contrast, respiration plays a role in "cyanotic breath-holding spells." Startle or sudden hurt causes a reflex to stop respiration in expiration involuntarily, with secondary circulatory impairment. Reports of pallid and cyanotic spells occurring in the same child suggest the two types are not mutually exclusive.[10]

There is no specific treatment for these breath-holding spells. A correct diagnosis and reassurance of the parents are all that is needed. Approximately 50% of the children have complete resolution of symptoms by age 4, and 100% of patients never experience further episodes after their eighth year. It has been reported, however, that up to 25% of people suffering breath-holding spells as children may develop NMS and concentration problems at a later stage of their life. This association has led some investigators to believe that these breath-holding spells are infantile forms of NMS.[82]

True short-lived LOC can occur in subarachnoid hemorrhage and other rare disorders in adults, but these are rare in childcare.

CONCLUSIONS

Syncope in the childhood period has a wide clinical spectrum. A hierarchical framework to diagnose syncope is presented, resting on the determination of first LOC and then TLOC, syncope, and the type of syncope. This framework, common to all specialties, encourages a broad diagnostic view, comprising all forms of syncope, epileptic seizures, and psychogenic TLOC. Understanding the mechanisms of syncopal symptoms and their underlying physiology is the first step toward diagnostic accuracy that can avoid the pitfalls during history taking. The vast majority of syncope in pediatrics is due to neurally mediated hypotension leading to NMS, but syncope can be the first presentation of a serious underlying medical condition. A detailed history and physical examination can identify a potential cause of syncope in many patients. The ECG can help screen for dangerous etiologies. The aim of this article is to present different types of syncope and to provide new practical clinical approaches to the diagnosis, investigation, and management of the pediatric population.

REFERENCES

1. Kapoor WN. Syncope. *N Engl J Med.* 2000;343(25):1856–1862.

2. Anderson JB, Czosek RJ, Knilans TK, Marino BS. The effect of paediatric syncope on health-related quality of life. *Cardiol Young.* 2012;22(5):583–538.

3. Kliegman RM, Toth H, Bordini BJ, Basel D. *Nelson Pediatric Symptom-Based Diagnosis*. Elsevier Health Sciences, 2022.

4. Massin MM, Bourguignont A, Coremans C, Comté L, Lepage P, Gérard P. Syncope in pediatric patients presenting to an emergency department. *J Pediatr*. 2004;145(2):223–228.

5. Zavala R, Metais B, Tuckfield L, DelVecchio M, Aronoff S. Pediatric syncope: a systematic review. *Pediatr Emerg Care*. 2020;36(9):442.

6. Fischer JW, Cho CS. Pediatric syncope: cases from the emergency department. *Emerg Med Clin*. 2010;28(3):501–516.

7. Brignole M, Moya A, De Lange FJ, et al. 2018 ESC guidelines for the diagnosis and management of syncope. *Kardiologia Polska (Polish Heart Journal)*. 2018;76(8):1119–1198.

8. Winder MM, Marietta J, Kerr LM, et al. Reducing unnecessary diagnostic testing in pediatric syncope: a quality improvement initiative. *Pediatr Cardiol*. 2021;42:942–950.

9. Van Dijk JG, Benditt DG, Fanciulli A, et al. Toward a common definition of syncope in children and adults. *Pediatr Emerg Care*. 2021;37(1):e66.

10. Stewart JM, van Dijk JG, Balaji S, Sutton R. A framework to simplify paediatric syncope diagnosis. *European J Pediatr*. 2023:1–10.

11. Stewart J, Boris J, Chelimsky G, et al. Pediatric disorders of orthostatic intolerance. Pediatrics. 2018;141(1):e20171673.

12. Shen W-K, Sheldon RS, Benditt DG, et al. 2017 ACC/AHA/HRS guideline for the evaluation and management of patients with syncope: a report of the American College of Cardiology/American Heart Association Task Force on Clinical Practice Guidelines and the Heart Rhythm Society. *J Am Coll Cardiol*. 2017;70(5):e39–e110.

13. Wieling W, Van Dijk N, De Lange FJ, et al. History taking as a diagnostic test in patients with syncope: developing expertise in syncope. *Eur Heart J*. 2015;36(5):277–280.

14. Moodley M. Clinical approach to syncope in children. *Semin Pediatr Neurol*. 2013;20(1):12–17.

15. Bayram AK, Pamukcu O, Per H. Current approaches to the clinical assessment of syncope in pediatric population. *Child's Nerv Syst*. 2016;32:427–436.

16. DiMario Jr FJ, Wheeler Castillo CS. Clinical categorization of childhood syncope. *J Child Neurol*. 2011;26(5):548–551.

17. Duplyakov D, Golovina G, Garkina S, Lyukshina N. Is it possible to accurately differentiate neurocardiogenic syncope from epilepsy? *Cardiol J*. 2010;17(4):420–427.

18. Stewart JM. Orthostatic intolerance in pediatrics. *J Pediatr*. 2002;140(4):404–411.

19. Kakavand B. Dizziness, syncope, and autonomic dysfunction in children. *Prog Pediatr Cardiol*. 2022;65:101512.

20. Rodday AM, Triedman JK, Alexander ME, et al. Electrocardiogram screening for disorders that cause sudden cardiac death in asymptomatic children: a meta-analysis. *Pediatrics*. 2012;129(4):e999–e1010.

21. Kenny RA, Bayliss J, Ingram A, Sutton R. Head-up tilt: a useful test for investigating unexplained syncope. *The Lancet*. 1986;327(8494):1352–1355.

22. Bartoletti A, Alboni P, Ammirati F, et al. 'The Italian Protocol': a simplified head-up tilt testing potentiated with oral nitroglycerin to assess patients with unexplained syncope. *EP Europace*. 2000;2(4):339–342.

23. Morillo CA, Klein GJ, Zandri S, Yee R. Diagnostic accuracy of a low-dose isoproterenol head-up tilt protocol. *Am Heart J*. 1995;129(5):901–906.

24. Zyśko D, Fedorowski A, Nilsson D, et al. Tilt testing results are influenced by tilt protocol. *EP Europace*. 2016;18(7):1108–1112.

25. Furukawa T, Maggi R, Solano A, Croci F, Brignole M. Effect of clinical triggers on positive responses to tilt-table testing potentiated with nitroglycerin or clomipramine. *Am J Cardiol*. 2011;107(11):1693–1697.

26. Kulkarni N, Mody P, Levine BD. Abolish the tilt table test for the workup of syncope! *Circulation*. 2020;141(5):335–337.

27. Chrysant SG. The tilt table test is useful for the diagnosis of vasovagal syncope and should not be abolished. *J Clin Hypertens*. 2020;22(4):686.

28. Thijs RD, Brignole M, Falup-Pecurariu C, et al. Recommendations for tilt table testing and other provocative cardiovascular autonomic tests in conditions that may cause transient loss of consciousness: consensus statement of the European Federation of Autonomic Societies (EFAS) endorsed by the American Autonomic Society (AAS) and the European Academy of Neurology (EAN). *Auton Neurosci*. 2021;233:102792.

29. Lisboa da Silva RMF, Oliveira PML, Tonelli HAF, Alves Meira ZM, Mota Cd CC. Neurally mediated syncope in children and adolescents: an updated narrative review. *Open Cardiovasc Med J*. 2022;16(1):10–19.

30. Stewart JM. Reduced iron stores and its effect on vasovagal syncope (simple faint). *J Pediatr*. 2008;153(1):9–11.

31. Steinberg LA, Knilans TK. Costs and utility of tests in the evaluation of the pediatric patients with syncope. *Prog Pediatr Cardiol*. 2001;13(2):139–149.

32. Jarjour IT, Jarjour LK. Low iron storage in children and adolescents with neurally mediated syncope. *J Pediat*. 2008;153(1):40–44.e1.

33. Anderson JB, Willis M, Lancaster H, Leonard K, Thomas C. The evaluation and management of pediatric syncope. *Pediatr Neurol*. 2016;55:6–13.

34. Sheldon R, Rose S, Ritchie D, et al. Historical criteria that distinguish syncope from seizures. *J Am Coll Cardiol*. 2002;40(1):142–148.

35. Del Rosso A, Ungar A, Maggi R, et al. Clinical predictors of cardiac syncope at initial evaluation in patients referred urgently to a general hospital: the EGSYS score. *Heart*. 2008;94(12):1620–1626.

36. Környei L, Szabó A, Róth G, Kardos A, Fogarasi A. Frequency of syncope as a presenting symptom in channelopathies diagnosed in childhood. Can the multivariable EGSYS score unmask these children? *Eur J Pediatr*. 2021;180:1553–1559.

37. Zhang Z, Jiang X, Han L, et al. Differential diagnostic models between vasovagal syncope and psychogenic pseudosyncope in children. *Front Neurol*. 2020;10:1392.

38. Li C, Zhang Y, Liao Y, et al. Differential diagnosis between psychogenic pseudosyncope and vasovagal syncope in children: a quantitative scoring model based on clinical manifestations. *Front Cardiovasc Med*. 2022;9:839183.

39. Jardine DL, Wieling W, Brignole M, Lenders JW, Sutton R, Stewart J. The pathophysiology of the vasovagal response. *Heart Rhythm*. 2018;15(6):921–929.

40. Kanjwal K, Calkins H. Syncope in children and adolescents. *Card Electrophysiol Clin*. 2013;5(4):443–455.

41. Joo B-E, Koo DL, Yim HR, Park J, Seo D-W, Kim JS. Seizure-like activities in patients with head-up tilt test-induced syncope. *Medicine*. 2018;97(51):e13602.

42. Brignole M, Menozzi C, Del Rosso A, et al. New classification of haemodynamics of vasovagal syncope: beyond the VASIS classification: analysis of the pre-syncopal phase of the tilt test without and with nitroglycerin challenge. *EP Europace*. 2000;2(1):66–76.

43. Masudi S. Syncope in children and adolescents. *Adolesc Med*. 2015;26:692–711.

44. Udyavar A, Deshpande S. Evaluation and management of reflex vasovagal syncope – A review. *Ind J Clin Cardiol*. 2022;3(1):34–46.

45. Wang Y, Wang Y, Li X, et al. Efficacy of increased salt and water intake on pediatric vasovagal syncope: a meta-analysis based on global published data. *Front Pediatr*. 2021;9:663016.

46. Tao C, Li X, Tang C, Jin H, Du J. Acceleration index predicts efficacy of orthostatic training on vasovagal syncope in children. *J Pediatr*. 2019;207:54–58.

47. Romano S, Branz L, Fondrieschi L, Minuz P. Does a therapy for reflex vasovagal syncope really exist? *High Blood Pressure & Cardiovascular Prevention*. 2019;26:273–281.

48. Sheldon RS, Grubb II BP, Olshansky B, et al. 2015 Heart rhythm society expert consensus statement on the diagnosis and treatment of postural tachycardia syndrome, inappropriate sinus tachycardia, and vasovagal syncope. *Heart Rhythm*. 2015;12(6):e41–e63.

49. Sheldon R, Raj SR, Rose MS, et al. Fludrocortisone for the prevention of vasovagal syncope: a randomized, placebo-controlled trial. *J Am Coll Cardiol*. 2016;68(1):1–9.

50. Yi S, Kong YH, Kim SJ. Fludrocortisone in pediatric vasovagal syncope: a retrospective, single-center observational study. *J Clin Neurol (Seoul, Korea)*. 2021;17(1):46.

51. Bagrul D, Ece I, Yılmaz A, Atik F, Kavurt AV. Midodrine treatment in children with recurrent vasovagal syncope. *Cardiol Young*. 2021;31(5):817–821.

52. Qingyou Z, Junbao D, Chaoshu T. The efficacy of midodrine hydrochloride in the treatment of children with vasovagal syncope. *J Pediatr*. 2006;149(6):777–780.

53. Lei LY, Raj SR, Sheldon RS. Pharmacological norepinephrine transporter inhibition for the prevention of vasovagal syncope in young and adult subjects: a systematic review and meta-analysis. *Heart Rhythm*. 2020;17(7):1151–1158.

54. Paech C, Wagner F, Mensch S, Antonin Gebauer R. Cardiac pacing in cardioinhibitory syncope in children. *Congenit Heart Dis*. 2018;13(6):1064–1068.

55. Linde C, Crijns HJ. Pacing for repeated vagal reflex-mediated syncope: an old problem with a solution. *Eur Heart J*. 2021;42(5):517–519.

56. Shah MJ, Silka MJ, Silva JNA, et al. 2021 PACES expert consensus statement on the indications and management of cardiovascular implantable electronic devices in pediatric patients: developed in collaboration with and endorsed by the Heart Rhythm Society (HRS), the American College of Cardiology (ACC), the American Heart Association (AHA), and the Association for European Paediatric and Congenital Cardiology (AEPC). Endorsed by the Asia Pacific Heart Rhythm Society (APHRS), the Indian Heart Rhythm Society (IHRS), and the Latin American Heart Rhythm Society (LAHRS). *Cardiol Young*. 2021;31(11):1738–1769.

57. Scanavacca M, Hachul D. Ganglionated plexi ablation to treat patients with refractory neurally mediated syncope and severe vagal-induced bradycardia. *Arquivos Brasileiros de Cardiologia*. 2019;112:709–712.

58. Lu Y, Wei W, Upadhyay GA, Tung R. Catheter-based cardio-neural ablation for refractory vasovagal syncope: first US report. *Case Rep*. 2020;2(8):1161–1165.

59. Aksu T, Guler TE, Bozyel S, Yalin K. Vagal responses during cardioneuroablation on different ganglionated plexi: is there any role of ablation strategy? *Int J Cardiol*. 2020;304:50–55.

60. Aksu T, Padmanabhan D, Shenthar J, et al. The benefit of cardioneuroablation to reduce syncope recurrence in vasovagal syncope patients: a case-control study. *J Interv Card Electrophysiol*. 2022;63:1–10.

61. Aksu T, Turagam M, Gautam S, et al. Effects of permanent cardiac pacing on ventricular repolarization when compared to cardioneuroablation. *J Electrocardiol*. 2021;67:13–18.

62. Freeman R, Wieling W, Axelrod FB, et al. Consensus statement on the definition of orthostatic hypotension, neurally mediated syncope and the postural tachycardia syndrome. *Auton Neurosci*. 2011;161(1–2):46–48.

63. Cheshire Jr WP. Clinical classification of orthostatic hypotensions. *Clin Auton Res*. 2017;27(3):133–135.

64. van Twist DJ, Harms MP, van Wijnen VK, et al. Diagnostic criteria for initial orthostatic hypotension: a narrative review. *Clin Auton Res*. 2021;31:1–14.

65. Benarroch EE. "Dysautonomia": a plea for precision. *Clin Auton Res*. 2021;31(1):27–29.

66. Rosen SG, Cryer PE. Postural tachycardia syndrome: reversal of sympathetic hyperresponsiveness and clinical improvement during sodium loading. *Am J Med*. 1982;72(5):847–850.

67. Conner R, Sheikh M, Grubb B. Postural orthostatic tachycardia syndrome (POTS): evaluation and management. *Br J Med Pract*. 2012;5(4):540.

68. Thieben MJ, Sandroni P, Sletten DM, et al. Postural orthostatic tachycardia syndrome: the Mayo clinic experience. In *Mayo Clinic Proceedings*, 2007: Elsevier. 82(3):308–13. doi: 10.4065/82.3.308.

69. Gaffney FA, Lane LB, Pettinger W, Blomqvist CG. Effects of long-term clonidine administration on the hemodynamic and neuroendocrine postural responses of patients with dysautonomia. *Chest*. 1983;83:436–438.

70. McDonald C, Frith J, Newton JL. Single centre experience of ivabradine in postural orthostatic tachycardia syndrome. *EP Europace*. 2011;13(3):427–430.

71. Bryarly M, Phillips LT, Fu Q, Vernino S, Levine BD. Postural orthostatic tachycardia syndrome: JACC focus seminar. *J Am Coll Cardiol*. 2019;73(10):1207–1228.

72. Varma N, Cygankiewicz I, Turakhia MP, et al. 2021 ISHNE/HRS/EHRA/APHRS expert collaborative statement on mHealth in arrhythmia management: digital medical tools for heart rhythm professionals: from the International Society for Holter and Noninvasive Electrocardiology/Heart Rhythm Society/European Heart Rhythm Association/Asia-Pacific Heart Rhythm Society. *Circ Arrhythm Electrophysiol*. 2021;14(2):e009204.

73. Krahn AD, Laksman Z, Sy RW, et al. Congenital long QT syndrome. *Clini Electrophysiol*. 2022;8(5):687–706.

74. Marsman EMJ, Postema PG, Remme CA. Brugada syndrome: update and future perspectives. *Heart*. 2022;108(9):668–675.

75. Bergeman AT, Wilde AA, van der Werf C. Catecholaminergic polymorphic ventricular tachycardia: a review of therapeutic strategies. *Card Electrophysiol Clin*. 2023;15:293–305.

76. Xia K, Sun D, Wang R, Zhang Y. Factors associated with the risk of cardiac death in children with hypertrophic cardiomyopathy: a systematic review and meta-analysis. *Heart & Lung*. 2022;52:26–36.

77. Kaski JP, Kammeraad JA, Blom NA, et al. Indications and management of implantable cardioverter-defibrillator therapy in childhood hypertrophic cardiomyopathy: a position statement from the AEPC Working Group on Basic Science, Genetics and Myocardial Disease and the AEPC Working Group on Cardiac Dysrhythmias and Electrophysiology. *Cardiol Young*. 2023;33(5):681–698.

78. Meliota G, Vairo U. Transcatheter interventions for neonates with congenital heart disease: a review. *Diagnostics*. 2023;13(16):2673.

79. Rosenzweig EB, Abman SH, Adatia I, et al. Paediatric pulmonary arterial hypertension: updates on definition, classification, diagnostics and management. *European Respiratory Journal*. 2019;53(1):1801916.

80. Lee JJ, Lin E, Widdifield J, et al. The long-term cardiac and noncardiac prognosis of Kawasaki disease: a systematic review. *Pediatrics*. 2022;149(3):e2021052567.

81. Bosman LP, Te Riele AS. Arrhythmogenic right ventricular cardiomyopathy: a focused update on diagnosis and risk stratification. *Heart*. 2022;108(2):90–97.

82. von Alvensleben JC. Syncope and palpitations: a review. *Pediatr Clin*. 2020;67(5):801–810.

11 Pseudosyncope and Ictal Syncope

Diagnosis and Management

Leonardo Calò, Marco Rebecchi, Pietro Desimone, Domenico Giamundo, Ermenegildo De Ruvo, and Antonella Sette

INTRODUCTION

Pseudosyncope is an apparent loss of consciousness in the absence of impaired cerebral perfusion. It is important to emphasize that pseudosyncope is not "malingering" in which the patient feigns an illness, greatly limiting their quality of life. These patients do not present structural heart disease, but very often, for the differential diagnosis with other forms, especially vasovagal syncope, tilt testing appears to be useful. The first-line treatment is definitely considered to be cognitive-behavioral therapy; in addition, a psychiatric evaluation should be performed, and finally, treatment with a low dosage of fludrocortisone may be recommended.

Ictal asystole, a most common form of ictal syncope, is a rare condition that consists of the absence of ventricular complexes for more than 4 seconds on the electrocardiogram, correlated by the onset of electroencephalographic alterations including seizures. In fact, it is well known that convulsive seizures can induce a number of transient cardiac effects, with an increased risk of tachyarrhythmias and bradyarrhythmias, such as atrioventricular blocks up to ictal asystole, through a sympathetic-vagal imbalance mechanism. Diagnosis is based on continuous video monitoring combined with electroencephalogram and telemetric electrocardiogram monitoring, implantable loop recorder in case of unexplained syncope. If drug therapy for epilepsy fails (primary therapy), cardiac pacing may be considered in selected cases. Finally, cardioneuroablation may be potentially considered an effective approach, although there is still no strong scientific data on this type of patient.

This chapter reviews pseudosyncope and ictal syncope based on a clinical literature review.

PSEUDOSYNCOPE

Definition and Epidemiology

Pseudosyncope, also known as psychogenic syncope, is the apparent loss of consciousness that occurs in the absence of impaired cerebral perfusion. It is more common among young individuals and women, with a prevalence of approximately 4% in patients evaluated for syncope.[1,2] Pseudosyncope may not always be preceded by prodromes, but when they do occur, they tend to be nonspecific, such as extreme weakness, dizziness, or a feeling of trembling in the legs.

Physiopathology and Symptoms

Clinically, pseudosyncope is characterized by recurrent episodes of loss of consciousness that last for a few minutes. Patients often exhibit a "bracing" response, preventing them from experiencing trauma. Episodes tend to occur in specific triggering contexts, for example, when in the presence of an audience. Other atypical triggers may also be involved, and it is common for patients to close their eyes during these episodes. Recovery from pseudosyncope can be marked by significant drowsiness.[3] The 2018 European Society of Cardiology guidelines for syncope diagnosis and management have identified other clinical features highly suggestive of pseudosyncope, such as body positioning resembling sleep with closed eyes, resistance to opening the eyes, eyelid flickering, eyeball movement, lack of response to speech or touch, and swallowing.[4] It is crucial to make an accurate differential diagnosis between pseudosyncope and other forms of syncope, especially cardiogenic, vasovagal, and neuromediated forms. While transient loss of consciousness is the primary clinical presentation of pseudosyncope, it can also be present in vasovagal syncope and seizures. Despite clear pathophysiological differences between vasovagal and pseudosyncope, such as transient cerebral hypoperfusion in vasovagal syncope and abnormal paroxysmal neuronal electrical discharges in seizures, the similarity in the clinical presentation can lead to a misdiagnosis rate of up to 30%.[5]

Diagnosis

Pseudosyncope typically occurs in patients with normal cardiological examinations and echocardiograms, as well as normal results from neurological imaging (CT and MRI) and hematochemical examinations. To aid in the differential diagnosis, tilt tests can be particularly useful (Figure 11.1).

DOI: 10.1201/9781003415855-13

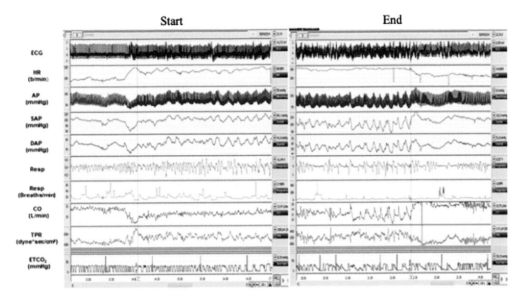

Figure 11.1 Representative example of multiparameter recording during a pseudosyncope attack in a young female undergoing a tilt test maneuver. The end graph (right panel) refers to the last 4 minutes of the pseudosyncope episode. Note the absence of alterations in the hemodynamics, i.e., heart rate and blood pressure, and in the respiratory rate during the attack (right panel). In addition, during tilt, there was a proper increase in heart rate and total peripheral resistance (TPR), blood pressure was unmodified, and cardiac output (CO) declined compared to the supine position, as expected. The only feature suggestive of the patient's distress was the respiratory pattern. Indeed, this latter was more irregular (see $ETCO_2$ trace, end-tidal carbon dioxide partial pressure) during pseudosyncope attack than in baseline supine position and during early tilt (left panel). Vertical dashed lines indicate the start (left) and the end (right) of the tilt maneuver. HR, heart rate; AP, arterial pressure; SAP, systolic arterial pressure; DAP, diastolic arterial pressure; Resp, respiratory activity.

In cases of pseudosyncope, there are no significant hemodynamic changes, with blood pressure and heart rate remaining relatively normal. In contrast, vasovagal syncope patients often exhibit a reduction in one or both of these parameters. Additionally, individuals with vasovagal syncope commonly experience classic triggers such as pain, intense emotions, recent meals, fear, and the sight of blood. Furthermore, vasovagal episodes are typically preceded by prodromes like blurred vision, nausea, sweating, and pallor.

The ACC/AHA/HRS 2017 guidelines suggested that, during a tilt test, additional monitoring with EEG (in addition to hemodynamic parameters) may help differentiate between pseudosyncope and seizures. In pseudosyncope, there are no changes in EEG activity, whereas in epilepsy, there is an electrical activity with a slow or slow–flat–slow pattern.[6] Near-infrared spectroscopy (NIRS) has been recently proposed as a simple, non-invasive instrument for continuous monitoring of cerebral perfusion during a tilt test. In cases of pseudosyncope, cerebral perfusion remains unchanged, unlike vasovagal syncope, where cerebral hypoperfusion is observed.[7] Pseudosyncope is also described in the fifth and last edition of DSM-5 (*Diagnostic and Statistical Manual of Mental Disorders*), where it is included in the diagnosis of conversion disorder under the category "somatic symptoms and related disorders." According to the diagnostic criteria of DSM-5, conversion disorder is characterized by the presence of one or more symptoms of impaired voluntary or sensory function not explained by other medical disorders (e.g., neurological or cardiac) or mental health issues and must cause clinically significant stress or impairment in the individual's social and professional activities.[8] It is important to emphasize that pseudosyncope is not a form of "malingering," where the patient pretends to have a disease. This highlights that pseudosyncope is a disorder with a significant impact on the patient's quality of life, and a delay in diagnosis can negatively affect the outcome of therapy.[9]

Treatment

The first-line treatment for pseudosyncope is cognitive-behavioral therapy (CBT), which combines cognitive therapy with behavioral therapy. CBT involves identifying and addressing faulty or maladaptive thought patterns, educating the patient about functional neurological disorders and stress responses, teaching stress management techniques, and helping the patient recognize and change unnecessary thought patterns that reinforce their symptoms.[10–12] Additionally, a psychiatric evaluation should be conducted to exclude and treat any psychiatric comorbidities such as anxiety, somatization, major depression, and panic attacks, which are more common in patients with pseudosyncope than in the general population.[13,14] As a pharmacological approach, treatment with low-dose fludrocortisone may be recommended to improve the pressure profile, reduce susceptibility to hypotension and syncope relapses, reassure the patient, and potentially improve functional symptoms.[15] In the case of vasovagal syncope, providing instruction on physical countermaneuvers and lifestyle advice may be sufficient to give the patient better control over their situation, reducing anxiety. However, the efficacy of physical countermaneuvers in pseudosyncope has not been definitively demonstrated.[16–20]

ICTAL SYNCOPE

Considerable interest has arisen in exploring the connections between the heart and the brain, especially regarding the influence and role of the central nervous system and the autonomic system on cardiac activity. The impact on cardiac function significantly affects the clinical course and prognosis of individuals with epilepsy. Seizures can induce various transient cardiac effects, particularly changes in heart rate variability (HRV), increasing the risk of tachyarrhythmias or bradyarrhythmias, atrioventricular blocks, and even ictal asystole. Cardiac alterations during and between seizures may play a significant role in the pathogenesis of sudden unexpected death in epilepsy (SUDEP), though its exact cause remains unknown.[21,22]

Incidence and Definition

Overall, individuals with epilepsy have a higher prevalence of arrhythmias compared to the general population. Among the various arrhythmias occurring during and after seizures, ictal asystole is the most common. Ictal asystole (IA) is a rare condition affecting 0.27%–0.4% of patients with refractory focal epilepsy undergoing video-EEG monitoring, primarily occurring in the context of temporal lobe epilepsy (80%) and less frequently in frontal lobe epilepsy (20%).[23] Ictal asystole involves the absence of ventricular complexes for more than 4 seconds on the ECG, accompanied by an electroencephalographic (EEG) seizure onset. IA is always accompanied by a diffuse slowing and flattening of electrical brain activity observed on the EEG, which potentially interrupts the ictal activity through an anoxic–ischemic mechanism. This autonomic dysregulation is reminiscent of vasovagal syncope, featuring a transient, progressive, and self-limiting slowing of the heart rate and a decrease in blood pressure. IA is often misdiagnosed as a primary cardiological phenomenon due to ECG documentation of marked bradyarrhythmia. Seizure-induced asystole may, therefore, be significantly underreported. The duration of asystole is strongly correlated with the duration of syncope, with longer asystole durations increasing the probability of developing ictal syncope.[24,25]

Physiopathology

The relationship between seizures and heart rate regulation is complex, with a major role played by the sympathetic and parasympathetic systems. The underlying mechanism could involve epileptic activity directly stimulating central autonomic networks; for instance, focal stimulation of parts of the limbic system can provoke asystole. Alternatively, seizure-induced fear and catecholamine release may trigger a vasovagal response, leading to cardioinhibition and vasodilatation. Increased sympathetic activity lowers the arrhythmic threshold. This, combined with genetic predispositions that result in heightened responses to autonomic innervation, such as in various disorders of ion channels like Long QT syndrome (LQTS), Brugada syndrome, and catecholaminergic polymorphic ventricular tachycardia, increases the risk of arrhythmias and sudden cardiac death[26] (Figure 11.2).

Furthermore, several genetic ion channel mutations are believed to be expressed not only in the heart but also in the brain. These mutations may potentially lead to both seizures and cardiac arrhythmias. For instance, mutations in the SCN5A gene, as well as pathogenic variants of RYR2 and HCN1–4, may predispose individuals to epilepsy and a higher risk of SUDEP. It is

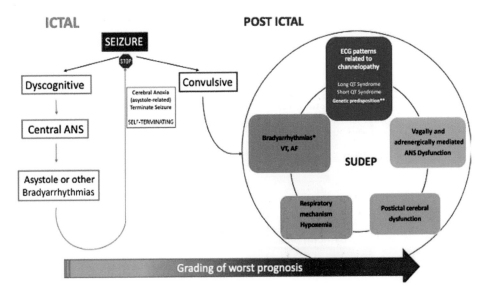

Figure 11.2 Different proarrhythmogenic mechanisms of dyscognitive and convulsive seizure. See the test for an explanation.

intriguing to examine the various clinical manifestations during the interictal, pre-ictal, ictal, and post-ictal phases, with a focus on heart rate variability (HRV) and the types of arrhythmias that occur.

HRV trends have been extensively studied as potential predictors of seizure severity and their potential role in the pathogenesis of SUDEP. HRV reflects the balance of autonomic outflow, with a decrease indicating sympathetic dominance. During the peri-ictal period, a significant reduction in HRV is observed, especially in individuals with temporal lobe epilepsy (TLE) and generalized tonic-clonic seizures (GTCS).[27] The enhanced sympathetic activity, along with the suppression of parasympathetic outflow, contributes to HRV changes in the post-ictal phase.

The effects of sympathetic dominance are also reflected in heart rate (HR), where up to 80% of patients show a continuous increase in HR from the pre-ictal to the ictal phase, with a reduced HR being less common. During the post-ictal period, patients may occasionally experience arrhythmias, including asystole, bradycardia, and AV block. There have also been reported cases of atrial flutter, atrial fibrillation, ventricular tachycardia, or ventricular fibrillation. Post-ictal arrhythmias are particularly common after GTCS and, in contrast to ictal arrhythmias, are often associated with a higher risk of near-SUDEP, necessitating medical intervention[28-30] (Figure 11.3).

Diagnosis

The most suitable diagnostic plan involves continuous video monitoring including interictal electroencephalogram and scalp topographical mapping combined with telemetry electrocardiogram monitoring. This diagnostic plan is important to formulate a differential diagnosis because in clinical practice marked fluctuations in heart rate, well documented in patients with reflex syncope, may also occur in patients with seizure disorders, ictal bradycardia, or asystole.[31] In addition, typical signs of temporal lobe epilepsy, such as motionless staring, automatic movements of the hand or mouth, communication disorders, and abnormal speech or behavior, are not always present or are not so clear, blurring the distinction between syncope and temporal lobe epilepsy.[32] In unexplained syncope, it could be used an implantable loop recorder to monitor heart rate variability and cardiac activity. They can consistently document a correlation between the presence of symptoms and arrhythmias, as well as exclude a causative role of heart rhythm disturbances in determining syncope or palpitations when they occur without any arrhythmia. Nevertheless, there are no clear guidelines on the use of implantable loop recorders in preventing death in high-risk epilepsy patients.[33]

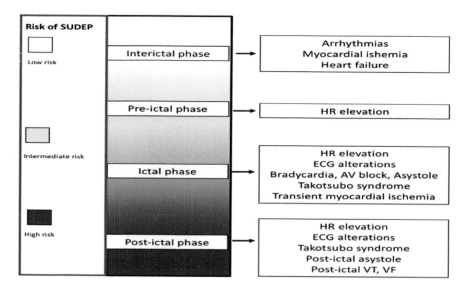

Figure 11.3 Cardiovascular involvement in epilepsy. The figure summarizes cardiac involvement in epileptic individuals, with a focus on the different clinical manifestations in the interictal period, pre-ictal, ictal, and post-ictal phases.

Therapy

Ictal asystole seizures are self-limited, as the global cerebral ischemia induced by the asystole ends the seizure. Although proper trials are lacking, retrospective studies suggest that improving seizure control may prevent ictal asystole.[34] Consequently, treatment is essential, and the primary approach should focus on optimizing seizure control with antiseizure medication or, if necessary and possible, epilepsy surgery.[35] However, pacemaker implantation may be considered if the primary treatment approach fails, especially in cases where cardioinhibition is the primary mechanism causing syncope. Nevertheless, several reports suggest that syncope in ictal asystole may also be primarily the result of vasodepression. This may explain why pacing sometimes fails to prevent syncope recurrences.[36] However, the contribution of cardiac pacing in the therapy of ictal asystole remains controversial.[37]

When complete abolishment of asystole occurs with anti-epileptic medication, it further confirms that asystole was caused by seizure activities. In some cases, a new treatment option could be considered, known as cardioneuroablation.[38] This procedure achieves partial parasympathetic denervation of the sinus and/or atrioventricular node, reducing the adverse parasympathetic influence on the heart. While there is limited evidence in the literature evaluating the efficacy of this method, it might represent a new treatment modality, especially for select pharmacoresistant patients with ictal asystole who are not eligible for surgery.[39] The correct approach to SUDEP is still uncertain. Refined SUDEP risk assessment scales may be useful in deciding which patients require a more aggressive approach, despite the risks associated with additional medication trials, surgery, or neuromodulation.[40]

REFERENCES

1. Walsh KE, Baneck T, Page RL, Brignole M, Hamdan MH. Psychogenic pseudosyncope: not always a diagnosis of exclusion. *Pacing Clin Electrophysiol.* 2018;41:480–486.

2. Raj V, Rowe AA, Fleisch SB, Paranjape SY, Arain AM, Nicolson SE. Psychogenic pseudosyncope: diagnosis and management. *Auton Neurosci.* 2014;184:66–72.

3. Blad H, Lamberts RJ, van Dijk GJ, Thijs RD. Tilt-induced vasovagal syncope and psychogenic pseudosyncope: overlapping clinical entities. *Neurology.* 2015;85:2006–2010.

4. Brignole M, Moya A, de Lange FJ, et al. and ESC Scientific Document Group. 2018 ESC guide-lines for the diagnosis and management of syncope. *Eur Heart J.* 2018;39:1883–1948

5. Leach JP, Lauder R, Nicolson A, Smith DF. Epilepsy in the UK: misdiagnosis, mistreatment, and undertreatment? The Wrexham area epilepsy project. *Seizure.* 2005;14:514–520.

6. Shen WK, Sheldon RS, Benditt DG, et al. 2017 ACC/AHA/HRS guideline for the evalu-ation and management of patients with syncope: executive summary: a report of the American College of Cardiology/American Heart Association Task Force on Clinical Practice Guidelines and the Heart Rhythm Society. *Circulation.* 2017;136:e25–e59.

7. Claffey P, Pérez-Denia L, Rivasi G, Finucane C, Kenny RA. Near-infrared spectroscopy in evaluating psychogenic pseudosyncope-a novel diagnostic approach. *QJM.* 2020;113:239–244.

8. American Psychiatric Association: *Diagnostic and Statistical Manual of Mental Disorders*, 5th ed (DSM5). Washington, DC: American Psychiatric Association, 2013.

9. McKenzie P, Oto M, Russell A, Pelosi A, Duncan R. Early outcomes and predictors in 260 patients with psychogenic nonepileptic attacks. *Neurology.* 2010;74:64–69.

10. Brown LB., Nicholson TR, Aybek S, Kanaan RA, David AS. Neuropsychological function and memory suppression in conversion disorder. *J Neuropsychol.* 2014;8:171–185.

11. Kozlowska K, Palmer DM, Brown KJ, et al. Conversion disorder in children and adolescents: a disorder of cognitive control. *J Neuropsychol.* 2015;9:87–108.

12. de Vroege L, Koppenol I, Kop WJ, Riem MME, van der Feltz-Cornelis CM. Neurocognitive functioning in patients with conversion disorder/functional neurological disorder. *J Neuropsychol.* 2021 Mar;15(1):69–87. https://doi.org/10.1111/jnp.12206. Epub 2020 Mar 29

13. Goldstein LH, Chalder T, Chigwedere C, et al. Cognitive behavioral therapy for psychogenic nonepileptic seizures: a pilot RCT. *Neurology.* 2010;74:1986–1994.

14. LaFrance WC Jr, Baird GL, Barry JJ, et al. and NES Treatment Trial (NEST-T) Consortium. Multicenter pilot treatment trial for psychogenic nonepileptic seizures: a randomized clinical trial. *JAMA Psychiatry.* 2014;71:997–1005.

15. Moya A, Permanyer-Miralda G, Sagrista-Sauleda J, et al. Limitations of head-up tilt test for evaluating the efficacy of therapeutic interventions in patients with vaso-vagal syncope: results of a controlled study of etilefrine versus placebo. *J Am Coll Cardiol.* 1995;25:65–69.

16. Krediet CT, van Dijk N, Linzer M, van Lieshout JJ, Wieling W. Management of vasovagal syncope: controlling or aborting faints by leg crossing and muscle tensing. *Circulation.* 2002;106:1684–1689.

17. Krediet CT, de Bruin IG, Ganzeboom KS, Linzer M, van Lieshout JJ, Wieling W. Leg crossing, muscle tensing, squatting, and the crash position are effective against vasovagal reactions solely through increases in cardiac output. *J Appl Physiol.* 2005;99:1697–1703.

18. Krediet CT, Go-Schön IK, van Lieshout JJ, Wieling W. Optimizing squatting as a physical maneuver to prevent vasovagal syncope. *Clin Auton Res.* 2008;18:179–186.

19. Raj V, Rowe AA, Fleisch SB, Paranjape SY, Arain AM, Nicolson SE. Psychogenic pseudosyn-cope: diagnosis and management. *Auton Neurosci.* 2014;184:66–72.

20. Sahota I, Sheldon R, Pournazari P. Clinical improvement of vasovagal syncope in the absence of specific therapies: the Seinfeld effect. *Cardiol J.* 2014;21:637–642.

21. Costagliola G, Orsini A, Coll M, Brugada R, Parisi P, Striano P. The brain-heart interaction in epilepsy: implications for diagnosis, therapy, and SUDEP prevention. *Ann Clin Transl Neurol.* 2021;8(7):1557–1568. https://doi.org/10.1002/acn3.51382.

22. Friedman D. Sudden unexpected death in epilepsy. *Curr Opin Neurol.* 2022;35(2):181–188. https://doi.org/10.1097/WCO.0000000000001034.

23. Enkiri SA, Ghavami F, Anyanwu C, Eldadah Z, Morrissey RL, Motamedi GK. New onset left frontal lobe seizure presenting with ictal asystole. *Seizure.* 2011;20(10):817–819. https://doi.org/10.1016/j.seizure.2011.07.012.

24. Khalil M, Shukralla AA, Kilbride R, et al. Ictal asystole during long-term video-EEG; semiology, localization, and intervention. *Epilepsy Behav Rep.* 2020;15:100416. https://doi.org/10.1016/j.ebr.2020.100416.

25. Bestawros M, Darbar D, Arain A, et al. Ictal asystole and ictal syncope: insights into clinical management. *Circ Arrhythm Electrophysiol.* 2015;8(1):159–164. https://doi.org/10.1161/CIRCEP.114.001667.

26. Allana SS, Ahmed HN, Shah K, Kelly AF. Ictal bradycardia and atrioventricular block: a cardiac manifestation of epilepsy. *Oxf Med Case Rep.* 2014;2014(2):33–35. https://doi.org/10.1093/omcr/omu015.

27. Fialho GL, Wolf P, Walz R, Lin K. SUDEP – more attention to the heart? A narrative review on molecular autopsy in epilepsy. *Seizure.* 2021 Apr;87:103–106. https://doi.org/10.1016/j.seizure.2021.03.010.

28. Duplyakov D, Golovina G, Lyukshina N, Surkova E, Elger CE, Surges R. Syncope, seizure-induced bradycardia and asystole: two cases and review of clinical and pathophysiological features. *Seizure.* 2014;23(7):506–511. https://doi.org/10.1016/j.seizure.2014.03.004.

29. Shmuely S, van der Lende M, Lamberts RJ, Sander JW, Thijs RD. The heart of epilepsy: current views and future concepts. *Seizure.* 2017;44:176–183. https://doi.org/10.1016/j.seizure.2016.10.001.

30. Rossetti AO, Dworetzky BA, Madsen JR, Golub O, Beckman JA, Bromfield EB. Ictal asystole with convulsive syncope mimicking secondary generalisation: a depth electrode study. *J Neurol Neurosurg Psychiatry.* 2005;76(6):885–887. https://doi.org/10.1136/jnnp.2004.051839.

31. Kohno R, Abe H, Akamatsu N, et al. Syncope and ictal asystole caused by temporal lobe epilepsy. *Circ J.* 2011;75(10):2508–2510. https://doi.org/10.1253/circj.cj-11-0261.

32. Giovannini G, Meletti S. Ictal asystole as the first presentation of epilepsy: a case report and systematic literature review. *Epilepsy Behav Case Rep.* 2014;2:136–141. https://doi.org/10.1016/j.ebcr.2014.06.001.

33. Nei M. Cardiac effects of seizures. *Epilepsy Curr.* 2009;9(4):91–95. https://doi.org/10.1111/j.1535-7511.2009.01303.x.

34. Casciato S, Quarato PP, Mascia A, et al. Ictal Asystole in drug-resistant focal epilepsy: two decades of experience from an epilepsy monitoring unit. *Brain Sci.* 2020;10(7):443. https://doi.org/10.3390/brainsci10070443.

35. Schuele SU, Bermeo AC, Locatelli E, Burgess RC, Lüders HO. Ictal asystole: a benign condition? *Epilepsia.* 2008;49(1):168–171. https://doi.org/10.1111/j.1528-1167.2007.01330.x.

36. Kepez A, Erdogan O. Arrhythmogenic epilepsy and pacing need: a matter of controversy. *World J Clin Cases.* 2015;3(10):872–875. https://doi.org/10.12998/wjcc.v3.i10.872.

37. Strzelczyk A, Cenusa M, Bauer S, et al. Management and long-term outcome in patients presenting with ictal asystole or bradycardia. *Epilepsia*. 2011;52(6):1160–1167. https://doi.org/10.1111/j.1528-1167.2010.02961.x.

38. van Westrhenen A, Shmuely S, Surges R, et al. Timing of syncope in ictal asystole as a guide when considering pacemaker implantation. *J Cardiovasc Electrophysiol*. 2021;32(11):3019–3026. https://doi.org/10.1111/jce.15239.

39. Rebecchi M, De Ruvo E, Sgueglia M, et al. Atrial fibrillation and sympatho-vagal imbalance: from the choice of the antiarrhythmic treatment to patients with syncope and ganglionated plexi ablation. *Eur Heart J Suppl*. 2023;25(Suppl C):C1–C6. https://doi.org/10.1093/eurheartjsupp/suad075.

40. Antolic B, Gorisek VR, Granda G, Lorber B, Sinkovec M, Zizek D. Cardioneuroablation in ictal asystole – new treatment method. *Heart Rhythm Case Rep*. 2018;4(11):523–526. https://doi.org/10.1016/j.hrcr.2018.07.018.

12 Other Neurological Conditions (Sleep Disorders, Autonomic Failure, and Structural Brain Lesions)

Ann-Kathrin Kahle, Katharina Scherschel, Fares-Alexander Alken, and Christian Meyer

INTRODUCTION

While the term neurocardiogenic syncope traditionally summarizes various syndromes with multiple underlying conditions and comorbidities, recent years and pathophysiologic insights have opened up new avenues for the understanding of diseases of the peripheral and central autonomic nervous system (ANS) (Figure 12.1). These include functional and morphological conditions predisposing to syncope, which are addressed in the following with a focus on primary and secondary autonomic failure (Figure 12.2).

SLEEP DISORDERS

The ANS is a key regulator of sleep and circadian pathophysiology, with sleep and consciousness being closely connected.[1] Obstructive sleep apnea (OSA) is the most common sleep disorder diagnosed in about 34% and 17% of middle-aged men and women. It is associated with an increased risk of cardiovascular diseases such as atrial fibrillation (AF), heart failure, and coronary artery disease, leading to higher all-cause and cardiovascular mortality.[2] Symptoms can vary especially in multimorbid or frail patients. Therefore, in-depth anamnesis is key in order to distinguish between syncope and sleepiness in some patients. Especially after traffic accidents, diagnosis can be challenging if third-party anamnesis is not possible.

Considering the pathophysiology of OSA, sympathetic activation due to intermittent apneas and hypopneas, and consequent compensatory hyperpneas, is well known. Simultaneously, increased parasympathetic activity is associated with long pauses and bradycardia (both sinus and conduction system-related). These may lead to chronic adaptations of the ANS favoring the occurrence of syncope during the daytime.[3,4] However, the pathophysiological mechanisms of a potential correlation between OSA and recurrent syncope are of multifactorial genesis, and to date, greater details are unknown. Evidence regarding the impact of OSA management on the incidence of syncopal episodes is limited, and randomized controlled trials are lacking. Continuous positive airway pressure as the therapy of choice is known to improve OSA-related symptoms, with a

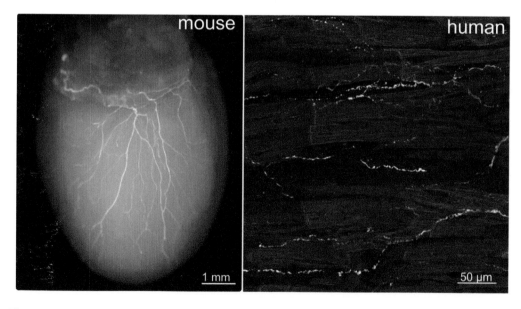

Figure 12.1 The intrinsic cardiac autonomic network. Sympathetic nerve fibers on the posterior mouse heart (left) and in the human left ventricle (right) illustrating the dense autonomic network of the heart innervating every single cardiomyocyte which is diminished in autonomic neuropathies.

DOI: 10.1201/9781003415855-14

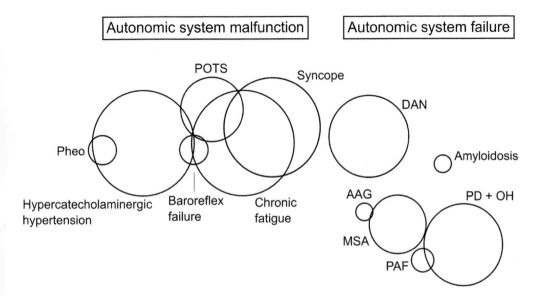

Figure 12.2   The Dysautonomia Universe. The expanding Dysautonomia Universe, as suggested by D. Goldstein, is illustrated indicating the growing number of syndromes and mechanistic understanding during the last two decades. Whereas in adults, dysautonomia usually represents functional malfunction of a generally intact autonomic nervous system, in the elderly, dysautonomia typically reflects a neurodegenerative disease. AAG, autoimmune autonomic ganglionopathy; DAN, diabetic autonomic neuropathy; MSA, multiple system atrophy; PAF, pure autonomic failure; PD+OH, Parkinson's disease with orthostatic hypotension; Pheo, pheochromocytoma; POTS, postural tachycardia syndrome.

reduction of bradycardia episodes by 72%–89%.[5] Therefore, it has been suggested that continuous positive airway pressure may effectively prevent recurrent syncopal episodes during the day.[3,4] Further treatment approaches for OSA include lifestyle interventions, weight loss, positional therapy, and oral appliances. The glucagon-like peptide-1 receptor agonist liraglutide has recently been shown to reduce OSA severity in combination with continuous positive airway pressure.[6] Interventional treatment approaches involve upper airway surgery, neurostimulation, and bariatric surgery.[7]

In patients with OSA, chronic recurrence of intermittent nocturnal hypoxia with acute alteration in intrathoracic pressure, oxidative stress, inflammation, and neurohumoral activation may lead to long-term atrial remodeling altering atrial electrophysiology.[7] These effects of the sympathetic and parasympathetic ANS result in a predisposition to AF and may be assessed by analysis of heart rate (HR) variability[8] and autonomic bedside testing.[9,10]

Patients with continuous positive airway pressure treatment are less likely to progress to more permanent forms of AF and have a reduced recurrence rate of AF both after cardioversion and catheter ablation.[11–13] Consequently, patients with AF and stable atrial tachycardia treated for OSA may be less likely to develop long pauses favoring the occurrence of a syncope. Otherwise, AF and atrial tachycardia treatment in patients with OSA may contribute to the improvement of some symptoms. Optimal therapy, especially in patients with long pauses, is under investigation (Figure 12.3). In the case of recurrent syncopal episodes and long pauses, a pacemaker often represents the treatment of choice.[5] If patients wish to avoid pacemaker implantation, pulmonary vein isolation may be considered. Whether accidental parasympathetic denervation may bring additional benefits is unclear.[14,15] To date, data comparing pulmonary vein isolation and cardiac pacing are sparse. A better understanding of the role of the ANS in the etiology of sleep disorders is needed to strengthen both diagnostic methods as well as non-invasive and interventional treatment options.

AUTONOMIC FAILURE
Epidemiological and pathophysiologic insights highlight the importance of diseases of the peripheral and central ANS in patients with syncope.[16] These include functional and

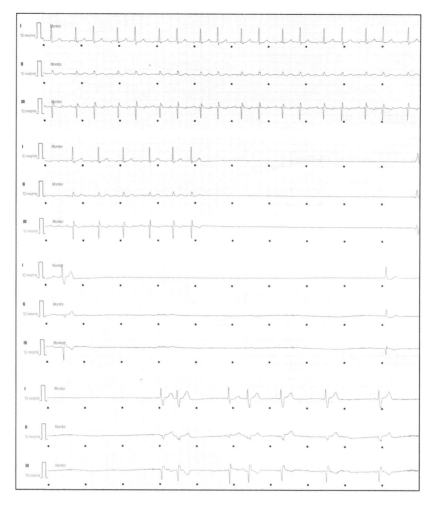

Figure 12.3 Long pauses in a patient with atrial fibrillation. Electrocardiogram (25 mm/s) of a female patient (58 years) with atrial fibrillation and prior pulmonary vein isolation two years ago. An ongoing stable atrial tachycardia converts into idioventricular rhythm with sinus beats. Following long pauses of 5.8 s and 2× 8.5 s, the patient received a dual-chamber pacemaker.

Table 12.1: Genesis of Autonomic Failure

Primary Autonomic Failure	Secondary Autonomic Failure
Pure autonomic failure	Diabetes
Multiple system atrophy	Amyloidosis
Parkinson's disease	Spinal cord injuries
Dementia with Lewy bodies	Auto-immune autonomic neuropathy
	Paraneoplastic autonomic neuropathy
	Kidney failure

morphological changes, which often manifest in different conditions of primary and secondary autonomic failure.[17] The primary causes of autonomic failure are neurodegenerative diseases, including pure autonomic failure and Parkinson's disease. Secondary autonomic failure may occur over time in patients with systemic diseases such as diabetes, amyloidosis, or advanced kidney failure (Figure 12.2 and Table 12.1).[17] Both conditions are highly prevalent but often unrecognized or misdiagnosed due to diverse and partly non-specific clinical presentations.

Orthostatic hypotension

Symptoms	Risk factors	Associated drugs
Chest pain	Aging	Beta-receptor blockers
Cognitive slowing	Alcohol drinking	Chemotherapeutic agents
Dizziness	Bed rest	Diuretics
Dyspnea	Deconditioning	Monoamine oxidase inhibitors
Fatigue	Fever	Narcotics
Gait disorders	Heat	Phenothiazines
Headache	Immobilisation	Sedatives
Leg buckling	Large and/or high-	Tranquilizers
Lightheadedness	carbohydrate meals	Tricyclic antidepressants
Nausea	Morning hours after waking	Vasodilators
Neck pain	Post-exercise time	
Nocturnal polyuria	Prolonged orthostatic stress	
Syncope	Sleep-disordered breathing	
Visual blurring		
Weakness		

Figure 12.4 Symptoms, risk factors, and drugs associated with orthostatic hypotension. Symptoms, risk factors, and drugs associated with the occurrence of orthostatic hypotension are listed in an alphabetical order. Pathophysiologically, orthostatic hypotension can be classified into structural and functional reasons of autonomic nervous system impairment. In this context, neurogenic orthostatic hypotension is a key manifestation of chronic autonomic failure in primary neurodegenerative disorders. Non-neurogenic orthostatic hypotension occurs due to functional impairment of the autonomic nervous system based, e.g., on different medications or an absolute or relative reduction in circulating blood volume.

The most prevalent symptoms are dizziness and lightheadedness upon standing. These prodromal signs may result in syncope, which is usually of gradual onset but may also occur suddenly. Importantly, especially with aging, co-morbidities should be determined in a detailed anamnesis (Figure 12.4).[18]

Pathophysiology

In autonomic failure, degeneration of central and/or peripheral autonomic pathways leads to an inadequate release of norepinephrine from sympathetic neurons.[19] Subsequent vasoconstrictor failure results in venous blood pooling below the diaphragm, followed by a reduction in venous return and cardiac output. A decrease in blood pressure (BP) upon standing may provoke the occurrence of syncope.[19] Orthostatic hypotension (OH), defined as a sustained reduction in systolic BP ≥20 mmHg or diastolic BP ≥10 mmHg within 3 minutes of active standing or head-up tilt table testing, represents the second most common etiology of syncope.[20] Pathophysiologically, OH can be divided into two categories. Neurogenic OH is the key manifestation of chronic autonomic failure involving structural causes of ANS impairment. Non-neurogenic OH is based on factors that may cause functional ANS failure, including various medications, absolute or relative reduction in circulating blood volume, venous pooling, and inotropic and/or chronotropic heart failure.[21] Based on temporal changes in orthostatic BP, three different clinical variants of OH have been proposed. Classical OH, as observed in autonomic failure, can be distinguished from initial and delayed OH. Initial OH is characterized by a time from an upright position to an abnormal BP response of ≤15 seconds based on a mismatch between cardiac output and peripheral vascular resistance. Delayed OH is observed when a BP reduction occurs after 3 minutes, probably due to a progressive fall in venous return and low cardiac output. It suggests an early manifestation of classical OH, potentially associated with incipient autonomic failure.[18]

Diabetic Autonomic Neuropathy

The leading cause of secondary autonomic failure is diabetic autonomic neuropathy (DAN), which has already been described five decades ago and is the most prevalent autonomic neuropathy today.[22] DAN affects the cardiovascular, urogenital, gastrointestinal, pupillomotor, thermoregulatory, and sudomotor systems.[23,24] The prevalence of cardiac autonomic neuropathy in patients with diabetes varies widely depending on the population studied and the tests and/or the diagnostic criteria used. An increase of up to 65% with age and diabetes duration and already approximately 15%–20% of asymptomatic patients with diabetes can be observed.[25,26] Simultaneously, aging itself causes declines in sympathetic, parasympathetic, and sensory fibers, leading to cardiac dysfunction.[27] Clinical predictors include glycemic control, diabetic polyneuropathy, and renal failure, as well as classic cardiovascular risk factors (Figure 12.5).[25] Symptomatic manifestations are sinus tachycardia due to parasympathetic dysfunction in the early phase, leading to impaired HR variability and exercise intolerance (Figure 12.6).[22] In the later disease stages, OH, present in up to 64% of diabetes patients, may result in recurrent syncopal episodes in up to 50% of patients[28,29] as well as silent myocardial ischemia due to sympathetic denervation.[18,30] Symptoms of ischemia in patients with diabetes mellitus are often non-specific. Screening for asymptomatic coronary artery disease in this population is controversial as multiple randomized controlled trials have not shown any differences in cardiovascular outcomes between patients who underwent routine screening compared with standard recommendations.[31] Selection of high-risk patients may therefore be necessary to adopt screening strategies.[32] In a meta-analysis of 15 studies, cardiac autonomic neuropathy has been reported to go along with an increased risk of mortality in patients with diabetes ranging from 27% to 56% over 5–10 years.[23,33] Consequently, lifestyle interventions including exercise and diet assessing diabetes as the underlying disease as well as conventional treatment approaches for OH should be pursued. In this context, sodium-glucose cotransporter two inhibitors have been suggested to reduce the risk of recurrent syncope based on the improvement of autonomic dysfunction and may potentially represent an important supplement in this population.[29]

Diagnostics

In most patients, basic diagnostics including anamnesis with medical history, physical examination with supine and standing BP measurements, and an electrocardiogram result in a high diagnostic yield. In others, advanced bedside testing is warranted to guide optimal therapeutic decision-making.[17,20,34] Considering the diagnosis of autonomic failure as the cause for recurrent syncope,[35] there are three available methods to assess the response to a change in posture from supine to erect. First, with a current class I indication, 24-hour ambulatory BP monitoring is recommended. It usually demonstrates a nocturnal non-dipping (mean BP falls <10% with respect to daytime) or reverse dipping (mean BP increases with respect to daytime) in patients with autonomic failure.[17] It further allows the determination of drug-induced hypotension or may be suggestive of additional disorders such as sleep apnea.[7] Still, there is limited evidence regarding the designation of the degree of OH. Therefore, further assessment to guide therapeutic

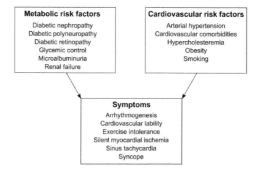

Figure 12.5 Cardiac autonomic neuropathy in patients with diabetes. Clinical metabolic and cardiovascular risk factors as well as symptoms of cardiac autonomic neuropathy in patients with diabetes are indicated. Current demographical changes and lifestyle-related health behaviors are often intertwined resulting in multimorbidity and frailty challenging the prevention, diagnosis, and treatment of cardiac autonomic neuropathy and related orthostatic hypotension and syncope.

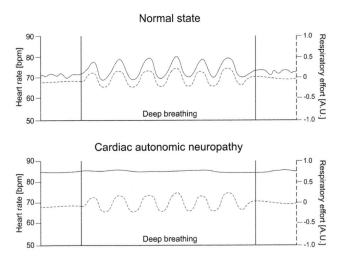

Figure 12.6 Reduced heart rate variability in cardiac autonomic neuropathy. Heart rate variability including respiratory sinus arrhythmia represents a measure of the oscillation in the intervals between consecutive heartbeats. Above, normal heart rate variability in response to deep breathing is illustrated. Caused by phasic changes of efferent vagal neural discharge directed to the sinus node, heart rate changes in synchrony with respiration shown in arbitrary units, with an increased heart rate during inspiration (positive respiratory effort) and a decreased heart rate during expiration (negative respiratory effort), defined as respiratory sinus arrhythmia. Below, reduced heart rate variability during deep breathing in a patient with diabetic neuropathy as an example for cardiac autonomic neuropathy characterized by widespread degeneration of both sympathetic and parasympathetic nerve fibers is illustrated. Impaired autonomic nervous system activity in diabetes patients with cardiac autonomic neuropathy results in reduced cardiac output and peripheral blood flow as well as an increased heart rate leading to limited exercise tolerance.

decision-making especially in patients who are strongly affected in daily life due to persistent and severe symptoms is needed. Second, active standing is used to distinguish syncope due to autonomic failure based on classical OH from other types of OH. The diagnosis can be determined with a sphygmomanometer, typically used for routine clinical testing because of its ubiquity and simplicity. Importantly, compensatory tachycardia can be seen during testing but may also be blunted or absent in more severe autonomic failure.[34] Third, during head-up tilt table testing, directly after head-up tilt, BP starts to decrease in patients with autonomic failure, with a decreasing rate of drop resulting in a concave curve. If HR control is still functional, an increase in HR occurs, attempting to compensate for low BP.[34] Head-up tilt table testing may be especially used for the reproduction of delayed OH, which cannot be detected by active standing because of its delayed onset. Whereas head-up tilt table testing, which is more time-consuming and resource-intensive than active standing, may further be helpful in some patients with recurrent vasovagal syncope, its meaning is limited in those with syncope of uncertain cause. Even for the differential diagnosis of postural tachycardia syndrome, an active standing test can be conclusive with an HR increase of >30 bpm or to >120 bpm without any relevant blood pressure drops within 10 minutes.[17] Moreover, a detailed patient history can be helpful since the onset of postural tachycardia syndrome is often precipitated by immunological stressors such as viral infection, vaccination, trauma, surgery, or psychosocial stress.[20]

Regarding further concepts of advanced testing, a Valsalva maneuver should be considered for patients with suspected autonomic failure as the absence of a BP overshoot and an HR increase during the Valsalva maneuver are strongly pathognomonic. In this context, the degree of hypotension and/or the lack of compensation during forced expiration correlates with the degree of autonomic dysfunction and related symptoms. Therefore, the Valsalva maneuver has an increased sensitivity for detecting milder forms of sympathetic impairment compared to tilt table testing.[34] Finally, in patients with autonomic failure, HR variability during deep breathing is blunted or even abolished due to the degeneration of parasympathetic fibers.[36] Deficient vascular sympathetic modulation is associated with a lack of oscillation in total peripheral resistance and non-neural respiratory-mediated fluctuations in BP and cardiac output (Figure 12.6).[17]

Besides the above-mentioned advanced autonomic testing techniques, a multidisciplinary diagnostic approach, e.g., neurological, psychiatric, and/or other additional evaluations, may further be required, depending on the underlying disease.[17]

Treatment

Treatment of autonomic failure mostly comprises non-pharmacological and pharmacological interventions.[17] Education and lifestyle modifications are suggested as first-line therapy in all cases elucidating awareness, the possible avoidance of triggers and situations (e.g., dehydration), and early recognition of prodromal signs (Figure 12.4). The expansion of extracellular volume should be pursued. In the absence of hypertension, patients should be assigned to have a sufficient salt and water intake, targeting 2–3 L of fluids per day and 10 g of sodium chloride supplementation.[37] Evaluation of discontinuation or reduction of vasoactive drugs should be considered as they increase the risk of recurrent syncopal episodes due to OH. In the case of persisting symptoms, counter-pressure maneuvers, abdominal binders and/or support stockings, training of active standing, and head-up tilt sleeping may be used to increase venous return and cardiac filling pressure.[19] Considering different pharmacological approaches, midodrine, an alpha-agonist, increases BP in the supine and upright position and improves symptoms of OH. A "pill-in-the-pocket" concept has been used successfully in some patients in situations when potential triggers cannot be avoided. However, it is neither helpful in all affected patients nor can it be regarded as a curing treatment and may further lead to pilomotor reactions.[38] Fludrocortisone, a mineralocorticoid stimulating renal sodium retention and expanding fluid volume, has little evidence, but some studies reported hemodynamic benefits and improvement of symptoms with a BP increase.[39] Regarding all possible treatment approaches, it should be mentioned that patients with primary autonomic failure often have supine hypertension, which can complicate the diagnosis and treatment of a syncope occurring due to OH and underlines the importance of conscientious evaluation. More in-depth evidence with prospective randomized controlled trials comparing different pharmacological agents as well as investigations of additional therapies are needed. This may involve, e.g., droxidopa, a centrally and peripherally acting alpha and beta-agonist, which so far has been shown to increase standing systolic BP in the short term but requires further investigation in the long term.[40,41] Interventional approaches used for the restoration of BP regulation have been conducted in some patients, including an implantable neuroprothesis stimulating the dorsal root entry zones of the thoracic spinal cord.[42] Considering adjunctive conservative treatment approaches, yoga has recently been reported to reduce the symptomatic burden and improve the quality of life in patients with recurrent vasovagal syncope compared to standard therapy alone.[43] Pathophysiologically, enhanced vascular and muscular tone mainly in the lower limbs both blunt the venodilation phase of a syncopal episode and accelerate the venous return. Yoga increases vagal tone and improves autonomic balance, while simultaneously reducing stress and anxiety. Consequently, relaxation techniques may prospectively be evaluated in patients with autonomic failure potentially expanding the current therapeutic armamentarium depending on the stage of the underlying disease.

STRUCTURAL BRAIN LESIONS

Structural brain lesions include areas of brain tissue that show damage from disease or injury. They may develop due to brain tumors, strokes, degenerative brain diseases occurring with aging such as Alzheimer's disease, immune and inflammatory conditions including multiple sclerosis or lupus erythematosus, congenital disorders, infections, epilepsy, traumatic brain injuries, and medical procedures. Depending on the localization and lesion dimension, ANS dysfunction additionally to other neurological impairments may be present. Primarily, interdisciplinary patient care with an emphasis on specialized neurological expertise is needed.

Considering the aging world population,[27] neurodegenerative disorders play an increasing role in daily life.[44] Syncope and falls represent a major cause of morbidity and mortality in elderly people,[45] and syncope is the primary reason for hospitalization in dementia patients.[46] Affected patients often present with non-specific symptoms without any prodromal signs.[47] Anamnesis may be difficult due to cognitive impairment as the majority of patients do not remember the dynamic of the syncope, which complicates both its diagnosis as well as management. Vascular aging contributes as the predominant mechanism to the occurrence of syncopal episodes in elderly people. Polypharmacy, as well as specific medications, e.g., cholinesterase inhibitors prescribed for Alzheimer's disease, further exacerbates the risk of bradyarrhythmia and hypotension potentially, resulting in syncope.[47,48] Consequently, adequate interdisciplinary management and treatment of elderly people with neurodegenerative disorders is needed to reduce syncopal events and falls, leading to trauma and major injuries such as subdural hematoma in a relevant number of patients.[47]

It should be considered that a subdural hematoma and syncope may be mutually dependent. According to the current guidelines, brain computed tomography or magnetic resonance imaging should be avoided in uncomplicated cases of syncope.[17] Nonetheless, neurologic imaging is recommended in the presence of novel neurologic deficits. In these situations, e.g., a subdural hematoma may be apparent elevating intracranial pressure, which temporarily impedes cerebral blood flow and therefore may cause recurrent episodes of syncope.[49]

As an important differential diagnosis to syncope associated with structural brain lesions, epileptic seizures should be kept in mind. They may be distinguished from syncope based on typical clinical characteristics. These include a rare nature of trigger, an epileptic aura specific for each patient, a synchronous, symmetrical, and hemilateral myoclonus, a memory deficit, and several minutes needed for the restoration of consciousness. In these patients, in whom transient loss of consciousness is suspected to be epilepsy, neurological evaluation with an electroencephalogram is indicated.[17]

Considering the pediatric population, syncope occurs commonly, affecting approximately 15% of children younger than 18 years. The most frequent underlying diagnoses for transient loss of consciousness are vasovagal syncope, OH, and (atypical) seizures, which characterize it as a benign event in the majority of patients.[50] Still, adolescents with concussions have been shown to experience symptoms of OH more frequently than healthy adolescents. However, they often do not meet the standard OH criteria, which underlines the importance of adequate assessment including anamnesis and suggests a possible adaptation of diagnostic tests.[51] In-depth evaluation should especially be considered in patients with syncope occurring during exercise, representing a potentially fatal condition, or with a family history of syncope, sudden death, myocardial disease, or arrhythmias.[52]

In conclusion, syncopal events in the presence of structural brain lesions may occur due to multiple causes implementing accurate (third-party) anamnesis as a key element of patient care. Detailed assessment of the timing of syncope, potential concomitant comorbidities, medication, and clinical investigation are needed to ensure adequate syncope treatment in these populations.

REFERENCES

1. Mehra R, Tjurmina OA, Ajijola OA, et al. Research opportunities in autonomic neural mechanisms of cardiopulmonary regulation: A report from the National Heart, Lung, and Blood Institute and the National Institutes of Health Office of the Director Workshop. *JACC Basic Transl Sci*. 2022;7:265–293.

2. Javaheri S, Barbe F, Campos-Rodriguez F, et al. Sleep apnea. *J Am Coll Cardiol*. 2017;69:841–858.

3. Puel V, Pepin JL, Gosse P. Sleep related breathing disorders and vasovagal syncope, a possible causal link? *Int J Cardiol*. 2013;168:1666–1667.

4. Willis FB, Isley AL, Geda YE, Quarles IV L, Fredrickson PA. Resolution of syncope with treatment of sleep apnea. *J Am Board Fam Med*. 2008;21:466–468.

5. Glikson M, Nielsen JC, Kronborg MB, et al. 2021 ESC guidelines on cardiac pacing and cardiac resynchronization therapy. *Eur Heart J*. 2021;42:3427–3520.

6. Jiang W, Li W, Cheng J, Li W, Cheng F. Efficacy and safety of liraglutide in patients with type 2 diabetes mellitus and severe obstructive sleep apnea. *Sleep Breath*. 2023;27:1687–1694.

7. Yeghiazarians Y, Jneid H, Tietjens JR, et al. Obstructive sleep apnea and cardiovascular disease: A scientific statement from the American Heart Association. *Circulation*. 2021;144:E56–E67.

8. Meyer C, Kahle AK. The autonomic nervous system as a piece of the mechanistic puzzle linking sleep and atrial fibrillation. *J Interv Card Electrophysiol*. 2023;66:815–822.

9. Eickholt C, Jungen C, Drexel T, et al. Sympathetic and parasympathetic coactivation induces perturbed heart rate dynamics in patients with paroxysmal atrial fibrillation. *Med Sci Monit*. 2018;24:2164–2172.

10. Apelt-Glitz K, Alken FA, Jungen C, Scherschel K, Klöcker N, Meyer C. Respiratory and heart rate dynamics during peripheral chemoreceptor deactivation compared to targeted sympathetic and sympathetic/parasympathetic (co-)activation. *Auton Neurosci*. 2022;241:103009.

11. Fein AS, Shvilkin A, Shah D, et al. Treatment of obstructive sleep apnea reduces the risk of atrial fibrillation recurrence after catheter ablation. *J Am Coll Cardiol*. 2013;62:300–305.

12. Naruse Y, Tada H, Satoh M, et al. Concomitant obstructive sleep apnea increases the recurrence of atrial fibrillation following radiofrequency catheter ablation of atrial fibrillation: Clinical impact of continuous positive airway pressure therapy. *Heart Rhythm*. 2013;10:331–337.

13. Neilan TG, Farhad H, Dodson JA, et al. Effect of sleep apnea and continuous positive airway pressure on cardiac structure and recurrence of atrial fibrillation. *J Am Heart Assoc*. 2013;2:e000421.

14. Jungen C, Scherschel K, Eickholt C, et al. Disruption of cardiac cholinergic neurons enhances susceptibility to ventricular arrhythmias. *Nat Commun*. 2017;8:14155.

15. Scherschel K, Hedenus K, Jungen C, et al. Cardiac glial cells release neurotrophic S100B upon catheter-based treatment of atrial fibrillation. *Sci Transl Med*. 2019;11:eaav7770.

16. Lovelace JW, Ma J, Yadav S, et al. Vagal sensory neurons mediate the Bezold-Jarisch reflex and induce syncope. *Nature*. 2023. https://doi.org/10.1038/s41586-023-06680-7.

17. Brignole M, Moya A, Lange De FJ, et al. 2018 ESC guidelines for the diagnosis and management of syncope. *Eur Heart J*. 2018;39:1883–1948.

18. Freeman R, Abuzinadah AR, Gibbons C, Jones P, Miglis MG, Sinn DI. Orthostatic hypotension: JACC state-of-the-art review. *J Am Coll Cardiol*. 2018;72:1294–1309.

19. Freeman R. Neurogenic orthostatic hypotension. *N Engl J Med*. 2008;358:615–624.

20. Freeman R, Wieling W, Axelrod FB, et al. Consensus statement on the definition of orthostatic hypotension, neurally mediated syncope and the postural tachycardia syndrome. *Auton Neurosci*. 2011;161:46–48.

21. Ricci F, Caterina De R, Fedorowski A. Orthostatic hypotension epidemiology, prognosis, and treatment. *J Am Coll Cardiol*. 2015;66:848–860.

22. Wheeler T, Watkins PJ. Cardiac denervation in diabetes. *Br Med J*. 1973;4:584–586.

23. Freeman R. Diabetic autonomic neuropathy. *Handb Clin Neurol*. 2014;126:63–79.

24. Chakraborty P, Farhat K, Po SS, Armoundas AA, Stavrakis S. Autonomic nervous system and cardiac metabolism. *J Am Coll Cardiol EP*. 2023;9:1196–1206.

25. Spallone V, Ziegler D, Freeman R, et al. Cardiovascular autonomic neuropathy in diabetes: Clinical impact, assessment, diagnosis, and management. *Diabetes Metab Res Rev*. 2011;27:639–653.

26. Goldberger JJ, Arora R, Buckley U, Shivkumar K. Autonomic nervous system dysfunction: JACC focus seminar. *J Am Coll Cardiol*. 2019;73:1189–1206.

27. Wagner JUG, Tombor LS, Malacarne PF, et al. Aging impairs the neurovascular interface in the heart. *Science*. 2023;381:897–906.

28. Sardu C, Paolisso P, Santamaria M, et al. Cardiac syncope recurrence in type 2 diabetes mellitus patients vs. normoglycemics patients: The CARVAS study. *Diabetes Res Clin Pract*. 2019;151:152–162.

29. Sardu C, Massimo Massetti M, Rambaldi P, et al. SGLT2-inhibitors reduce the cardiac autonomic neuropathy dysfunction and vaso-vagal syncope recurrence in patients with type 2 diabetes mellitus: The SCAN study. *Metabolism*. 2022;137:155243.

30. Vinik AI, Ziegler D. Diabetic cardiovascular autonomic neuropathy. *Circulation*. 2007;115:387–397.

31. Marx N, Federici M, Schütt K, et al. 2023 ESC guidelines for the management of cardiovascular disease in patients with diabetes. *Eur Heart J*. 2023;44:4043–4140.

32. Young LH, Wackers FJT, Chyun DA, et al. Cardiac outcomes after screening for asymptomatic coronary artery disease in patients with type 2 diabetes the DIAD study: A randomized controlled trial. *JAMA*. 2009;301:1547–155.

33. Maser RE, Mitchell BD, Vinik AI, Freeman R. The association between cardiovascular autonomic neuropathy and mortality in individuals with diabetes a meta-analysis. *Diab Care*. 2003;26:1895–1901.

34. Brignole M, Moya A, Lange De FJ, et al. Practical instructions for the 2018 ESC guidelines for the diagnosis and management of syncope. *Eur Heart J*. 2018;39:e43–e80.

35. Jones PK, Gibbons CH. The role of autonomic testing in syncope. *Auton Neurosci*. 2014;184:40–45.

36. Jungen C, Alken FA, Eickholt C, et al. Respiratory sinus arrhythmia is reduced after pulmonary vein isolation in patients with paroxysmal atrial fibrillation. *Arch Med Sci*. 2019;16:1022–1030.

37. Schroeder C, Bush VE, Norcliffe LJ, et al. Water drinking acutely improves orthostatic tolerance in healthy subjects. *Circulation*. 2002;106:2806–2811.

38. Low PA. Efficacy of midodrine vs placebo in neurogenic orthostatic hypotension. *JAMA*. 1997;277:1046.

39. Lieshout Van JJ, Derk A, Harkel Ten J, Wieling W. Fludrocortisone and sleeping in the head-up position limit the postural decrease in cardiac output in autonomic failure. *Auton Res*. 2000;10:35–42.

40. Elgebaly A, Abdelazeim B, Mattar O, Gadelkarim M, Salah R, Negida A. Meta-analysis of the safety and efficacy of droxidopa for neurogenic orthostatic hypotension. *Clin Auton Res*. 2016;26:171–180.

41. Hauser RA, Favit A, Hewitt LA, et al. Durability of the clinical benefit of droxidopa for neurogenic orthostatic hypotension during 12 weeks of open-label treatment. *Neurol Ther*. 2022;11:459–469.

42. Squair JW, Berney M, Castro Jimenez M, et al. Implanted system for orthostatic hypotension in multiple-system atrophy. *N Engl J Med*. 2022;386:1339–1344.

43. Sharma G, Ramakumar V, Sharique M, et al. Effect of yoga on clinical outcomes and quality of life in patients with vasovagal syncope (LIVE-Yoga). *J Am Coll Cardiol EP*. 2022;8:141–149.

44. Cortes-Canteli M, Iadecola C. Alzheimer's disease and vascular aging: JACC focus seminar. *J Am Coll Cardiol*. 2020;75:942–951.

45. Tinetti ME, Williams CS. Falls, injuries due to falls, and the risk of admission to a nursing home. *J Am Coll Cardiol*. 1997;337:1279–1284.

46. Rudolph JL, Zanin NM, Jones RN, et al. Hospitalization in community-dwelling persons with Alzheimer's disease: Frequency and causes. *J Am Geriatr Soc*. 2010;58:1542–1548.

47. Ungar A, Mussi C, Nicosia F, et al. The "syncope and dementia" study: A prospective, observational, multicenter study of elderly patients with dementia and episodes of "suspected" transient loss of consciousness. *Aging Clin Exp Res*. 2015;27:877–882.

48. Kim DH, Brown RT, Ding EL, Kiel DP, Berry SD. Dementia medications and risk of falls, syncope, and related adverse events: Meta-analysis of randomized controlled trials. *J Am Geriatr Soc*. 2011;59:1019–1031.

49. Bruner DI, Jamros C, Cogar W. Subdural hematoma presenting as recurrent syncope. *J Emerg Med*. 2015;49:e65–e68.

50. Pratt JL, Fleisher GR. Syncope in children and adolescents. *Pediatr Emerg Care*. 1989;5:80–82.

51. Haider MN, Patel KS, Willer BS, et al. Symptoms upon postural change and orthostatic hypotension in adolescents with concussion. *Brain Inj*. 2021;35:226–232.

52. Driscoll DJ, Jacobsen SJ, Porter CJ, Wollan PC, Cardiology P. Syncope in children and adolescents. *J Am Coll Cardiol*. 1997;29:1039–1045.

13 Management of Reflex Syncope

13A Management of Reflex Syncope

Non-Pharmacological and Pharmacological

Giulia Rivasi and Artur Fedorowski

PART A. NON-PHARMACOLOGICAL MEASURES

Non-pharmacological interventions represent the mainstay of treatment in patients with non-cardiac syncope. These interventions are based on three pillars: reassurance of the benign nature of symptoms, education regarding triggers and strategies to avoid them, and lifestyle measures.[1] Patients should be informed that their condition is benign and usually self-limited, which helps to reduce anxiety, and education should be implemented in every patient.[2] Patients should be encouraged to identify their own triggers (e.g., prolonged standing, high ambient temperature or humidity, rapid posture changes, physiological activities such as micturition, especially in the morning or during the night) and manage their daily routine to minimize exposure. Moreover, it is crucial that an awareness of warning symptoms be developed, allowing for early recognition and intervention by the patient to abort syncope and prevent injuries. Awareness of prodromal symptoms and related management strategies may give empowerment and confidence, thus limiting psychosocial limitations caused by syncope propensity.

Easy-to-apply lifestyle measures should be promoted to minimize orthostatic stress, e.g., patients should be advised to stand up slowly from supine/sitting to upright positions and avoid prolonged standing, particularly if motionless and/or in warm and crowded environments. Moreover, patients should be advised to pause in the sitting position for some minutes after waking while performing thigh, buttock, or calf contractions (Figure 13.1), since orthostatic symptoms are more likely to occur after nocturnal sleeping.

Patients should be educated to perform physical counterpressure maneuvers (PCPM), i.e., isometric contractions including leg-crossing, arm tensing, and hand-gripping (Figure 13.2), which might allow them to abort (or delay) vasovagal and orthostatic hypotension-related syncope by increasing systemic blood pressure (BP).[1] The increase in BP is presumed to be due to both mechanical compression of the venous vascular bed and reflex increase in systemic vascular resistance caused by the activation of muscle mechanosensitive receptors. PCMs should be performed as soon as warning signs are present, thereby counteracting venous pooling and the vasodepressor effect that leads to reflex syncope. Although supported by low level of evidence,[3] PCPM is a risk-free, easy-to-perform, and low-cost treatment that can be proposed as a first-line strategy for patients who are able to recognize prodromal symptoms before syncope.[4,5] The major limitation to the use of PCPM is that they can only be implemented by patients with a recognizable prodrome, but they are not useful to avoid syncope in patients with no or very short prodromes. However, PCPM and other maneuvers, such as toe raises and stepping on the place, are also helpful as preventive measures when applied pre-emptively to increase BP when standing. PCPM may be difficult to perform or less effective in older patients and in those with low muscle strength, motor disabilities, or impaired balance.[6,7]

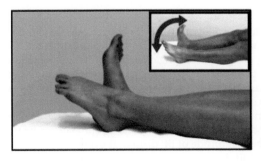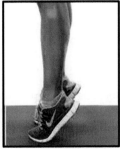

Figure 13.1 Muscle contractions to be performed in the supine and sitting position to prevent symptoms of orthostatic intolerance on standing.

DOI: 10.1201/9781003415855-15

135

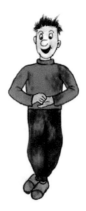

Figure 13.2 Physical counterpressure maneuvers.

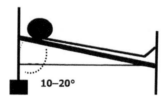

Figure 13.3 Head-up sleeping.

Adequate water intake (min 2 L/day) is recommended to avoid hypovolemia, particularly in patients with orthostatic hypotension (OH).[1,8] The water bolus, i.e., the rapid ingestion of approximately 500 mL of water, may be helpful to prevent BP falls in predisposing situations and during exercise.[9] Water bolus elicits within a few minutes a systolic BP increase of approximately 30 mmHg, which is probably mediated by the activation of a sympathetic reflex and might alleviate symptoms of orthostatic intolerance. In patients with low BP values, increasing daily diet salt intake can be suggested (2.3–4.6 g of salt per day). Caution in water and salt supplementation should be used in patients with known heart, kidney, or liver failure. Alcohol intake should be avoided due to the associated vasodilation.

High-thigh compression stockings may be useful to reduce venous pooling on standing in patients with OH and other forms of orthostatic intolerance.[8] Yet, they are difficult to apply and uncomfortable to wear, especially in older people, making compliance with their use frequently low. As most of the pooling occurs in the splanchnic circulation, abdominal binders may offer better efficacy and tolerability,[9] while knee-high stockings are not as effective.

Good effects on orthostatic tolerance may be derived from lower body muscle strengthening. Indeed, this improves the efficacy of the "muscle pump" that empties venous vessels, favoring venous return to the heart and preventing venous pooling in the lower body.[10] Reclining exercises that are not gravitationally challenging, e.g., recumbent or semi-recumbent cycling or rowing, are preferable in patients with severe OH. As post-exercise hypotension can predispose susceptible individuals to syncope, patients should be well hydrated prior to exercise and should be careful when standing after an exercise session.

Tilt training consists of maintaining upright posture against a wall for longer and longer periods and may progressively enhance patients' ability to tolerate orthostatic stress. It can be recommended in well-motivated patients with recurrent orthostatic syncope, but long-term compliance is poor.[1,11]

As an additional measure, head-up sleeping may be beneficial in patients with OH. Sleeping at a 10°–20° full-body head-up tilt position (Figure 13.3) permits gravitation stress, which reduces nocturnal BP and pressure natriuresis and maintains activation of the renin–angiotensin–aldosterone system during sleep, thus reducing the magnitude of BP drop in the morning.[12]

Post-prandial hypotension can be minimized by eating smaller and more frequent meals with a lower carbohydrate content and avoiding alcohol intake. Patients should be advised against sudden standing or physical activity immediately after eating.[12]

Non-pharmacological treatment strategies reduce syncope recurrences and significantly improve the quality of life in most patients with non-cardiac syncope.[13] Their efficacy may be more limited in patients with a greater syncope burden (i.e., a higher number of syncope episodes and/or a longer duration of syncope history).[13] However, these interventions have no side effects and do not incur additional costs. Therefore, non-pharmacological measures represent a valuable first-line treatment approach to be implemented in every patient with non-cardiac syncope.

PART B. PHARMACOLOGICAL PREVENTION OF SYNCOPE RECURRENCES

Intensive BP lowering is known to increase the risk of hypotension and syncope.[14] In particular, literature data indicate that hypotensive risk increases at low BP values, being more relevant at systolic BP <120 mmHg.[15] Therefore, strict BP control should preferably be avoided in hypertensive patients with a history of severe and/or recurrent hypotensive syncope and withdrawal or dose reduction of hypotensive medications may be appropriate to prevent symptom recurrence.[15] However, also uncontrolled hypertension has been demonstrated to favor hypotension, with a reported increase of OH incidence from 5% to 19%, which is likely attributable to pressure natriuresis.[16,17] Therefore, patients with syncope should not be denied antihypertensive treatment, but more prudent BP lowering targeting systolic BP values of 130–140 mmHg are advisable, to minimize the risk of hypotension-related adverse events.[15] This mainly applies to older adults, who typically show a higher risk of syncope and falls due to the coexistence of multiple age-related factors predisposing to hypotension.[15,18] In older patients with a history of vasodepressor reflex syncope, the reduction of antihypertensive treatment to target a systolic BP of 140 mmHg was found to result in a 63% decrease in syncopal recurrences, with no increase in cardiovascular risk.[19] In the discontinuation of antihypertensive treatment in elderly people (DANTE) study, deprescribing of antihypertensive medications in older adults with mild cognitive impairment and a mean BP of 149/82 mmHg resulted in a 45% increased probability of recovery from OH.[20] Therefore, in older people the lowest risk of hypotension corresponds to higher BP values than in younger adults, with a minimum hypotensive risk at a systolic BP of approximately 140 mmHg.[15] Deprescribing, i.e., progressive reduction or withdrawal of antihypertensive medications, should thus be considered in younger syncope patients (<65 years) with systolic BP <120 mmHg or in older syncope patients with systolic BP <130 mmHg.[21] Higher BP values—up to a systolic BP of 160 mmHg—can be accepted in individuals with severe frailty or disability, since the risk of hypotension and falls is extremely high, while the benefits of antihypertensive treatment remain doubtful.[18] Deprescribing should be considered also in patients with recurrent/severe syncope and hypotensive episodes on ABPM. Indeed, recent data indicate a linear association between the increase in 24-hour systolic BP and the reduction of hypotensive episodes, with modest systolic BP increases (i.e., +7 mmHg) resulting in a 61% reduction in the number of hypotensive episodes <90 mmHg. Although available evidence on deprescribing is limited to date, discontinuation of antihypertensive medications does not seem to increase the risk of mortality and cardiovascular events and can be safely performed if BP control is deemed excessive.[22,23]

Hypotensive effects are not equivalent among antihypertensive drug classes, and specific medications can exacerbate the predisposition to hypotension in susceptible individuals (Figure 13.4).

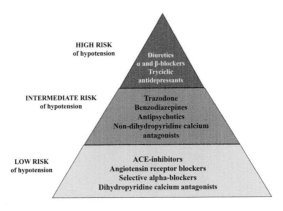

Figure 13.4 Hypotensive risk profile of major antihypertensive and psychoactive drug classes.

These mainly include medications that interfere with autonomic compensatory responses to standing and those causing volume depletion (e.g., diuretics) or venous pooling (e.g., vasodilators such as α-adrenergic receptor blockers).[24] Loop diuretics seem to be more prone than thiazide diuretics to cause hypovolemia and should be avoided as antihypertensive treatment in frail older patients, unless specifically indicated (e.g., for severe renal impairment or heart failure).[25] Similarly, the use of α-blockers as a treatment for high BP should be discouraged in older people due to their recognized impact on orthostatic BP, which may be even more pronounced at advanced age.[25] In older male adults with obstructive symptoms related to prostatic hypertrophy, molecules with higher uroselective and minor hypotensive effects are recommended as the first choice, e.g., silodosin and tamsulosin. Prazosin, terazosin, and doxazosin should be avoided, due to the increased risk of OH.[24] Also, beta-blockers may impair the BP response to standing, due to their negative inotropic and chronotropic effects,[26] and prescriptions should be limited to patients with specific indications.[25] By contrast, ACE inhibitors and angiotensin receptor blockers are known to be associated with a very low risk of hypotension or even mild protective effects.[24] Medical therapy optimization in patients with syncope should thus include a careful review of antihypertensive drug classes, giving preference to those at the lowest risk of hypotensive adverse events. Bedtime administration of antihypertensive medications might be considered, particularly in the presence of a non-dipping or reverse-dipping nocturnal BP pattern.

In addition to antihypertensives, some psychoactive medications may likewise induce hemodynamic effects and predispose to hypotension.[24] OH is reported to occur in 10%–50% of patients taking tricyclic antidepressants, due to vasodilating effects deriving from α-receptor blockade. A similar mechanism is described for trazodone and antipsychotics, with a higher OH incidence at advanced age. Finally, benzodiazepines have been reported to significantly impair the BP response to standing, particularly in older, deconditioned individuals.[27,28] The use of prolonged release formulations or fractioned doses may be considered to minimize the risk of hypotension.

Despite optimal non-pharmacological treatment and medication review, debilitating symptoms may persist in a non-negligible proportion of patients. Pharmacological treatment options are limited but can be considered in individuals who continue to suffer recurrent hypotensive symptoms despite education, lifestyle modifications, and deprescribing of hypotensive medications. This mainly applies to patients with constitutional hypotension (i.e., systolic BP <105 mmHg in males and <98 mmHg in females) or patients with recurrent hypotensive episodes despite normal mean BP values.[1] It is important to bear in mind that pharmacological strategies should not aim to achieve pre-defined BP values but should rather target the improvement of patients' symptoms and quality of life.[29] Consequently, pharmacological treatment should be managed on an individual basis and progressively titrated to reach the lowest effective dose. Higher doses might be necessary in patients with neurogenic OH. Available pharmacological treatment options are detailed in Table 13.1.

Table 13.1: Pharmacological Treatment Options for Patients with Non-cardiac Syncope and Persisting Symptoms Despite Non-pharmacological Treatment

	Mechanism of Action	Dosage	Side Effects	Contraindications
Midodrine	Selective alpha-receptor agonist inducing arterial and venous vasoconstriction	2.5–10 mg twice to three times per day	Pilomotor reactions, chills, urinary retention, supine hypertension	Heart failure/coronary artery disease, urinary retention, glaucoma, peripheral artery disease
Fludrocortisone	Mineralocorticoid inducing renal water and sodium reabsorption	Initial dose 0.1–0.2 mg daily, to be titrated (max 0.3 mg daily)	Hypokalemia, supine hypertension, volume overload, headache	Heart failure, severe renal impairment
Atomoxetine	Norepinephrine transporter inhibition	Initial dose 20 mg daily Max dose 40 mg daily	Palpitations and insomnia	Cardiac diseases
Droxidopa	Synthetic norepinephrine prodrug promoting vasoconstriction	Initial dose 100 mg tid Max dose 600 mg tid	Supine hypertension, headache, dizziness, nausea	Cardiac diseases, patients receiving drugs increasing NE levels

Midodrine is a prodrug and selective alpha-receptor agonist that induces arterial and venous vasoconstriction, leading to reduced venous pooling and increased peripheral resistance.[29] Randomized, double-blind trials support the use of midodrine (2.5–30 mg/day) in patients with autonomic failure and neurogenic OH, showing significant improvement of standing BP and orthostatic tolerance.[30] Moreover, the randomized, placebo-controlled, double-blind Prevention of Syncope Trial IV[31] demonstrated that midodrine reduces the risk of recurrences by 39% in patients with vasovagal syncope. Midodrine is characterized by a short half-life, which requires frequent dosing and may limit long-term compliance. It is usually administered at an initial dose of 2.5–10 mg twice to three times a day and then titrated, as tolerated, up to a maximum dose of 30 mg/day.[2] The most common adverse effects are pilomotor reactions, chills, and urinary retention, which require special caution in older males.[8]

Fludrocortisone is a synthetic mineralocorticoid, which expands intravascular volume by increasing renal water and sodium reabsorption.[29] In the randomized placebo-controlled double-blind Prevention of Syncope Trial II (POST2),[32] fludrocortisone was administered in vasovagal syncope patients at a dose of 0.2 mg daily, showing a significant reduction of recurrence risk. Moreover, fludrocortisone has been shown to improve standing BP in small-sized, open-label studies involving patients with neurogenic OH associated with diabetes and Parkinson's disease.[24] Fludrocortisone is usually administered at the initial dose of 0.1–0.2 mg/day and then gradually increased up to 0.3–0.4 mg/day.[2] Common side effects include hypokalemia, supine hypertension, volume overload, and headaches. Given the risk of fluid overload, heart failure and renal impairment are relative contraindications to the prescription of fludrocortisone.[8]

Droxidopa is a synthetic norepinephrine prodrug that is converted into norepinephrine by aromatic l-amino acid (DOPA) decarboxylase in both the central nervous system and peripheral tissues, thus promoting vasoconstriction.[29] Randomized placebo-controlled trials have shown beneficial effects of droxidopa on standing BP and orthostatic tolerance in patients with neurogenic OH, resulting in a reduction of symptom impact on daily activities and quality of life.[33,34] Droxidopa is usually administered at an initial dose of 100 mg three times per day and is then titrated until symptom reduction occurs to a maximum dose of 600 mg three times per day. Typical adverse effects include headaches, dizziness, and nausea, which are often dose-dependent.[8] Droxidopa may exacerbate symptoms in patients with heart failure, arrhythmias, and ischemic heart disease. Caution is also recommended in patients receiving other medications increasing norepinephrine levels (e.g., α1-agonists and α2-agonists).

Recently, norepinephrine transporter (NET) inhibitors have emerged as an additional promising treatment option for reflex syncope.[2] Norepinephrine that is released at synapses is either cleared by diffusion or reuptake through active transport into terminals by the presynaptic NET, which recaptures as much as 90% of released norepinephrine. The rationale for the use of NET inhibitors is that they tend to raise synaptic norepinephrine concentrations and may prevent or reduce the loss of sympathetic tone at the onset of vasovagal syncope. Inhibition of the NET protein (e.g., with the selective inhibitor atomoxetine) may therefore be helpful to maintain cardiac output and BP during orthostatic stress, preventing hypotension, bradycardia, and syncope. NET inhibition mainly acts through eliciting a significant HR increase which preserves mean arterial pressure. Indeed, NET inhibitors were found to reduce the likelihood of tilt-induced vasovagal syncope mainly by blunting reflex bradycardia, thereby preventing final falls in cardiac index and BP.[35] Atomoxetine does not prevent the development of the vasovagal reflex but may prevent the progression of presyncope to syncope. Similarly, atomoxetine was found to increase seated and standing systolic BP in patients with central autonomic failure with orthostatic hypotension.[35]

REFERENCES

1. Brignole M, Moya A, De Lange FJ, et al. 2018 ESC Guidelines for the diagnosis and management of syncope. *Eur Heart J.* 2018;39:1883–1948.

2. Fedorowski A, Kulakowski P, Brignole M, et al. Twenty-five years of research on syncope. *Europace.* 2023.

3. Dockx K, Avau B, De Buck E, Vranckx P, Vandekerckhove P. Physical manoeuvers as a preventive intervention to manage vasovagal syncope: A systematic review. *PLoS One.* 2019.

4. Brignole M, Croci F, Menozzi C, et al. Isometric arm counter-pressure maneuvers to abort impending vasovagal syncope. *J Am Coll Cardiol.* 2002.

5. van Dijk N, Quartieri F, Blanc JJ, et al. Effectiveness of physical counterpressure maneuvers in preventing vasovagal syncope. The physical counterpressure manoeuvres trial (PC-trial). *J Am Coll Cardiol.* 2006.

6. Croci F, Brignole M, Menozzi C, et al. Efficacy and feasibility of isometric arm counter-pressure manoeuvres to abort impending vasovagal syncope during real life. *Europace.* 2004.

7. Tomaino M, Romeo C, Vitale E, et al. Physical counter-pressure manoeuvres in preventing syncopal recurrence in patients older than 40 years with recurrent neurally mediated syncope: A controlled study from the Third International Study on Syncope of Uncertain Etiology (ISSUE-3). *Europace.* 2014.

8. Ricci F, De Caterina R, Fedorowski A. Orthostatic hypotension: Epidemiology, prognosis, and treatment. *J Am Coll Cardiol.* 2015.

9. Newton JL, Frith J. The efficacy of nonpharmacologic intervention for orthostatic hypotension associated with aging. *Neurology.* 2018.

10. Hatoum T, Raj S, Sheldon RS. Current approach to the treatment of vasovagal syncope in adults. *Intern Emerg Med.* 2023.

11. Tan MP, Newton JL, Chadwick TJ, Gray JC, Nath S, Parry SW. Home orthostatic training in vasovagal syncope modifies autonomic tone: results of a randomized, placebo-controlled pilot study. *Europace.* 2010.

12. Fanciulli A, Leys F, Falup-Pecurariu C, Thijs R, Wenning GK. Management of orthostatic hypotension in Parkinson's disease. *J Parkinsons Dis.* 2020.

13. Romme JJ, Reitsma JB, Go-Schön IK, et al. Prospective evaluation of non-pharmacological treatment in vasovagal syncope. *Europace.* 2010.

14. Rivasi G, Ceolin L, Capacci M, Matteucci G, Testa GD, Ungar A. Risks associated with intensive blood pressure control in older patients. *Kardiol Pol.* 2023.

15. Rivasi G, Brignole M, Rafanelli M, et al. Blood pressure management in hypertensive patients with syncope: how to balance hypotensive and cardiovascular risk. *J Hypertens.* 2020.

16. Di Stefano C, Milazzo V, Totaro S, et al. Orthostatic hypotension in a cohort of hypertensive patients referring to a hypertension clinic. *J Hum Hypertens.* 2015.

17. Kamaruzzaman S, Watt H, Carson C, Ebrahim S. The association between orthostatic hypotension and medication use in the British Women's Heart and Health Study. *Age Ageing.* 2009.

18. Rivasi G, Tortu V, D'Andria MF. Hypertension management in frail older adults: a gap in evidence. *J Hypertens.* 2021.

19. Solari D, Tesi F, Unterhuber M, et al. Stop vasodepressor drugs in reflex syncope: A randomised controlled trial. *Heart.* 2017.

20. Moonen JE, Foster-Dingley JC, de Ruijter W, van der Grond J, de Craen AJ, van der Mast RC. Effect of discontinuation of antihypertensive medication on orthostatic hypotension in older persons with mild cognitive impairment: The DANTE Study Leiden. *Age Ageing.* 2016.

21. Sheppard JP, Burt J, Lown M, et al. Effect of antihypertensive medication reduction vs usual care on short-term blood pressure control in patients with hypertension aged 80 years and older: the optimise randomized clinical trial. *JAMA.* 2020.

22. Iyer S, Naganathan V, McLachlan AJ, Le Conteur DG. Medication withdrawal trials in people aged 65 years and older: A systematic review. *Drugs Aging.* 2008.

23. Rivasi G, Rafanelli M, Mossello E, Brignole M, Ungar A. Drug-related orthostatic hypotension: beyond anti-hypertensive medications. *Drugs Aging.* 2020.

24. Williams B, Mancia G, Spiering W, et al. 2018 practice guidelines for the management of arterial hypertension of the European society of cardiology and the European society of hypertension ESC/ESH task force for the management of arterial hypertension. *Eur Heart J.* 2018.

25. Canney M, O'Connell MD, Murphy CM, et al. Single agent antihypertensive therapy and orthostatic blood pressure behaviour in older adults using beat-to-beat measurements: the Irish longitudinal study on ageing. *PLoS One.* 2016.

26. Rivasi G, Kenny RA, Ungar A, Romero-Ortuno R, et al. Effects of benzodiazepines on orthostatic blood pressure in older people. *Eur J Intern Med.* 2020.

27. Shi SJ, Garcia KM, Meck JV. Temazepam, but not zolpidem, causes orthostatic hypotension in astronauts after spaceflight. *J Cardiovasc Pharmacol.* 2003.

28. Eschlböck S, Wenning G, Fanciulli A. Evidence-based treatment of neurogenic orthostatic hypotension and related symptoms. *J Neural Transm.* 2017.

29. Izcovich A, González Malla C, Manzotti M, Catalano HN, Guyatt G, et al. Midodrine for orthostatic hypotension and recurrent reflex syncope: A systematic review. *Neurology.* 2014.

30. Sheldon R, Faris P, Tang A. Midodrine for the prevention of vasovagal syncope. *Ann Intern Med.* 2021.

31. Sheldon R, Raj SR, Rose MS, et al. Fludrocortisone for the prevention of vasovagal syncope a randomized, placebo-controlled trial. *J Am Coll Cardiol.* 2016.

32. Kaufmann H, Freeman R, Biaggioni I, et al. Droxidopa for neurogenic orthostatic hypotension: A randomized, placebo-controlled, phase 3 trial. *Neurology.* 2014.

33. Keating GM. Droxidopa: A review of its use in symptomatic neurogenic orthostatic hypotension. *Drugs.* 2015.

34. Sheldon RS, Lei L, Guzman JC, et al. A proof of principle study of atomoxetine for the prevention of vasovagal syncope: the prevention of syncope trial VI. *Europace.* 2019.

35. Shibao C, Raj SR, Gamboa A, et al. Norepinephrine transporter blockade with atomoxetine induces hypertension in patients with impaired autonomic function. *Hypertension.* 2007.

13B Management of Reflex Syncope

Cardioneuroablation

Tolga Aksu, Jeanne M. Du-Fay-de-Lavallaz, Asad Khan, and Henry Huang

INTRODUCTION

Vasovagal syncope (VVS) is a clinical condition caused by sudden-onset and prolonged brady-cardia (cardioinhibitory response) and hypotension (vasodepressor response). However, both of these responses eventually contribute to the loss of consciousness to a certain extent.[1] The current European guidelines recommend dual-chamber pacing (DDD) in patients >40 years of age with severe, unpredictable, and recurrent syncope and symptomatic asystolic pause(s) >3 seconds or asymptomatic pause(s) >6 seconds due to sinus arrest or atrioventricular block as diagnosed by an implantable loop recorder or during head-up tilt testing (HUT) (class I). These recommendations, especially the 40 years age cutoff, are supported by randomized controlled trials (RCT) in the field. The ISSUE-3 study[2] randomized such a cohort of patients (>40 years, with recurrent asystolic syncope and non-syncopal asystole >6 seconds), where all patients (mean age 63 years) with a DDD pacemaker (PPM) to pacing vs sensing only and showed a significant reduction in syncope recurrences in patients with active pacemakers. In the VPS II and the SYNPACE double-blinded RCTs, patients aged more than 18 years (mean age 50 and 52 years, respectively) were random-ized to "pacemaker on" or to "pacemaker off" cross-over arms. These two trials demonstrated no benefit of pacing in relatively younger patients.[3,4] The more recently published RCTs, SPAIN and BIO Sync CLS Study trials, recruited patients ≥40 years of age with a mean age of 56 and 62 years, respectively.[5,6] We are therefore currently lacking randomized data on the benefit of pacing in VVS patients <40 years of age and the data on patients <60 years of age remains limited.

A novel treatment strategy, namely, radiofrequency catheter ablation of parasympathetic gan-glionated plexi (GPs) located close to the sinus and atrioventricular nodes, has been proposed to eliminate vagal efferent output during VVS.[7-10] The investigators who first applied this technique named it cardioneuroablation (CNA).[11] Due to the small size of primarily observational studies, CNA treatment strategy was not included in the 2018 European Society of Cardiology (ESC) or 2017 American Heart Association, American College of Cardiology, and Heart Rhythm Society syncope guidelines for treatment of these patients.[1,12] Nevertheless, in recent years, the adoption of CNA in clinical practice as an alternative to PPM placement especially in younger patients with cardioin-hibitory syncope has grown. A recent meta-analysis of observational studies that included a total of 465 patients (mean age between 33 and 50 years) and one RCT (mean age 38 years) demonstrated that freedom from syncope after CNA was higher than 90% during a 2-year follow-up.[13,14] In the present chapter, we aim to explore the potential impact of CNA in patients with VVS.

ANATOMY OF THE CARDIAC AUTONOMIC NERVOUS SYSTEM FOR CARDIONEUROABLATION

The cardiac autonomic nervous system (ANS) consists of parasympathetic and sympathetic sys-tems that can further be divided into extrinsic and intrinsic parts. The extrinsic elements of the cardiac ANS arise from the brain cortex, brainstem, spinal cord, and preganglionic sympathetic axons with the postganglionic sympathetic neurons located in the sympathetic chain ganglia. Preganglionic parasympathetic axons of the vagus nerve synapse with autonomic ganglia of the parasympathetic division, which are distributed mainly within the epicardium and cluster in anatomically well-defined areas known as the ganglionated plexus (GP).[15] Myocardial and endo-cardial post-ganglionated efferent nerves extend toward the sinoatrial node (SAN), the atrioven-tricular node (AVN), the roots of the caval and pulmonary veins, and the ventricular regions.[16] Because atrial GPs integrate autonomic innervation into the SAN and AVN, GPs may serve as potential targets for parasympathetic denervation.

The concept of GP was defined by Armour et al. in humans in 1997.[15] According to the concept, the following atrial regions, which contain most of the autonomic parasympathetic ganglia, are defined as GP: superior (anterior) right atrial GP (RSGP); inferior (posterior) right atrial GP (RIGP); superior left atrial GP (LSGP); posterolateral (inferior) left atrial GP (LIGP); and posteromedial left atrial GP (PMLGP). Because parasympathetic fibers from the vein of Marshall innervate surround-ing left atrial structures and the coronary sinus, the vein of Marshall may also be considered part of the cardiac ANS and is often referred to as the Marshal Tract (GP-MTGP).[17] Figure 13.1 schematically

DOI: 10.1201/9781003415855-16

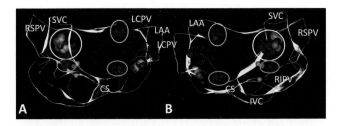

Figure 13.1   Schematic view of ganglionated plexi (GPs) distribution.

illustrates the distribution of major atrial GPs, which are usually targeted during cardioneuroablation. Based on a combination of anatomical and physiological experiments, it is currently believed that the largest number and density of autonomic ganglia which supply nerves to the SAN neural network are usually located at the RSGP, post-ganglionated nerves from the PMLGP, and RIGP and that the MTGP extends toward the interatrial septum and presumably supplies the AVN region.[16–20]

MAPPING AND ABLATION OF GANGLIONATED PLEXUS

Three approaches can be used for the identification of GPs: first, an anatomical approach; second, an approach using high-frequency stimulation (HFS); last, an approach focusing on electrogram analysis.[20] In brief, in a purely anatomic-guided approach, extensive regional radiofrequency energy ablation is delivered at the presumed anatomic sites of the GP. When using HFS, sites with a positive vagal response with different high-frequency delivery stimulation protocols are tagged as potential GP sites. In the electrogram-guided strategy, areas demonstrating fragmentation are targeted. According to a recently published meta-analysis, the technique utilized by operators for mapping GP to guide CNA did not carry a significant effect on freedom from syncope (P=0.206).[21]

The optimal approach for mapping and the number of GPs to be targeted remain unclear. In the great majority of studies, GPs were targeted via a left atrial or bi-atrial approach.[7,8,10,11] In a recently published study, limited right atrial ablation for RSGP appeared to reduce the risks associated with transseptal puncture and manipulation in the left atrium.[9] However, CNA limited to right atrial ablation was associated with significantly lower freedom from syncope (81.5%; 95% CI 51.9%–94.7%; p for comparison between right and left/bi-atrial approaches<0.001) vs left atrial ablation only (94.0%; 95% CI 88.6%–96.9%) and bi-atrial ablation (92.7%; 95% CI 86.8%–96.1%).[21]

As CNA target sites are anatomically similar to those for atrial fibrillation ablation during pulmonary vein isolation, operators need to be mindful of the potential for thermal collateral injury of the esophagus and phrenic nerve and take appropriate precautions. As autonomic neurons in GP are epicardially embedded, it is likely transmural radiofrequency lesions are required to achieve clinical efficacy. Currently, the optimal endpoint of each radiofrequency application is yet to be determined. Elimination of all targeted electrograms or of the vagal responses at a given GP site may serve as reasonable endpoints. Pachon et al.[22] suggested the use of extracardiac vagal stimulation (ECVS), which evaluates parasympathetic innervation to the sinoatrial and atrioventricular nodes, as a procedural endpoint. However, ECVS requires specialized equipment and may sometimes trigger atrial fibrillation unexpectedly, which may prolong procedure time.

CARDIONEUROABLATION IN VASOVAGAL SYNCOPE

In the first report of CNA in patients with pure VVS published in 2011, 43 patients with a significant cardioinhibitory response to the head-up tilt table test (HUT) (18 women, 33±15 years of age) underwent bi-atrial ablation by using spectral atrial potential-guided CNA. During 45±22 months of follow-up, only 3 of 18 patients had recurrent syncope.[23]

In a follow-up study published in 2016, 57 VVS patients (aged 43.2±13.4 years; 35 women) with a positive response to HUT were enrolled, and high-frequency stimulation and anatomically guided left atrial GP ablation were performed in 10 and 47 cases, respectively.[24] No significant differences were found between HFS and anatomically guided ablation, either in freedom from syncope (100% versus 89.4%, P=0.348) or in recurrent prodromes (50% versus 76.6%, P=0.167). In subsequent work from the same group, Hu et al.[25] retrospectively assessed the results of left atrial CNA in 115 patients (42.9±17.9 years) enrolled between 2015 and 2018 with positive HUT (cardioinhibitory response in 11.3%, mixed response in 74.8%, and vasodepressor response in 13.9%, respectively). They observed 92.2% freedom from syncope over a median follow-up of 18 months.

Aksu et al.[26] compared the 2019 bi-atrial electrogram-guided CNA (12 patients) with a hybrid approach in which a combination of HFS and spectral analysis (eight patients) in patients with VVS. There were no syncopal recurrences in any case at the end of the 6-month follow-up. In the combined approach group, syncope recurred in two cases after a 12-month follow-up. The same group published in 2022 the first case-control study in patients with cardioinhibitory responses to HUT.[27] Fifty-one patients (50.4%) underwent CNA, and 50 (49.6%) patients received conventional treatment. A survival analysis was performed on 19 pairs of propensity-matched patients: During a median follow-up of 22 months (IQR 13–35), the four-year syncope-free rate estimate was 0.86 (95% CI, 0.63–1.00) for the CNA group and 0.50 (95% CI, 0.30–0.82) for the conventional treatment group in the matched cohort.[28] A subsequent study evaluated the efficacy of CNA in preventing a positive response to HUT.[28] Fifty-one patients with VVS were included in the study. After confirmation of >3 seconds of asystole on HUT, all patients underwent CNA. HUT was repeated one month after CNA. During a median follow-up period of 11 months (interquartile range 3–27 months), all but 3 (5.8%) of 51 patients were free of syncope. Repeated HUTs were negative in 44 (86.2%) patients.

The efficacy of CNA through a right-sided approach was reported by Debruyne et al.[29] in 2021 that included 31 patients with cardioinhibitory[11] or mixed type[20] responses on HUT. After limited anatomically guided ablation supported by the computed tomography scan merged with the electroanatomic map, one patient was considered to have a treatment failure and underwent pacemaker implantation. The remaining 9 patients with syncope recurrence accumulated 17 episodes during the 12 months after the procedure compared with 254 episodes at baseline, reflecting a significant burden reduction in the 12 last months preceding CNA (–93%; $P=0.008$). A purely empirical right atrial anatomical approach was reported by Calo et al.[30] in 2021 in a cohort of 18 VVS patients (mean age 36.9±11.2 years). With a mean follow-up of 34.1±6.1 months, three (16.6%) patients experienced syncopal episodes and five patients (27.7%) experienced only prodromal episodes.

A meta-analysis of all available observational data up to February 2022 found a 92% freedom of syncope after CNA with no differences identified among different CNA techniques; however, a higher syncope recurrence rate was observed with a right atrial-only approach when compared with left atrial or bi-atrial approaches.[13] Finally, in the first randomized controlled trial of CNA published in 2023, 48 patients with treatment-refractory cardioinhibitory responses to HUT were randomized to receive CNA or not.[14] After a 2-year follow-up, CNA was associated with a significant decrease in syncope (CNA group: 8% vs control group: 54%) and improved quality of life.

PATIENT SELECTION

As discussed in other relevant chapters, nonpharmacologic treatments including education, lifestyle modification, and physical counterpressure maneuvers remain the cornerstone of the management of VVS patients and should be suggested first in all cases before any invasive intervention is discussed. CNA should only be considered for patients with severe syncope forms, such as very frequent VVS affecting quality of life; recurrent syncope without prodromal symptoms, which exposes the patient to a risk of trauma; and syncope occurring during a high-risk activity and only in cases of nonpharmacological treatment failure.[1] While almost all previous studies assessing patients with CNA recruited VVS cases based on HUT results, asystole documented by an implantable cardiac monitor (ICM) has recently been suggested as a convenient tool to not only select symptomatic patients likely to benefit from a CNA but also to evaluate the absolute long-term efficacy of this intervention.[31] Hence, employing a comparable method exploiting symptom-ECG correlation as the one used to select patients for cardiac pacing could also serve as a guiding principle in identifying suitable candidates for CNA.

Despite the absence of confirmed benefits from randomized controlled trials (RCTs) regarding pacemaker implantation for Vasovagal Syncope (VVS) in patients under 40, the prevailing cardioinhibitory response characterizing VVS suggests the potential efficacy of a pacemaker in averting syncopal episodes, akin to its impact on older patients. Yet, introducing a device in this younger demographic poses concerns, including the necessity for frequent generator changes, infection risks, vascular occlusion, and lead failure, raising skepticism about the genuine advantage of pacemakers within this age range.

Given the absence of a satisfactory therapeutic option in these younger patients and the high risk for long-term complications associated with pacemaker implantation, CNA studies mainly focused on patients <40 years of age, and recommending this procedure in that age group may be

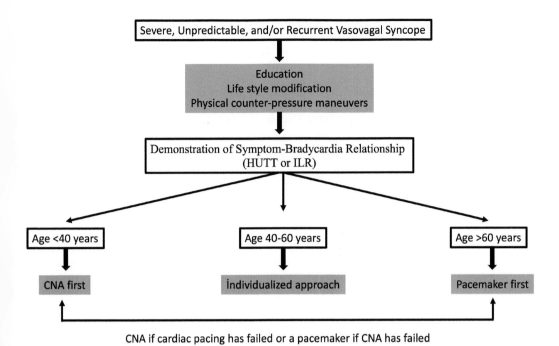

Figure 13.2 Practical decision pathway for the management of vasovagal syncope.

reasonable. The experience with CNA is limited to a few anecdotal cases in patients >60 years of age, and the efficacy of CNA seems to decrease with increasing age.[32] In the older population, given the concurring comorbidities and mechanisms responsible for sinus bradycardia, atrioventricular block, and syncope, the implantation of a DDD-CLS pacemaker device should be considered as the first option. For patients between 40 and 60 years, a patient-specific personalized approach between CNA and pacemaker implantation should be considered, and this subgroup should be studied in RCTs. A staged approach of CNA followed by observation and delayed pacemaker implantation if necessary may be preferred after 60 years, if the patient prefers initially to undergo ablation, especially in the context of a positive response to atropine. In contrast, in patients <40 years of age, unresponsiveness to atropine may be accepted as an indicator for the existence of intrinsic sinus node disease or sinus node-atrial conduction abnormality, disqualifying these patients from CNA and favoring pacing as a first-line therapy. In patients, in whom both interventional modalities have failed, the vasodepressor response might be the culprit requiring appropriate investigation and treatment. A practical decision pathway is summarized in Figure 13.2.

FUTURE DIRECTIONS
It should be emphasized that the potential for a placebo effect of invasive procedures on patients with VVS, as revealed by the VPS and VPS II trials,[3,33] needs to be considered when designing future RCTs. The VPS trial demonstrated an 85.4% relative risk reduction of syncope when patients were randomized to pacemaker implantation vs. no implantation.[33] Additionally, VVS is most prevalent in young patients. Its severity often diminishes with age, reflecting a status of autonomic dysregulation that may correct itself with time. It is known that the parasympathetic system has an anti-inflammatory and protective effect in the presence of myocardial ischemia. Parasympathetic denervation by CNA may introduce a lifetime sympathetic dominant state, which may be unfavorable in patients with cardiovascular diseases. Finally, the optimal lesion set and ablation endpoints of CNA are yet to be defined by RCTs and appropriate long-term follow-up. Randomized, sham-controlled clinical trials are needed to determine the magnitude of placebo effects and the long-term benefits of this attractive treatment strategy.

REFERENCES

1. Brignole M, Moya A, de Lange FJ, et al. 2018 ESC guidelines for the diagnosis and management of syncope. *Eur Heart J.* 2018;39:1883–1948.

2. Brignole M, Menozzi C, Moya A, et al. Pacemaker therapy in patients with neurally mediated syncope and documented asystole: Third International Study on Syncope of Uncertain Etiology (ISSUE-3): A randomized trial. *Circulation.* 2012;125:2566–2571.

3. Connolly SJ, Sheldon R, Thorpe KE, et al. Pacemaker therapy for prevention of syncope in patients with recurrent severe vasovagal syncope: Second Vasovagal Pacemaker Study (VPS II): A randomized trial. *JAMA.* 2003;289:2224–2229.

4. Raviele A, Giada F, Menozzi C, et al. A randomized, double-blind, placebo-controlled study of permanent cardiac pacing for the treatment of recurrent tilt-induced vasovagal syncope. The vasovagal syncope and pacing trial (SYNPACE). *Eur Heart J.* 2004;25:1741–1748.

5. Brignole M, Russo V, Arabia F, et al. Cardiac pacing in severe recurrent reflex syncope and tilt-induced asystole. *Eur Heart J.* 2021;42:508–516.

6. Baron-Esquivias G, Morillo CA, Moya-Mitjans A, et al. Dual-chamber pacing with closed loop stimulation in recurrent reflex vasovagal syncope: The SPAIN study. *J Am Coll Cardiol.* 2017;70:1720–1728.

7. Pachon JC, Pachon EI, Cunha Pachon MZ, Lobo TJ, Pachon JC, Santillana TG. Catheter ablation of severe neurally meditated reflex (neurocardiogenic or vasovagal) syncope: Cardioneuroablation long-term results. *Europace.* 2011;13:1231–1242.

8. Hu F, Zheng L, Liang E, et al. Right anterior ganglionated plexus: The primary target of cardioneuroablation? *Heart Rhythm.* 2019;16:1545–1551.

9. Debruyne P, Rossenbacker T, Janssens L. Durable physiological changes and decreased syncope burden 12 months after unifocal right-sided ablation under computed tomographic guidance in patients with neurally mediated syncope or functional sinus node dysfunction. *Circ Arrhythm Electrophysiol.* 2021;14:e009747.

10. Aksu T, Padmanabhan D, Shenthar J, et al. The benefit of cardioneuroablation to reduce syncope recurrence in vasovagal syncope patients: A case–control study. *J Interv Card Electrophysiol.* 2022;63:77–86.

11. Pachon JC, Pachon EI, Pachon JC, et al. "Cardioneuroablation" – new treatment for neurocardiogenic syncope, functional AV block and sinus dysfunction using catheter RF-ablation. *Europace.* 2005;7:1–13.

12. Shen WK, Sheldon RS, Benditt DG, Cohen MI, Forman DE, Goldberger ZD. 2017 ACC/AHA/HRS guideline for the evaluation and management of patients with syncope: A report of the American College of Cardiology/American Heart Association Task Force on Clinical Practice Guidelines and the Heart Rhythm Society. *J Am Coll Cardiol.* 2017;70:e39–110.

13. Vandenberk B, Lei LY, Ballantyne B, et al. Cardioneuroablation for vasovagal syncope: A systematic review and meta-analysis. *Heart Rhythm.* 2022:S1547-5271(22)02088-4.

14. Piotrowski R, Baran J, Sikorska A, Krynski T, Kulakowski P. Cardioneuroablation for reflex syncope: Efficacy and effects on autonomic cardiac regulation – a prospective randomized trial. *JACC Clin Electrophysiol.* 2023;9:85–95.

15. Armour JA, Murphy DA, Yuan BX, Macdonald S, Hopkins DA. Gross and microscopic anatomy of the human intrinsic cardiac nervous system. *Anat Rec.* 1997;247:289–298.

16. Pauza DH, Skripka V, Pauziene N, Stropus R. Morphology, distribution, and variability of the epicardiac neural ganglionated subplexuses in the human heart. *Anat Rec.* 2000;259:353–382.

17. Ulphani JS, Arora R, Cain JH, et al. The ligament of Marshall as a parasympathetic conduit. *Am J Physiol Heart Circ Physiol.* 2007;293:H1629–H1635.

18. Randall WC, Ardell JL, O'Toole MF, Wurster RD. Differential autonomic control of SAN and AVN regions of the canine heart: Structure and function. *Prog Clin Biol Res.* 1988;275:15–31.

19. Billman GE, Hoskins RS, Randall DC, Randall WC, Hamlin RL, Lin YC. Selective vagal postganglionic innervation of the sinoatrial and atrioventricular nodes in the non-human primate. *J Auton Nerv Syst.* 1989;26:27–36.

20. Aksu T, Gopinathannair R, Gupta D, Pauza DH. Intrinsic cardiac autonomic nervous system: What do clinical electrophysiologists need to know about the "heart brain"? *J Cardiovasc Electrophysiol.* 2021;32(6):1737–1747.

21. Vandenberk B, Lei LY, Ballantyne B, et al. Cardioneuroablation for vasovagal syncope: A systematic review and meta-analysis. *Heart Rhythm.* 2022;19(11):1804–1812.

22. Pachon M JC, Pachon M EI, Santillana P TG, et al. Simplified method for vagal effect evaluation in cardiac ablation and electrophysiological procedures. *JACC Clin Electrophysiol.* 2015;1:451–460.

23. Pachon JC, Pachon EI, Cunha Pachon MZ, Lobo TJ, Pachon JC, Santillana TG. Catheter ablation of severe neurally meditated reflex (neurocardiogenic or vasovagal) syncope: Cardioneuroablation long-term results. *Europace.* 2011;13(9):1231–1242.

24. Sun W, Zheng L, Qiao Y, et al. Catheter ablation as a treatment for vasovagal syncope: Long-term outcome of endocardial autonomic modification of the left atrium. *J Am Heart Assoc.* 2016;5(7):e003471.

25. Hu F, Zheng L, Liang E, et al. Right anterior ganglionated plexus: The primary target of cardioneuroablation? *Heart Rhythm.* 2019;16(10):1545–1551.

26. Aksu T, Guler TE, Mutluer FO, Bozyel S, Golcuk SE, Yalin K. Electroanatomic-mapping-guided cardioneuroablation versus combined approach for vasovagal syncope: A cross-sectional observational study. *J Interv Card Electrophysiol.* 2019;54 (2):177–188.

27. Aksu T, Padmanabhan D, Shenthar J, et al. The benefit of cardioneuroablation to reduce syncope recurrence in vasovagal syncope patients: A case–control study. *J Interv Card Electrophysiol.* 2022;63(1):77–86.

28. Aksu T, Guler TE, Bozyel S, Yalin K, Gopinathannair R. Usefulness of post-procedural heart rate response to predict syncope recurrence or positive head up tilt table testing after cardioneuroablation. *Europace.* 2020;22(9):1320–1327.

29. Debruyne P, Rossenbacker T, Janssens L, et al. Durable physiological changes and decreased syncope burden 12 months after unifocal right-sided ablation under computed tomographic guidance in patients with neurally mediated syncope or functional sinus node dysfunction. *Circ Arrhythm Electrophysiol.* 2021;14(6):e009747.

30. Calo L, Rebecchi M, Sette A, et al. Catheter ablation of right atrial ganglionated plexi to treat cardioinhibitory neurocardiogenic syncope: A long-term follow-up prospective study. *J Interv Card Electrophysiol.* 2021;61(3):499–510.

31. Aksu T, Guler TE, Saygı S, Yalin K. Usage of implantable loop recorder to evaluate absolute effectiveness of cardioneuroablation. *J Cardiovasc Electrophysiol.* 2019;30(12):2986–2987.

32. Qin M, Zhang Y, Liu X, Jiang WF, Wu SH, Po S. Atrial ganglionated plexus modification: A novel approach to treat symptomatic sinus bradycardia. *JACC Clin Electrophysiol.* 2017;3:950–959.

33. Connolly SJ, Sheldon R, Roberts RS, Gent M. The North American Vasovagal Pacemaker Study (VPS). A randomized trial of permanent cardiac pacing for the prevention of vasovagal syncope. *J Am Coll Cardiol.* 1999;33:16–20.

13C Management of Reflex Syncope

Cardiac Pacing in Reflex Syncope

Michael Liu, Dan Sorajja, and Win-Kuang Shen

VASOVAGAL SYNCOPE

Three small, randomized, unblinded trials showed positive results for pacing versus medication or no treatment in VVS.[1-3] VPS was a 54-patient study using rate-drop-response that found an 85% reduction in risk of syncope and was terminated early due to efficacy for 46 patients.[1] VASIS was a 42-patient study that found syncope recurrence of 5% in the pacemaker arm versus 61% in the no-pacemaker arm. The authors concluded that the greater the cardioinhibitory component of VVS is, the higher the likelihood that pacing therapy may be effective. Ammirati et al. conducted a 93-patient study using rate-drop-response and found a syncope recurrence rate of 4.3% in the pacemaker arm versus 25.5% in the medical therapy arm. These trials were markedly flawed by their design that was unblinded and not compared to a true placebo control group.

Another three placebo-controlled randomized trials were then performed in which patients were implanted with a pacemaker with pacing therapy programmed "off." The SYNPACE and the VPS II trials were negative studies, suggesting there may have been a significant placebo effect in previous studies.[4,5] SYNPACE was terminated early due to ethical concerns as VPS II was a negative study, although VPS II had a short follow-up, being six months or until first recurrence. While these studies did not support the role of DDD pacing with a rate-drop-response algorithm, some investigators have pointed out the lack of demonstrated cardioinhibitory VVS prior to the implantation of the pacemakers.

In contrast to SYNPACE and VPS II, the International Study of Syncope of Unknown Etiology (ISSUE)-3 demonstrated a significant reduction in the syncope recurrence rate using pacing in patients ≥40 years and cardioinhibitory VVS.[6] To have a pacemaker implantation, these patients had to have documented asystole of ≥3 seconds during syncope or ≥6 seconds on an implantable cardiac monitor (ICM), and carotid sinus hypersensitivity patients were excluded. In ISSUE-3, 77 patients of age 40 years or older with three or more episodes of neurally mediated syncope with documented asystolic pause on ICM were randomized to receive a dual chamber permanent pacemaker programmed to either DDDR plus rate-drop-response or ODO (sensing only). This was a multicenter, prospective, double-blinded trial with a follow-up of up to 24 months. The primary endpoint was a comparison of the number of patients with syncopal recurrence and comparison of cumulative risk of syncope between treatment groups. 19 of 39 patients with pacemakers off had recurrence versus 8 of 38 patients with pacemakers on. The estimated syncope recurrence rate in the control group was 37% at one year and 57% at two years. In the group with the pacemaker turned on, the estimated recurrence rate was 25% at one year and 25% at two years. Interestingly, among the many patients in ISSUE-3 who underwent tilt-table testing, there appeared to be more benefit from a pacemaker in those patients who were tilt-negative. It is unknown whether the patients with abnormal tilt testing were more predisposed to hypotension, making high-rate pacing unlikely or not effective enough to increase cardiac output. Of note, in many tilt tests, the presence of asystole or a cardioinhibitory response occurs after the blood pressure has approached the nadir.[7] Similar findings were also seen in the observational Syncope Unit Project (SUP)-2 study.[8] In the SUP-2 study, cardioinhibition had to be observed on testing performed in a stepwise manner, including carotid sinus massage, tilt testing, and the ILR. Again, the rate of syncope was significantly decreased with the pacemaker implanted, and there was more benefit in tilt-negative patients.

More recently, closed-loop stimulation (CLS) has been studied and has been found to have significantly decreased the syncope recurrence rate with the pacing therapy turned on (see Programmable Algorithms). In the SPAIN trial, 46 patients aged 40 years or older with at least five VVS episodes and two episodes in the last year with cardioinhibitory response on tilt-table testing were studied in a randomized, double-blind, multicenter, crossover trial comparing DDD-CLS pacing (CLS rate of 110 bpm and lower rate limit of 45 bpm) with sham DDI pacing at a backup rate of 30 beats per minute.[9] The pacing intervention occurred much earlier than in prior studies. The rate of recurrent VVS was 8.7% with DDD-CLS versus 46% with DDI 30 bpm. There were a greater proportion of patients with at least a 50% reduction in syncopal episodes (72% vs 28%), as

DOI: 10.1201/9781003415855-17

149

well as a greater time to first syncope (29.2 months vs 9.3 months).[9] In BioSync CLS, 127 patients with an syncope with asystolic pause of greater than 3 seconds on tilt-table testing were randomized to pacing with CLS turned on versus pacing turned off. The CLS pacing group had a syncope recurrence rate of 10/63 (16%) of the pacing group versus 34/64 (53%) of the control group [HR, 0.23 (95% CI: 0.11–0.47)].[10] The CLS rate was 120 bpm with a medium CLS rate-adaptive response, while devices were programmed ODO in the pacing off and CLS off cohorts.

ACC/AHA/HRS guidelines from 2017 give a IIb recommendation for dual chamber pacing in a select population of patients 40 years of age or older with recurrent VVS and prolonged spontaneous pauses, largely driven by ISSUE-3 data.[11]

ESC guidelines from 2018 give an IIa recommendation for documented symptomatic asystolic pauses greater than 3 seconds or asymptomatic pauses greater than 6 seconds due to sinus arrest or AV block.[12] There is a IIb recommendation to reduce syncope recurrence with a tilt-induced asystolic response or adenosine-sensitive syncope. This recommendation is based on one small, preliminary, randomized controlled trial that suggests possible adenosine-sensitive syncope.[13]

PROGRAMMABLE ALGORITHMS
Rate-Drop-Response
Medtronic

Rate-drop-response (RDR) is a specific feature on Medtronic devices that will provide rapid pacing when the heart rate is detected below a certain limit. The RDR algorithm searches for heart rate change over a time duration window, with the window height (top rate minus bottom rate) and window width (how many beats) being programmable. If patients experience cardioinhibitory vasovagal syncope, the pacemaker will detect the decreased heart rate and provide a short period of rapid pacing therapy, such as 90–120 bpm, to try and prevent symptoms. However, there are limitations as the device tries to differentiate rate falls that occur with VVS from the fluctuating decreases in heart rate associated with activity level and circadian rhythm. Due to the overlap between these conditions, unnecessary pacing interventions can occur.

There has been promise with RDR, as an earlier study showed that the rate-drop feature could decrease syncope burden from 1.2 events/month to 0.3 events/month.[14] Prior studies have shown more benefit in pacing support for tilt-negative patients, and these results suggest RDR would benefit those patients with a largely cardioinhibitory response alone. As noted above, there are patients in whom the presence of the cardioinhibitory response occurs minutes after the vasodepressor response has progressed to the point that pacing is ineffective to increase cardiac output (ISSUE-3, SUP-2). If RDR is programmed on, it should be noted that one small study showed no benefit in pacing faster at 120 bpm rather than 80–90 bpm[15] (Tables 13.2 and 13.3).

Five randomized controlled trials used rate-drop-response algorithms in their study design. The positive results of SAFE PACE for pacing in CSS are questionable as the primary endpoint was the reduction in the number of falls. Syncope was a secondary endpoint and occurred in a low percentage of patients (16% of participants). Paced patients did not have a significant reduction in syncope than controls (see Table 13.4).

Rate-drop-response for VVS appears to be effective based on the results of VPS and Ammirati et al. (see Table 13.1).

The question of the efficacy of RDR in younger patients is not definitely known. Many of the early pacing studies used an inclusion criteria of greater than 35–40 years,[3,6] and these younger patients were subsequently excluded from future studies. Interestingly, in VPS, the pacemaker intervention group has an average age of 46 years versus 40 years in the no-pacemaker group.[1] In their Cox model, age <40 versus ≥40 years had no effect on the benefit of a pacemaker. While there is no clear data regarding pacing recommendations for younger patients with VVS, the pathophysiology is similar. Importantly, the lifetime risk of complications from pacemaker implantation should be considered.[16] However, if implanted, it is possible that a pacemaker with RDR may benefit younger patients as they are more likely to have cardioinhibitory syncope.[17]

Closed-Loop Stimulation
Biotronik Inc. (Biotronik GmbH, Berlin, Germany)

The benefits of closed-loop stimulation (CLS) were first suggested in the preliminary results from Kanjwal et al.[18] In CLS, the right ventricular lead impedance, measured from the electrode tip to the pulse generator, was taken as a surrogate marker of right ventricular preload. Contractility of the right ventricular plays a role, and so an intracardiac impedance curve is generated for each

Table 13.1: Evidence of Randomized Controlled Trials for Pacing in Vasovagal Syncope

Author/Year	Sample Size/Inclusion	Study Methods	Study Outcome	Comments
Connolly 1999[1] VPS	*Number of patients:* 54 *Inclusion criteria:* at least six syncopal spells Positive tilt-table test with syncope or presyncope and relative bradycardia	*Type of study:* single-center, randomized, prospective, unblinded *Follow-up:* varying lengths of time up to 15 months *Primary endpoint(s):* first recurrence of syncope *Secondary endpoint(s):* occurrence of presyncope	*Outcome:* reduction in risk of syncope by 85.4% (95% CI 59.7%–94.7%) Recurrent syncope in 19/27 patients (70%) of no pacemaker and 6/27 (22%) in PPM Time from randomization to syncope: 54 days in no PPM, 112 days in PPM	Rate-drop-response Early termination for efficacy for 46 patients
Sutton et al. 2000[2] VASIS	*Number of patients:* 42 *Inclusion criteria:* ≥3 syncopes over last two years with last episode within six months and interval between first and last episode of >6 months and positive cardioinhibitory response to tilt testing age >40 years or if <40 years proven refractoriness to conventional drug therapy	*Type of study:* multicenter, prospective, randomized, unblinded *Follow-up:* minimum one year, maximum 6.7 years, mean 3.7 years±2.2 years *Primary endpoint(s):* reduce interval to first recurrence of syncope *Secondary endpoint(s):* reduce total burden of syncopal recurrences	*Outcome:* syncope 1/19 (5%) with PPM 14/23 (61%) with no PPM Difference ($p=0.0006$) First recurrence of syncope after 1, 3, and 5 years was 0%, 6%, and 6% in PPM. 39%, 50%, and 75% in no PPM	Rate hysteresis The greater the cardioinhibitory component is, the higher likelihood that pacing therapy may be effective
Ammirati et al. 2001[3]	*Number of patients:* 93 *Inclusion criteria:* age >35 years ≥3 syncopal episodes in last two years with most recent episode in last 6 months Positive response to tilt-table testing with syncope occurring in association with relative bradycardia	*Type of study:* multicenter, prospective, randomized unblinded with parallel groups comparing atenolol 10mg vs DDD pacemaker with RDR *Follow-up:* every three months, mean follow-up 520±266 days *Primary endpoint(s):* first recurrence of syncope	*Outcome:* PPM arm syncope recurrence 4.3% (2/46 pts) Beta-blocker arm: 25.5% (12/47 pts) Significant difference ($p=0.004$) Kaplan Meier PPM: first recurrence after 6, 12, 24, 36 months were 0%, 3.3%, 7.2%, 7.2% Beta-blocker: 14.1%, 24.1%, 33.9%, 33.9%	Rate-drop-response Positive study Comparison with beta-blocker

(Continued)

151

Table 13.1: (*Continued*) Evidence of Randomized Controlled Trials for Pacing in Vasovagal Syncope

Author/Year	Sample Size/Inclusion	Study Methods	Study Outcome	Comments
Connolly 2003 VPS II[4]	*Number of patients:* 100 *Inclusion criteria:* older than 19 years, typical history of recurrent vasovagal syncope with at least six lifetime episodes, or at least three episodes in two prior years to enrollment Positive tilt-table test	*Type of study:* multicenter, prospective, double-blind, randomized *Follow-up:* six months or up to time of occurrence of first episode of recurrent syncope *Primary endpoint(s):* comparison of cumulative risk of syncope *Secondary endpoint(s):* number of patients with presyncope	*Outcome:* ODO; 22/52 patients syncope DDD 16/48 pts Risk of syncope in ODO 40% (95% CI, 25%–52%) vs 31% (95% CI, 17%–43%) in DDD RRR in time to syncope with DDD was 30% (95% CI, –33% to 63%) (p=0.14) ODO 49/52 (94%) had presyncope vs DDD 46/48 (96%) Median episodes of presyncope per 100 days of follow-up: 16 days ODO vs 13 days DDD	Comments: negative study Rate-drop-response one episode of tamponade in DDD one episode of infection requiring reimplantation ODO
Raviele et al. 2004[5] SYNPACE	*Number of patients:* 29 *Inclusion:* frequently recurrent syncope and positive head-up tilt testing and asystolic or mixed response, at least six syncopal episodes in patient's lifetime, the last occurring no more than six months before enrollment At least one recurrence within 12 months following positive head-up tilt testing Exclusion of any other cause of syncope Age >18 years	*Type of study:* multicenter, prospective, randomized double-blinded *Follow-up:* clinical diary Minimum of four months, median 715 days *Primary endpoint(s):* syncope recurrence and median time to first syncope recurrence *Secondary endpoint(s):* syncope rate Pre-syncopal recurrences Syncope recurrence in Mixed and Asystolic groups	*Outcome:* PPM ON: syncope recurrence 8/16 pts (50%) PPM OFF: Syncope recurrence 5/13 pts (38%) Median time to syncope recurrence ON vs OFF: 97 [38–144] vs 20 [4–302] days (p=0.38) Probability of remaining syncope-free at year was similar 44% vs 31% in PPM ON vs OFF (p=0.58)	Negative study Terminated early due to ethical concerns as VPS II showed negative study Subgroup analysis of mixed group vs asystolic group

(*Continued*)

Table 13.1: (Continued) Evidence of Randomized Controlled Trials for Pacing in Vasovagal Syncope

Author/Year	Sample Size/Inclusion	Study Methods	Study Outcome	Comments
Brignole et al. 2012[6] ISSUE-3	*Number of patients:* 77 *Inclusion:* ≥40 years old ≥3 episodes of likely neurally mediated syncope (defined as any form of reflex syncope with exception of carotid sinus syndrome Received ILR, documented asystolic pause (sinus arrest or AV block) ≥3 seconds at time of syncope or asymptomatic/presyncopal episodes with documented asystolic pause ≥6 seconds	*Type of study:* multicenter, prospective, randomized, double-blind *Follow-up:* 24 months or up to first episode of recurrence of syncope *Primary endpoint(s):* Comparison of number of patients with syncopal recurrence Comparison of cumulative risk of syncope between treatment groups with use of log-rank test	*Outcome:* 19/39 patients with pacemaker off had recurrence vs 8/38 patients with pacemaker on Estimated product-limit syncope recurrence rate was 37% (95% CI, 24–55) at one year and 57% (95% CI, 40–74) at 2 years in pacemaker off arm 25% (95% CI, 13–45) at 1 year and 25% (95% CI, 13–45) at 2 years in pacemaker on arm (p=0.039) Risk reduction of 57% (95% CI, 4–81)	Positive double-blind randomized trial PPM is effective in reducing recurrence of syncope Used ILR to document pauses which may contribute to positive trial
Baron-Esquivias 2017[7] SPAIN	*Number of patients:* 46 *Inclusion:* age ≥40 years At least five VVS episodes and two within the last year Tilt test with cardioinhibitory response	*Type of study:* randomized, prospective, double-blind, multicenter, crossover *Follow-up:* 24 months *Primary endpoint(s):* Proportion of patients who reduced total number of syncopal episodes by ≥50% Time to first syncope	*Outcome:* proportion of patients with ≥50% reduction in syncopal episodes was 72% (95% CI: 47–90%) with DDD-CLS compared with 28% (95% CI: 9.7–53%) with sham DDI (p-0.017) Time to first syncope was 29.2 months versus 9.3 months (OR 0.11 [95% CI: 0.03 to 0.37; p<0.0001]	Closed-loop stimulation Compared DDD-CLS vs sham DDI at 30 bpm
Brignole et al., 2021[10] BioSync CLS	*Number of patients:* 127 *Inclusion:* age ≥40 years At least two episodes of severe reflex syncope in the past year Syncope with asystolic pause >3 seconds induced by tilt-table testing	*Type of study:* multicenter, prospective, randomized, placebo-controlled, patient-blinded, and outcome-assessor blinded *Follow-up:* 24 months *Primary endpoint(s):* Time to first recurrence of syncope *Secondary endpoint(s):* first recurrence of syncope or presyncope	*Outcome:* syncope in 10/63 (16%) of pacing group vs 34/64 (53%) of the control group [HR, 0.23 (95% CI: 0.11–0.47)] NNT 2.2 Combined endpoint of syncope or presyncope in 23/63 (37%) of pacing group vs 40/64 (63%) in the control group [HR, 0.44 (95% CI: 0.26–0.73)]	Closed-loop stimulation

Abbreviations: CI, confidence interval; PPM, permanent pacemaker; RDR, rate-drop-response; RRR, relative risk reduction; ILR, implantable loop recorder; VVS, vasovagal syncope; CLS, closed-loop stimulation; HR, hazard ratio; NNT, number needed to treat; Bpm, beats per minute; OR, odds ratio.

153

Table 13.2: Randomized Controlled Trials Using Rate-Drop-Response

Author/Year	Patient Population	Outcomes
Connolly 1999, VPS[1]	VVS	Positive study
Ammirati et al. 2001[3]	VVS	Positive study
Kenny 2001, SAFE PACE[26]	CSS	Positive study
Connolly 2003, VPS II[4]	VVS	Negative study
Ryan 2010, SAFE PACE[27]	CSS	Negative study

Abbreviations: VVS, vasovagal syncope; CSS, carotid sinus syndrome.

Table 13.3: Randomized Controlled Trials Using Closed-Loop Stimulation

Author/Year	Patient Population	Outcomes
Occhetta 2004[38]	VVS	Positive study
Russo et al. 2013[21]	VVS	Positive study
Baron-Esquivias 2017[9]	VVS	Positive study
Palmisano 2018[39]	VVS	Positive study
Brignole et al. 2021[10]	VVS	Positive study

Abbreviations: VVS, vasovagal syncope; CSS, carotid sinus syndrome.

cardiac cycle. When impedance suddenly changes, as shown by a change in the shape of the impedance curve during systole, the CLS then detects the decrease in right ventricular return and correspondingly triggers a higher pacing rate.[19,20] The CLS triggers pacing much earlier than the RDR algorithm. By introducing pacing when the stroke volume is more adequate, the increase in heart rate from pacing is more likely to affect mean arterial pressure.[7] In the retrospective Kanjwal study, syncope recurrence was 83% in patients with rate-drop programmed on versus only 59% in the dual chamber CLS pacemakers.[18]

Russo et al. then investigated CLS in a 50-patient randomized, single-center, prospective, single-blind, crossover trial. Inclusion criteria were age >40 years and cardioinhibitory VVS associated with asystole of greater than 3 seconds during tilt-table testing. The primary endpoints were the number of syncopal episodes with CLS turned on versus CLS turned off. There was a difference in the number of syncope episodes: 1 of 50 patients (2%) experienced syncope with CLS turned on versus 8 of 50 patients (16%) with CLS turned off ($p = 0.004$).[21] Additionally, a meta-analysis involving six trials, including four randomized controlled trials, involving 224 patients with VVS implanted with CLS and 163 patients implanted with conventional pacing found that CLS significantly reduced recurrent VVS events (pooled OR 0.23, 95% CI 0.13–0.39).[22]

In the SPAIN study as described above, CLS was studied in a randomized, double-blind, controlled study with patients over 40 years old along with frequent syncope and cardioinhibitory responses on the tilt test.[9] These patients had implantation with a CLS pacemaker programmed with CLS on for 12 months with a crossover to CLS off for another 12 months. With the group programmed DDD-CLS, the proportion of patients with ≥50% reduction in syncope was 72%, while the group programmed DDI-30 only saw 28% of patients have a similar reduction in syncope. The time to first recurrence of syncope was sevenfold longer in those patients programmed with DDD-CLS.

In a similarly designed study, Brignole et al. looked at patients ≥40 years with frequent syncope and tilt-table testing showing syncope with an asystolic pause ≥3 seconds.[10] In this BioSync CLS study, patients had a syncope recurrence of 19% at one-year follow-up and 22% at two-year follow-up with the pacemaker programmed with pacing on and CLS on. In contrast, those patients with the pacemakers as ODO (non-pacing) and CLS off had syncope recurrences of 53% at one-year follow-up and 68% at two-year follow-up.

Table 13.4: Evidence of Clinical Trials for Pacing in Carotid Sinus Syndrome

Author/Year	Sample Size/Inclusion	Study Methods	Study Outcome	Comments
Brignole 1992[24]	*Number of patients:* 60 *Inclusion criteria:* history of recurrent episodes of syncope or presyncope that had caused major trauma or judged to involve risk of future trauma or death or caused patient discomfort and interfered with daily activity reproduction of spontaneous symptoms by means of carotid sinus massage that caused ventricular asystole ≥3 seconds which was reproducible within a few days no other identifiable cause of symptoms	*Type of study:* randomized, prospective, comparative study, nonblinded *Follow-up:* 34±10 months *Primary endpoint(s):* recurrence of syncope *Secondary endpoint(s):* recurrence of any symptom (syncope+minor symptoms) Difference between mixed and cardioinhibitory CSS	*Outcome:* difference between paced and nonpaced patients Lower recurrence of symptoms in the paced group 3/32 pts (8%) vs 16/28 pts (57%) (p=0.0002) Rate of syncope in the paced group after one, two, three, and four years were 100%, 97%, 93%, and 84%, respectively, vs in nonpaced 64%, 54%, 38%, and 38% (p=0.0001) Difference persisted when subdivided into cardioinhibitory vs mixed Absence of any symptoms in paced: 66%, 43%, 27%, and 27% vs 21%, 14%, 7%, and 7% (p=0.002)	Positive study Included both cardioinhibitory and mixed CSS
Kenny 2001 SAFE PACE[26]	*Number of patients:* 175 *Inclusion criteria:* age ≥50 years ED visit for non-accidental fall Cardioinhibitory response to CSM	*Type of study:* randomized, nonblinded *Follow-up:* 12 months *Primary endpoint(s):* number of falls during year after randomization *Secondary endpoint(s):* number of syncopal episodes and number of injurious events	*Outcome:* paced patients less likely to fall (OR 0.42, 95% CI: 0.23–0.75) Paced patients reported episode of syncope similar to nonpaced (OR 0.53, 95% CI: 0.23, 1.2) Syncope: no significant difference between paced patients (11%) and controls (22%) who reported syncope (OR 0.53, 95% CI: 0.23, 1.20)	Makes assumption that carotid sinus syndrome is cause of falls For syncope endpoint, not statistically significant Rate-drop-response

(Continued)

Table 13.4: (Continued) Evidence of Clinical Trials for Pacing in Carotid Sinus Syndrome

Author/Year	Sample Size/Inclusion	Study Methods	Study Outcome	Comments
Claesson 2007[25]	*Number of patients:* 60 *Inclusion criteria:* at least one episode of syncope or presyncope and induced cardioinhibitory CSS (asystole lasting ≥3 seconds in response to carotid sinus stimulation)	*Type of study:* single-center, nonblinded, randomized *Follow-up:* 12 months *Primary endpoint(s):* patients with syncope at 12 months *Secondary endpoint(s):* patients with presyncope at 12 months	Outcome: pacing: syncope 3/30 patients (10%) vs no pacing 12/30 patients (40%) ($p=0.008$) Presyncope 8/30 pts (27%) vs 2/30 (7%) no pacing	Cardioinhibitory CSS 10 patients crossed over to pacing group Positive study
Ryan 2010 SAFE PACE 2[27]	*Number of patients:* 141 *Inclusion criteria:* age >65 years Cardioinhibitory carotid hypersensitivity, two unexplained falls, and/or one syncope in the past year >3 seconds asystole in response to CSM	*Type of study:* multicenter, double-blind (used ILR as control), randomized *Follow-up:* 24 months *Primary endpoint(s):* number of falls Episodes of syncope *Secondary endpoint(s):* episodes of syncope and falls before and after implantation of device	*Outcome:* RR of falling 0.79 (95% CI 0.41–1.5) Number of episodes of syncope (mean): PPM 0.42 vs ILR 0.66 RR 0.87 (95% CI 0.3–2.48) RR of fall after implantation of device RR 0.23 (95% CI 0.15–0.37) Less likely to report syncope (95% CI 0.26–0.86) Number of syncopal events RR 0.52 (95% CI 0.29–0.95)	Rate-drop-response Patients had less severe cardioinhibitory CSS than SAFE PACE (RR interval was 4.37 sec in SAFE PACE and 3.12 seconds in SAFE PACE 2) Number of episodes of syncope was not significantly different between groups, was only significantly different when comparing patients before and after device implantation

Abbreviations: CSS, carotid sinus syndrome; ED, emergency department; CSM, carotid sinus massage; OR, odds ratio; CI, confidence interval; ILR, implantable loop recorder; RR, relative risk; PPM, permanent pacemaker.

For patients with chronotropic incompetence in the setting of impending VVS, the CLS mechanism remains at an advantage compared to RDR. However, patients with a vasodepressor-predominant mechanism for the VVS remain at risk for syncope.[23]

RECOMMENDATION

Pacing has been demonstrated to be an effective therapy for refractory vasovagal syncope in select patient populations. Specifically, ICM use to identify significant cardioinhibitory syncope can help identify which patients may benefit the most. CLS and rate-drop-response are two effective pacing algorithms. A shared decision-making approach is warranted to balance the risks of procedural complications with lifestyle benefits.

CAROTID SINUS SYNDROME

Pacing for CSS was studied in four randomized clinical trials.[24-27] Brignole and Claesson published two positive studies, although both were not double-blinded. SAFE PACE and SAFE PACE 2 did not demonstrate any benefit; furthermore, the primary clinical endpoint was a reduction in the number of falls. The reduction in syncope was not significant in either study. Overall, the cardioinhibitory type of CSS likely will benefit the most from pacing support.

ESC guidelines downgraded their level of recommendation from class I to IIa for pacing in dominant cardioinhibitory CSS, due to its similar outcomes as vasovagal syncope. ACC/AHA/HRS guidelines also give an IIa recommendation for pacing in CSS that is cardioinhibitory or mixed.

RECOMMENDATION

Pacing in CSS can be reasonable if cardioinhibitory CSS is demonstrated to correlate with symptoms. The data are somewhat mixed, but overall, they would be reasonable to pursue in patients with cardioinhibitory or mixed CSS with severe symptoms. A shared decision-making approach is warranted to balance the risks of procedural complications with lifestyle benefits.

E. Others

Counter Maneuvers

Physical counterpressure maneuvers are simple and effective ways to reduce the burden of syncope. These are movements to recruit skeletal muscle to increase vascular tone and blood pressure, inhibiting the vasodilatory component of reflex syncope. There is one randomized controlled trial demonstrating this effect,[28] as well as several smaller non-randomized trials.[29-31] The PC-Trial (Physical Counterpressure Manoeuvres Trial) was a multicenter, prospective, randomized trial with 106 patients randomized to conventional therapy plus training in counterpressure maneuvers versus 117 patients with conventional therapy alone.[28] The yearly syncope burden, syncope recurrence, and actuarial recurrence-free survival were improved in the counterpressure maneuver group with a relative risk reduction of 39% (95% CI 11%–53%).

The American Heart Association describes various maneuvers such as leg crossing with muscle tensing, squatting, arm tensing, isometric handgrip, and neck flexion for the prevention of orthostatic symptoms. https://cpr.heart.org/en/resuscitation-science/first-aid-guidelines/first-aid/description-of-recommended-physical-counterpressure-maneuvers

Tilt-Table Training

Tilt training is another modality that exposes the body to progressively longer periods in the upright position. Two randomized trials reported no benefit.[32,33] Furthermore, there is low compliance among patients prescribed tilt-table training.[34] ESC guidelines do not recommend tilt-table training due to insufficient evidence of efficacy with this modality,[12] while ACC/AHA/HRS guidelines state that the usefulness of orthostatic training is uncertain.[11]

Yoga

There has been some evidence to suggest that yoga can decrease the burden of syncope. Yoga was first postulated to have benefits for VVS in 2015 in an observation study of 44 patients. In the yoga group of 21 patients, there was an improvement in the number of episodes of syncope and presyncope, as well as an improvement in the syncope functional status questionnaire score (SFSQS). In the yoga intervention group, 15 of the 21 patients no longer had a positive head-up tilt-table study.[35]

Shenthar et al. published a trial of 97 symptomatic VVS patients randomized to guideline-directed therapy versus yoga therapy. The group randomized to yoga therapy had a lower syncope burden.[36]

Sharma et al. demonstrated in LIVE-Yoga, which was a 55-patient randomized control study, a decreased number of syncopal or presyncopal events, with more patients that were symptom-free and had an improvement in quality of life.[37]

REFERENCES

1. Connolly SJ, Sheldon R, Roberts RS, Gent M. The North American Vasovagal Pacemaker Study (VPS). A randomized trial of permanent cardiac pacing for the prevention of vasovagal syncope. *J Am Coll Cardiol.* 1999;33(1):16–20.

2. Sutton R, Brignole M, Menozzi C, et al. Dual-chamber pacing in the treatment of neurally mediated tilt-positive cardioinhibitory syncope: pacemaker versus no therapy: a multicenter randomized study. The Vasovagal Syncope International Study (VASIS) Investigators. *Circulation.* 2000;102(3):294–299.

3. Ammirati F, Colivicchi F, Santini M. Permanent cardiac pacing versus medical treatment for the prevention of recurrent vasovagal syncope: a multicenter, randomized, controlled trial. *Circulation.* 2001;104(1):52–57.

4. Connolly SJ, Sheldon R, Thorpe KE, et al. Pacemaker therapy for prevention of syncope in patients with recurrent severe vasovagal syncope: Second Vasovagal Pacemaker Study (VPS II): a randomized trial. *JAMA.* 2003;289(17):2224–2229.

5. Raviele A, Giada F, Menozzi C, et al. A randomized, double-blind, placebo-controlled study of permanent cardiac pacing for the treatment of recurrent tilt-induced vasovagal syncope. The vasovagal syncope and pacing trial (SYNPACE). *Eur Heart J.* 2004;25(19):1741–1748.

6. Brignole M, Menozzi C, Moya A, et al. Pacemaker therapy in patients with neurally mediated syncope and documented asystole: Third International Study on Syncope of Uncertain Etiology (ISSUE-3): a randomized trial. *Circulation.* 2012;125(21):2566–2571.

7. van Dijk JG, Ghariq M, Kerkhof FI, et al. Novel methods for quantification of vasodepression and cardioinhibition during tilt-induced vasovagal syncope. *Circ Res.* 2020;127(5):e126–e38.

8. Brignole M, Arabia F, Ammirati F, et al. Standardized algorithm for cardiac pacing in older patients affected by severe unpredictable reflex syncope: 3-year insights from the Syncope Unit Project 2 (SUP 2) study. *Europace.* 2016;18(9):1427–1433.

9. Baron-Esquivias G, Morillo CA, Moya-Mitjans A, et al. Dual-chamber pacing with closed loop stimulation in recurrent reflex vasovagal syncope: the SPAIN study. *J Am Coll Cardiol.* 2017;70(14):1720–1728.

10. Brignole M, Russo V, Arabia F, et al. Cardiac pacing in severe recurrent reflex syncope and tilt-induced asystole. *Eur Heart J.* 2021;42(5):508–516.

11. Shen WK, Sheldon RS, Benditt DG, et al. 2017 ACC/AHA/HRS guideline for the evaluation and management of patients with syncope: Executive summary: A report of the American College of Cardiology/American Heart Association Task Force on Clinical Practice Guidelines and the Heart Rhythm Society. *Circulation.* 2017;136(5):e25–e59.

12. Brignole M, Moya A, de Lange FJ, et al. 2018 ESC guidelines for the diagnosis and management of syncope. *Eur Heart J.* 2018;39(21):1883–1948.

13. Flammang D, Antiel M, Church T, et al. Is a pacemaker indicated for vasovagal patients with severe cardioinhibitory reflex as identified by the ATP test? A preliminary randomized trial. *EP Europace.* 1999;1(2):140–145.

14. Benditt DG, Sutton R, Gammage M, et al. "Rate-drop response" cardiac pacing for vasovagal syncope. Rate-Drop Response Investigators Group. *J Interv Card Electrophysiol.* 1999;3(1):27–33.

15. Kurbaan AS, Franzén AC, Stack Z, Heaven D, Mathur G, Sutton R. Determining the optimal pacing intervention rate for vasovagal syncope. *J Interv Card Electrophysiol.* 2000;4(4):585–9.

16. Ozcan KS, Osmonov D, Altay S, et al. Pacemaker implantation complication rates in elderly and young patients. *Clin Interv Aging.* 2013;8:1051–1054.

17. Kochiadakis GE, Papadimitriou EA, Marketou ME, Chrysostomakis SI, Simantirakis EN, Vardas PE. Autonomic nervous system changes in vasovagal syncope: is there any difference between young and older patients? *Pacing Clin Electrophysiol.* 2004;27(10):1371–1377.

18. Kanjwal K, Karabin B, Kanjwal Y, Grubb BP. Preliminary observations on the use of closed-loop cardiac pacing in patients with refractory neurocardiogenic syncope. *J Interv Card Electrophysiol.* 2010;27(1):69–73.

19. Morillo CA, Brignole M. Pacing for vasovagal syncope: tips for use in practice. *Auton Neurosci.* 2022;241:102998.

20. Ruzieh M, Ammari Z, Dasa O, Karim S, Grubb B. Role of closed loop stimulation pacing (CLS) in vasovagal syncope. *Pacing Clin Electrophysiol.* 2017;40(11):1302–1307.

21. Russo V, Rago A, Papa AA, et al. The effect of dual-chamber closed-loop stimulation on syncope recurrence in healthy patients with tilt-induced vasovagal cardioinhibitory syncope: a prospective, randomised, single-blind, crossover study. *Heart.* 2013;99(21):1609–1613.

22. Rattanawong P, Riangwiwat T, Chongsathidkiet P, et al. Closed-looped stimulation cardiac pacing for recurrent vasovagal syncope: a systematic review and meta-analysis. *J Arrhythm.* 2018;34(5):556–564.

23. Palmisano P, Pellegrino PL, Ammendola E, et al. Risk of syncopal recurrences in patients treated with permanent pacing for bradyarrhythmic syncope: role of correlation between symptoms and electrocardiogram findings. *Europace.* 2020;22(11):1729–1736.

24. Brignole M, Menozzi C, Lolli G, Bottoni N, Gaggioli G. Long-term outcome of paced and nonpaced patients with severe carotid sinus syndrome. *Am J Cardiol.* 1992;69(12):1039–1043.

25. Claesson JE, Kristensson BE, Edvardsson N, Währborg P. Less syncope and milder symptoms in patients treated with pacing for induced cardioinhibitory carotid sinus syndrome: a randomized study. *Europace.* 2007;9(10):932–936.

26. Kenny RA, Richardson DA, Steen N, Bexton RS, Shaw FE, Bond J. Carotid sinus syndrome: a modifiable risk factor for nonaccidental falls in older adults (SAFE PACE). *J Am Coll Cardiol.* 2001;38(5):1491–1496.

27. Ryan DJ, Nick S, Colette SM, Roseanne K. Carotid sinus syndrome, should we pace? A multi-centre, randomised control trial (Safepace 2). *Heart.* 2010;96(5):347–351.

28. van Dijk N, Quartieri F, Blanc JJ, et al. Effectiveness of physical counterpressure maneuvers in preventing vasovagal syncope: the Physical Counterpressure Manoeuvres Trial (PC-Trial). *J Am Coll Cardiol.* 2006;48(8):1652–1657.

29. Brignole M, Croci F, Menozzi C, et al. Isometric arm counter-pressure maneuvers to abort impending vasovagal syncope. *J Am Coll Cardiol.* 2002;40(11):2053–2059.

30. Krediet CT, van Dijk N, Linzer M, van Lieshout JJ, Wieling W. Management of vasovagal syncope: controlling or aborting faints by leg crossing and muscle tensing. *Circulation.* 2002;106(13):1684–1689.

31. Kim KH, Cho JG, Lee KO, et al. Usefulness of physical maneuvers for prevention of vasovagal syncope. *Circ J.* 2005;69(9):1084–1088.

32. Duygu H, Zoghi M, Turk U, et al. The role of tilt training in preventing recurrent syncope in patients with vasovagal syncope: a prospective and randomized study. *Pacing Clin Electrophysiol.* 2008;31(5):592–596.

33. Foglia-Manzillo G, Giada F, Gaggioli G, et al. Efficacy of tilt training in the treatment of neurally mediated syncope. A randomized study. *Europace.* 2004;6(3):199–204.

34. Reybrouck T, Heidbüchel H, Van De Werf F, Ector H. Long-term follow-up results of tilt training therapy in patients with recurrent neurocardiogenic syncope. *Pacing Clin Electrophysiol.* 2002;25(10):1441–1446.

35. Gunda S, Kanmanthareddy A, Atkins D, et al. Role of yoga as an adjunctive therapy in patients with neurocardiogenic syncope: a pilot study. *J Interv Card Electrophysiol.* 2015;43(2):105–110.

36. Shenthar J, Gangwar RS, Banavalikar B, Benditt DG, Lakkireddy D, Padmanabhan D. A randomized study of yoga therapy for the prevention of recurrent reflex vasovagal syncope. *Europace.* 2021;23(9):1479–1486.

37. Sharma G, Ramakumar V, Sharique M, et al. Effect of yoga on clinical outcomes and quality of life in patients with vasovagal syncope (LIVE-Yoga). *JACC Clin Electrophysiol.* 2022;8(2):141–149.

38. Occhetta E, Bortnik M, Audoglio R, Vassanelli C. Closed loop stimulation in prevention of vasovagal syncope. Inotropy Controlled Pacing in Vasovagal Syncope (INVASY): a multicentre randomized, single blind, controlled study. *Europace.* 2004;6(6):538–547.

39. Palmisano P, Dell'Era G, Russo V, et al. Effects of closed-loop stimulation vs. DDD pacing on haemodynamic variations and occurrence of syncope induced by head-up tilt test in older patients with refractory cardioinhibitory vasovagal syncope: the Tilt test-Induced REsponse in Closed-loop Stimulation multicentre, prospective, single blind, randomized study. *Europace.* 2018;20(5):859–866.

14 The Legal Aspects of Syncope

Frederik J. de Lange and Robert S. Sheldon

ABBREVIATIONS

MVA: Motor Vehicle Accident
CCS: Canadian Cardiovascular Society
QoL: Quality of Life

CONSEQUENCES OF SYNCOPE TO PATIENTS AND BYSTANDERS

Over 50% of people faint at some time in their lives, and we now recognize that the predilection to vasovagal syncope can last a lifetime.[1-5] Although it is rarely fatal, syncope does cause injury, and for this, the risk needs to be both estimated and reduced. This chapter reviews the legal consequences of syncope. In general, this is about estimating the prediction of *risk*, defined as the likelihood of *recurrence* of syncope and the likelihood of *harm* by syncope.

For the person who faints, the risks with possible legal implications include personal injury, exclusion from educational opportunities, danger at work, and the risk of motor vehicle accidents. Factors to be considered include the magnitude of the harm, the person who is harmed, the legal consequences of the harm, and how to prevent the harm. For the employer, there exists not only human concern for employees but also the legal liability of foreseeable, preventable injury due to fainting in potentially dangerous situations. For society as a whole, there is the risk of motor vehicle accidents causing serious injury, death, and financial loss.

Finally, in some jurisdictions physicians who care for syncope patients share both professional responsibility and legal liability for adverse outcomes of syncope. This is especially true in Canada. At the First International Workshop on Syncope Risk Stratification in the Emergency Department in Gargnano, Italy, in 2013, 96% of physicians stated that work aspects should be considered by the ED physician when managing a syncope patient.

Regardless of risk and harm, syncope directly reduces quality of life (QoL). The QoL in patients with recurring syncope is substantially reduced, and in many cases, it is similar to severe rheumatoid arthritis and chronic low back pain, with high levels of somatization, anxiety, and depression comparable to those of psychiatric inpatients.[6,7] Although it is an intermittent disorder, its impact on daily life is similar to that of a chronic disorder.

Syncope usually is first assessed in emergency departments or family practices. International guidelines call for first-encounter attempts at establishing both diagnosis and risk.[8,9] This should include assessing the patient's risk at work and while driving and advising when to return to work and driving.

CONSEQUENCES OF SYNCOPE WHILE AT WORK

Syncope is particularly significant in hazardous work settings. The most dangerous jobs can be classified based on the number of associated fatalities (Table 14.1, adopted from Barbic et al.[10]). Even vasovagal syncope could become the cause of major morbidity or mortality in one of these jobs. There are robust data that report that injury occurs in 15% of faints,[4,5] and although most injuries are simply contusions and abrasions, this does provide a quantitative estimate of the likelihood of adverse consequences of syncope. About one faint in seven results in injury, and the consequences could be serious in an intrinsically dangerous environment. Patients with these jobs may benefit from clinical and psychological support.

Risk assessment of the work environment entails understanding factors that might increase the likelihood of syncope, or increase the magnitude of the consequences. Factors in the work environment that might predispose to syncope include prolonged standing by cashiers and servers, an overly warm environment, frequent changes of posture that might trigger initial orthostatic hypotension, and the use of heavy protective clothing that by reducing body heat loss may induce dehydration and vasodilatation.[10]

There are many factors in the work environment that might worsen the consequences. These include short-order cooks working near hot oil pots, roofers, power-line workers, wind turbine maintenance workers, exposed construction workers, police and firemen, and of course commercial drivers and pilots. Risk is inevitable and cannot be completely avoided, and a dangerous environment with a highly unlikely risk of syncope might actually be acceptable to some.

DOI: 10.1201/9781003415855-18

Table 14.1: The 10 Most Dangerous Jobs Based on Number of Fatalities and the Main Cause of Deaths by US Bureau of Labor Statistics (www.bls.gov) in 2012

Job Description	Main Cause of Death
Timber and logging workers	Contact with objects and equipment
Fishermen and related fish industry workers	Transportation incidents
Aircraft pilot and flight engineers	Transportation incidents
Structural iron and steel workers	Contact with objects and equipment
Farmers and ranchers	Transportation incidents
Roofers and linemen	Falls
Electrical power-line installers and repairers	Harmful substance exposure/environment
Drivers and truck drivers	Transportation incidents
Refuse and recyclable material collectors	Transportation incidents
Military and police personnel	Transportation incidents
Construction laborers	Falls
Firefighters	Fires and explosions
Helpers, construction trades	Falls
Grounds maintenance workers	Falls

Most risk assessments can be managed routinely in the clinic, but occasionally consultative help is needed. A discussion between a syncope expert and an occupational health physician may provide a wise, individualized balance between optimal safety and undue restrictions from driving and work.

Empiric risk models have been proposed to help stratify the risk of patients with syncope in relation to different jobs. However, they require validation by prospective and structured studies. The accuracy of these models should address three main questions:

1. Can work be safely resumed?

2. Under what environmental conditions can work be safely resumed?

3. How long without syncope is required before work can be safely resumed?

PREDICTING THE LIKELIHOOD OF SYNCOPE

Assessing the risk of syncope in dangerous environments requires being able to predict the likelihood of recurrent syncope. This is difficult, given the wide range of ages, genders, provoking settings and situations, and syncope frequency. Some factors are now clear. The predilection to syncope lasts many years,[2,11] and given the genetic basis of vasovagal syncope, it may last a lifetime.[12] Vasovagal syncope occurs in clusters in many patients,[13] and the duration of clusters ranges from days to decades.[13] Within clusters, the days in which syncope occurs are randomly distributed. Patients often present with a worsening of frequency compared to previous years.[14] Finally, after specialist assessment the likelihood of syncope recurring drops dramatically in the range of 50%–75%.[15]

Data from numerous clinical trials provide estimates of the likelihood of recurrence. Almost all the predictive power is the syncope frequency in the one year before the presentation.[14] People who have only fainted once in the previous year have an approximate 5% risk of syncope in the next year, and the risk increases with an increased prior year frequency (Figure 14.1). Patients who have fainted at least four times in the previous year have a 50%–60% likelihood of a recurrence.[16] Therefore, patients with a very sparse history of syncope are at very low risk, while care must be taken with patients who faint frequently. A recent cross-over administrative dataset analysis reported that an emergency visit for syncope did not increase the risk of subsequent traffic collision.[17]

HISTORY OF CANADIAN DRIVING SCORE: When Fit to Drive?

The CCS Consensus Guidelines on Fitness to Drive introduced the Risk of Harm (RH) formula,[18] which quantifies the risk of serious harm or death due to syncope while driving with the following equation.

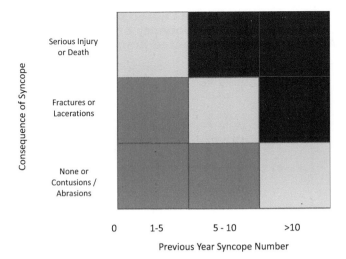

Figure 14.1 A heat map for risk assessment syncope at work and in the car. Patients in the red zone should not be driving, while those in the green zone should be free to drive. The likelihood of syncope (on the horizontal axis) can be estimated from available literature, while estimations of the consequence of syncope may be more subjective.

$$RH = TD \times SCI \times V \times AC,$$

where

- TD (time driving)=fractional time spent driving
- SCI (sudden cardiac incapacitation)=the time-dependent likelihood of syncope
- V=type of vehicle
- AC (accident consequences)=probability that a syncope spell during driving results in a fatal or injury-producing accident.

The CCS estimated V=0.28 for private drivers, V=1.0 for commercial drivers, and AC=0.02 per spell. Based on existing but sparse societal data in 1993, the acceptable RH was estimated to be 0.005% per person-year. From this, the theoretical Risk of Harm can be calculated as follows: (faints while driving per driving-year)=(0.02×0.28). The original CCS driving guidelines[18] assumed that the Canadian population tolerated a risk of serious injury or death due to a syncope causing a motor vehicle accident of <1/20,000 or 0.005% per year. The theoretical model led to an estimate of a societal risk tolerance of <1% per year for a risk of syncope while driving.

Nearly 40 years later, the question is whether the estimate of societal tolerance of the risk of death and serious injury was accurate, and there is recent evidence that the underlying assumption was overly strict. More recent estimates of societal risk acceptance of serious injury or death due to syncope causing an MVA are available in large datasets from the UK, the USA, and Canada from 2009 to 2013.[19] Data retrieved from the Internet reported[19] a mean risk of serious injury or death while driving to be 0.067% in the general population (Table 14.2). Similarly, data from Washington State in 1987–1988 estimated[20] that in individuals >65 years old the risk of serious injury due to an MVA was 0.08%. The US national estimate[19] was >0.013%. Taken together, the average from these data is 0.075% per year. Societies appear to tolerate a 15-fold higher risk than was assumed by the CCS guideline authors. The risks are even higher in young men and women, who continue to cause highway carnage without driving restrictions.

What is the currently acceptable risk of causing a motor vehicle accident? The yearly risks of an MVA (Table 14.2) in Canada,[19] the USA,[19] the UK,[19] and Denmark[21] were 0.56%, 2.29%, 0.49%, and 1.21%. The mean is 1.14% per year, very similar to the CCS Guideline risk tolerance of <1% per year.

The difficulty in assessing this risk is that all the data were administrative data, providing only compiled risks, and none reported the risk of syncope itself. These estimates are available from the first 2 Prevention of Syncope Trials (POST 1–2),[22,23] which included 418 patients with an average of

Table 14.2: Estimated Risk of Harm Caused by Syncope While Driving Compared with the Frequency of MVAs and Injuries in Alberta, Canada, the United Kingdom, and the United States

Location, Year (Ref. #)	MVAs, %	Injuries, %	Serious Injury, %	Death, %	Serious Injury and Death, %
Canada, 2012	0.56 (est)	0.51	0.044	0.009	0.053
United States, 2009	2.29	0.63	NR	0.013	>0.013
United Kingdom, 2013	0.4	0.52	0.078	0.0044	0.082
Country averages	1.11±1.02	0.55 ± 0.07	0.061 (exc USA)	0.009±0.004	0.067 (exc USA)
CCS guidelines	<1	N/A	<0.005	<0.005	<0.005
Syncope	0.31	N/A	≤0.0017 (est)	≤0.0017 (est)	≤0.0017 (est)

The rates are expressed as the likelihood of an event per 100 driver-years, denoted as %.
MVA, motor vehicle accident; CCS, Canadian Cardiovascular Society; Est, estimated; exc, excluding; MVA, motor vehicle accident; NR, not reported.

10 lifetime syncopal episodes and a median of three syncopal episodes in the prior year.[19] The rigorously collected data led to an estimated likelihood of syncopal episodes while driving of 0.62% per driver-year, and there were no serious injuries. The risk of serious harm was estimated to be <0.0035% per driver-year. This is a high-risk population: 40% fainted in the year while in the study and many had several syncope recurrences.

Are these estimates externally valid?

In four administrative or observational studies[19,24–26] of patients with syncope, the yearly likelihood of fainting while driving (Table 14.2) was 0.62%, 0.33%, 0%, and 1% (mean 0.32%). In five observational or administrative studies[19,21,24–27] of patients with syncope, the yearly likelihood of fainting while driving causing an MVA was 0.62%, 0%, 0.26%, 0%, 1.06%, and 2.2% (mean 0.69%). In the same five studies,[19,21,24–27] the yearly risk of a syncope-associated MVA causing serious injury or death was 0%, 0%, 0%, 0%, and 0.007% (mean 0.0015%).

Overall, the compiled data on the risk of MVAs in patients with syncope and recent estimates of societal risk tolerance suggest that current guidelines substantially overestimate the risk of serious injury or death due to syncope causing an MVA. The risk of serious injury or death per year due to a syncope-associated MVA after assessment is 0.0015%, 50-fold less than the societally tolerated risk of 0.075% and the historical CCS benchmark of less than <0.005%. Therefore, the CCS Guidelines overestimated the likelihood that syncope while driving causes serious injury or death. In particular, patients with only 1 recent syncopal spell, those who faint only while standing or exercising, and those with reliable and prolonged pre-syncopal prodromes should be permitted to continue to drive.

PHYSICIANS AND THE LAW

Should the physician inform the patient about fit to drive? One of several problems faced by physicians is that there is considerable variation among national and subnational jurisdictions in guidelines for driver restrictions and the duty of physicians to report. All countries have regulations regarding the ability to drive patients with a predilection to syncope, but there is a wide range of reporting requirements and regulations about driving.

Current Italian legislation does not include specific prescriptions in case of syncope in truck drivers. This lack of guidance for occupational physicians impairs the ability to advise patients on work fitness. The judgment of work fitness for truck drivers can be especially complex, and cooperation is needed between occupational health physicians and syncope specialists.

In the United States, regulations for commercial drivers are set federally, while regulations for private drivers are set by individual states. In contrast, in Canada, all driving regulations are set provincially with interprovincial variability of driving regulations and duty to report. Some provinces such as Ontario have very aggressive reporting guidelines, while others such as Alberta have no mandatory reporting guidelines, even for commercial drivers. Both the US and Canadian guidelines are mainly aimed at non-arrhythmic syncope.

Canada has some of the more stringent expectations. In 70% of provinces, physicians are expected to report patients to provincial authorities if the patients have a history of syncope. Whether this does any good is debatable, partly because of its impracticality and of the common sense of physicians. Simpson et al. reported that over 90% of Ontario physicians routinely ignored the law[28] in a startling act of civil disobedience.

In most other countries, healthcare professionals are not obliged to inform their patients regarding fit to drive. The Austroads guidelines published recently state that health professionals should maintain an awareness of any changes in health care and health technology that may affect their assessment of drivers. Health professionals should also maintain an awareness of changes in the law that may affect their legal responsibilities.

The holder of the driving license is obliged to inform their selves about the legal regulations concerning fitness to drive. That is, the legal responsibility and liability lie with the patient and not with the physician. However, it is not forbidden to advise a patient not to drive when the safety of public traffic is at stake. Physicians can advise a patient not to drive according to local regulations. This is made more difficult by the absence of any particular specialty that has taken ownership of syncope management. In contrast, neurologists usually have a firm grasp of driving guidelines for epileptics and cardiologists understand driving recommendations for patients with ventricular tachycardia. This is not the case for every patient with syncope, especially non-cardiac syncope, because syncope does not belong to any one particular specialty. The FAST II database reported that less than 20% of physicians discuss fit to drive, but 40% of the patients found themselves not fit.[29]

SUMMARY AND RECOMMENDATIONS

Syncope in the acute setting is usually addressed for the first time at the emergency department. The initial evaluation results in either a certain or highly likely diagnosis and an estimated prognosis. A risk stratification should be performed upon the initial evaluation. Dealing with the legal aspects of syncope with respect to driving and working is about predicting the *risk*, defined as the likelihood of *recurrence* of syncope and the likelihood of *harm* by syncope.[30] Most regulations concerning returning to work and driving are too strict. Physicians assessing a syncope patient should consider whether the patient is fit to drive or can resume work.

REFERENCES

1. Olde Nordkamp LR, van Dijk N, Ganzeboom KS et al. Syncope prevalence in the ED compared to general practice and population: A strong selection process. *Am J Emerg Med.* 2009;27:271–279.

2. Serletis A, Rose S, Sheldon AG, Sheldon RS. Vasovagal syncope in medical students and their first-degree relatives. *Eur Heart J.* 2006;27:1965–1970.

3. Jorge J, Raj S, Liang Z, Sheldon R. Quality of life and injury due to vasovagal syncope. *Clin Auton Res.* 2022;32:147–149.

4. Jorge JG, Raj SR, Teixeira PS, Teixeira JAC, Sheldon RS. Likelihood of injury due to vasovagal syncope: A systematic review and meta-analysis. *Europace.* 2021;23:1092–1099.

5. Jorge JG, Pournazari P, Raj SR, Maxey C, Sheldon RS. Frequency of injuries associated with syncope in the prevention of syncope trials. *Europace.* 2020;22:1896–1903.

6. Linzer M, Pontinen M, Gold DT, Divine GW, Felder A, Brooks WB. Impairment of physical and psychosocial function in recurrent syncope. *J Clin Epidemiol.* 1991;44:1037–1043.

7. van Dijk N, Sprangers MA, Colman N, Boer KR, Wieling W, Linzer M. Clinical factors associated with quality of life in patients with transient loss of consciousness. *J Cardiovasc Electrophysiol.* 2006;17:998–1003.

8. Brignole M, Moya A, de Lange FJ et al. 2018 ESC guidelines for the diagnosis and management of syncope. *Eur Heart J.* 2018;39:1883–1948.

9. Shen WK, Sheldon RS, Benditt DG et al. 2017 ACC/AHA/HRS guideline for the evaluation and management of patients with syncope: Executive summary: A report of the American College of Cardiology/American Heart Association Task Force on Clinical Practice Guidelines and the Heart Rhythm Society. *J Am Coll Cardiol.* 2017;70:620–663.

10. Barbic F, Casazza G, Zamuner AR et al. Driving and working with syncope. *Auton Neurosci.* 2014;184:46–52.

11. Ganzeboom KS, Mairuhu G, Reitsma JB, Linzer M, Wieling W, van Dijk N. Lifetime cumulative incidence of syncope in the general population: A study of 549 Dutch subjects aged 35–60 years. *J Cardiovasc Electrophysiol.* 2006;17:1172–1176.

12. Sheldon RS, Gerull B. Genetic markers of vasovagal syncope. *Auton Neurosci.* 2021;235:102871.

13. Sahota IS, Maxey C, Pournazari P, Sheldon RS. Clusters, Gaps, and randomness: Vasovagal syncope recurrence patterns. *JACC Clin Electrophysiol.* 2017;3:1046–1053.

14. Sumner GL, Rose MS, Koshman ML, Ritchie D, Sheldon RS. Recent history of vasovagal syncope in a young, referral-based population is a stronger predictor of recurrent syncope than lifetime syncope burden. *J Cardiovasc Electrophysiol.* 2010;21:1375–1380.

15. Pournazari P, Sahota I, Sheldon R. High remission rates in vasovagal syncope. *JACC: Clinical Electrophysiology.* 2017;3:384–392.

16. Sheldon R, Faris P, Tang A et al. Midodrine for the prevention of vasovagal syncope: A randomized clinical trial. *Ann Intern Med.* 2021;174:1349–1356.

17. Staples JA, Erdelyi S, Merchant K et al. Syncope and traffic crash: A population-based case-crossover analysis. *Can J Cardiol.* 2024;40:554–561.

18. Simpson C, Dorian P, Gupta A, et al. Assessment of the cardiac patient for fitness to drive: Drive subgroup executive summary. *Can J Cardiol.* 2004;20:1314–1320.

19. Tan VH, Ritchie D, Maxey C, Sheldon R. Prospective assessment of the risk of vasovagal ayncope during driving. *JACC Clin Electrophysiol.* 2016;2:203–208.

20. Koepsell TD, Wolf ME, McCloskey L et al. Medical conditions and motor vehicle collision injuries in older adults. *J Am Geriatr Soc.* 1994;42:695–700.

21. Nume AK, Gislason G, Christiansen CB et al. Syncope and motor vehicle crash risk: A Danish nationwide study. *JAMA Intern Med.* 2016;176:503–510.

22. Sheldon R, Connolly S, Rose S et al. Prevention of syncope trial (POST): A randomized, placebo-controlled study of metoprolol in the prevention of vasovagal syncope. *Circulation.* 2006;113:1164–1170.

23. Sheldon R, Raj SR, Rose MS et al. Fludrocortisone for the prevention of vasovagal syncope: A randomized, placebo-controlled trial. *J Am Coll Cardiol.* 2016;68:1–9.

24. Sheldon R, Koshman ML. Can patients with neuromediated syncope safely drive motor vehicles? *Am J Cardiol.* 1995;75:955–956.

25. Folino AF, Migliore F, Porta A, Cerutti S, Iliceto S, Buja G. Syncope while driving: Pathophysiological features and long-term follow-up. *Auton Neurosci.* 2012;166:60–65.

26. Maas R, Ventura R, Kretzschmar C, Aydin A, Schuchert A. Syncope, driving recommendations, and clinical reality: Survey of patients. *BMJ*. 2003;326:21.

27. Silva M, Godinho A, Freitas J. Transient loss of consciousness assessment in a University Hospital: From diagnosis to prognosis. *Porto Biomed J*. 2016;1:118–123.

28. Simpson CS, Klein GJ, Brennan FJ, Krahn AD, Yee R, Skanes AC. Impact of a mandatory physician reporting system for cardiac patients potentially unfit to drive. *Can J Cardiol*. 2000;16:1257–1263.

29. Snijders Blok MR, de Lange FJ, Thijs RD, van Dijk JG, Wieling W, van Dijk N. Driving status of syncope patients is not part of standard advice. *Ned Tijdschr Geneeskd*. 2017;161:D1328.

30. Barbic F, Dipaola F, Casazza G et al. Syncope in a working-age population: Recurrence risk and related risk factors. *J Clin Med*. 2019;8:150.

15 Syncope and Falls in Older Adults

Desmond O'Donnell and Rose Anne Kenny

INTRODUCTION

Often an isolated condition in younger patients, syncope in older patients is frequently multifactorial, with more than one attributable cause present in up to one-third. History taking is therefore more challenging in older patients and is further complicated by atypical or absent prodromes, amnesia for loss of consciousness, and difficulty obtaining informant accounts. As frailty, physical and cognitive comorbidities are common, a comprehensive geriatric assessment is recommended, incorporating physical, functional, social, environmental, and psychological assessments, as well as a detailed medication review.

Epidemiology

Syncope is the seventh most common reason for emergency admission of patients older than 65 years.[1] The prevalence of syncope is trimodal—with peaks in late teens, later mid-life, and the oldest old.[2] While often seen as a condition of younger people, 10%–15% of individuals have their first faint after the age of 65 years.[3] From the age of 70, its incidence increases rapidly, up to 81.2 per 1,000 patient years ≥80 years of age.[2] The true prevalence of syncope is likely underestimated due to amnesia for transient loss of consciousness (TLOC) and lack of witness accounts for events in older patients.

Causes of Syncope in Older Adults

Reflex syncope is the most common cause of syncope across all age groups; however, orthostatic hypotension (OH) and cardiogenic causes of syncope become more common with age.[4,5] In older patients, more than one cause of syncope may be present.[1,4,6] Multimorbidity, frailty, and polypharmacy add to the complexity of identifying an attributable cause of events.[7]

Pathophysiology

Several age-related pathophysiological changes increase susceptibility to changes in total peripheral vascular resistance or cardiac output. These include increased left ventricular hypertrophy, loss of myocytes and collagen, fibrotic infiltration, autonomic dysfunction, and reduced baroreflex sensitivity. Additionally, older adults are prone to reduced blood volume due to excessive salt wasting by the kidneys,[8] and this, together with age-related diastolic dysfunction and inadequate heart rate responses to stress, increases susceptibility to OH and vasovagal syncope (VVS).[9] Changes in vascular stiffness and pulse pressure can result in altered cerebral blood flow and pre-dispose to OH.[10] Syncope in older patients may thus result from single or multiple processes, each contributing to reduced cerebral oxygen delivery below the level required for maintenance of consciousness.

Evaluation

The starting point for the evaluation of syncope is a careful history (including a witness account of events where possible), physical examination, 12-lead electrocardiogram (ECG), and measurement of orthostatic blood pressure.[7] Further investigations will be informed by the outcome of this initial assessment. Specific consideration should be given to whether there is a cardiac or neurologic cause or whether the cause is multifactorial.[11,12]

History may not always be reliable, as the older patient may present with atypical features, may have cognitive issues affecting recall, is less likely to have a prodrome, and commonly has amnesia for either prodrome or TLOC (up to 40% with reflex syncope).[7,13,14] An approach to diagnosis that incorporates overlapping clinical syndromes, like that in frailty, is therefore appropriate for syncope in older adults.

Syncope Units

To increase diagnostic accuracy, personalize management, and reduce unnecessary testing, dedicated syncope units are recommended. These units provide specialist, structured diagnostics and evidence-based treatment and are frequently led by geriatricians given the high prevalence of syncope in older persons.[15] Given the increased risk of unexplained falls seen in those with

DOI: 10.1201/9781003415855-19

asymptomatic hypotensive disorders such as OH, these units should provide care for older adults presenting with unexplained falls as well as those with syncope.[16]

REFLEX SYNCOPE
Vasovagal Syncope
Pathophysiology

The mechanisms underlying VVS in older adults remain poorly understood, as most research has focused on younger adults.[17] In VVS, the responses to prolonged orthostasis result in stimulation of ventricular mechanoreceptors and activation of the Bezold–Jarisch reflex, leading to paradoxical peripheral vasodilation, hypotension, and bradycardia. Due to an age-related decline in baroreceptor sensitivity, the paradoxical responses to orthostasis (as in VVS) can be less marked in older adults.[17] However, polypharmacy, comorbidities, and impaired baroreflex sensitivity can precipitate dysautonomic responses during prolonged orthostasis and render older adults susceptible to VVS.[17]

Presentation

The most common triggers in older adults are prolonged standing, dehydration, and vasodilator medications. Some patients experience symptoms precipitated by micturition, defecation, or coughing. Prodromal symptoms include fatigue, dizziness, weakness, diaphoresis, nausea, visual and auditory disturbances, vertigo, headache, and abdominal discomfort. Prodromal duration varies greatly, and older patients may have poor recall of these symptoms.[7] Loss of consciousness is usually brief, during which some patients develop involuntary movements,[18] usually myoclonic jerks, but tonic-clonic movements also occur. Thus, VVS may masquerade as a seizure or an unexplained fall. Recovery is usually rapid, but older patients can experience protracted symptoms such as confusion, disorientation, nausea, headache, and dizziness.

Evaluation

Using head-up tilting, VVS can be reproduced in susceptible individuals.[19] A test is diagnostic if symptoms are reproduced, with a decline in blood pressure (BP) of greater than 50 mmHg or systolic blood pressure less than 90 mmHg.[20] The cardioinhibitory response is defined as asystole in excess of 3 seconds or heart rate (HR) slowing to less than 40 beats/min for a minimum of 10 seconds.[21] In contrast to younger patients, for older patients, the hemodynamic response induced during head-up tilt is more likely to be indicative of real-time events and patients respond well to treatment with cardiac pacing or medications as indicated.[22]

Carotid Sinus Syndrome and Carotid Sinus Hypersensitivity
Pathophysiology

Carotid sinus hypersensitivity (CSH) is defined as an exaggerated hypotensive or bradycardiac response to carotid sinus massage (CSM).[12] Carotid sinus syndrome (CSS) is defined as CSH with syncope during CSM and is a frequently overlooked cause of syncope in older adults. Abnormal responses to CSM are asystole exceeding 3 seconds (cardioinhibitory), a fall in systolic BP exceeding 50 mmHg in the absence of cardio-inhibition (vasodepressor/hypotensive), or a combination of the two (mixed).[12] CSS is virtually unknown before the age of 50 years; its incidence increases with age thereafter.[12]

Presentation

Syncope is usually precipitated by stimulation of the carotid sinus, such as by head turning or tight neckwear, or by vagal triggers such as prolonged standing, dehydration, and fasting. In a significant number of patients, no trigger is identified and CSH presents as unexplained falls in one-third of cases.[23]

Evaluation

Performing supine and upright CSM increases the likelihood of symptom reproduction, but testing should be confined to supine CSM in frail older persons suspected of compromised cerebral perfusion and risk of neurological sequelae.[24] The traditional diagnosis of CSM combines diagnostic CSM criteria, coupled with symptom reproduction; however, in older patients with amnesia, the latter characteristic may be absent.[25] Implantable loop recorders should be considered if CSM is contra-indicated or cannot be completed.

Management

It is advisable to treat all patients with a history of two or more symptomatic episodes, but the need for intervention in those with a solitary event should be assessed on an individual basis. Dual-chamber cardiac pacing is the treatment of choice in patients with symptomatic cardioinhibitory CSS, and with appropriate pacing, syncope is abolished in 85%–90% of patients.[23] Treatment of vasodepressor CSS focuses on modification of vasodepressor medications, while treatment with fludrocortisone can also be considered.[26]

ORTHOSTATIC HYPOTENSION

Epidemiology/Pathophysiology

OH is common, although the prevalence depends on the characteristics of the cohort (10% community adults treated for hypertension, 65% nursing home residents) and the method of assessment (two to three times higher if phasic BP measurement is used rather than oscillometric).[27] Population-based studies have demonstrated a significant age gradient for orthostatic BP, showing that 7% of 50- to 55-year-old BPs failed to stabilize by 2 minutes after standing compared with 41% of those aged 80 and older.[28]

Causative Factors

OH is caused by age-related vascular and baroreflex changes or autonomic neuropathy. In older adults with hypertension and cardiovascular disease and those on vasoactive drugs, circulatory adjustments to orthostatic stress are disturbed, rendering them particularly vulnerable to OH.[29]

Autonomic neuropathy, either primary or secondary (diabetes, multisystem atrophy, Lewy body dementia, Parkinson's disease, amyloidosis), is more common with age.

Medications

Medications at the highest risk of precipitating OH include cardiovascular medications (e.g., diuretics, nitrates, β- and α-receptor blockers) and medications acting on the central nervous system (e.g., antidepressants, antipsychotics, trazodone, and benzodiazepines).[30] Recent reports suggest that tighter control of BP reduces cardiovascular events and reduces the future incidence of OH.[31] However, non-judicious use of antihypertensive agents in frail older patients increases the risk of OH.[32]

Evaluation

Orthostatic hypotension is diagnosed by a sustained reduction in systolic blood pressure of at least 20 mmHg or diastolic blood pressure of 10 mmHg within 3 minutes of standing or head-up tilt.[12] The reproducibility of OH depends on the time of measurement and on autonomic function. It should be repeated in the morning after the older adult maintains a supine posture for at least 10 minutes. Phasic BP measurements are more sensitive for the detection of transient falls in BP.[33] Ambulatory BP will detect postprandial hypotension as well as orthostatic hypotensive and supine hypertensive periods and guide the timing of medications.[34]

Management

The goal of therapy for symptomatic OH is to improve cerebral perfusion. Nonpharmacologic interventions should be tried initially, including avoidance of precipitating factors, maintenance of adequate hydration, elevation of the head of the bed, and application of graduated pressure from an abdominal support garment or compression stockings, although compliance with these is often limited.[34] Medications known to contribute to OH should be discontinued or reduced. Bolus intake of 500 mL of fluid in advance of the trigger may help.[34] Recently, continuous positive airway pressure has been shown to benefit hemodynamics by reducing supine hypertension and orthostatic hypotension.[35]

Postprandial hypotension often coexists with OH in older patients and can be detected by BP readings within 90 minutes of a meal seated and then standing, as well as with ambulatory BP monitoring.[34] It is managed by tailoring the timing of hypotension-inducing medications and intake of small, frequent, low-carbohydrate meals.

Numerous drugs have been used to raise BP in OH, with fludrocortisone and midodrine the most commonly used. Adverse effects of fludrocortisone include hypertension, cardiac failure, edema, and hypokalemia, while midodrine can precipitate hypertension, pilomotor erection, and gastrointestinal symptoms.[34] Other medications include acarbose (used primarily for postprandial hypotension as it reduces carbohydrate absorption from the gut), atomoxetine, and pyridostigmine.[34]

CARDIAC SYNCOPE

One-third of cases of syncope in older patients are caused by cardiac disorders.[4] Cardiac syncope is characterized by little or no hypotensive prodrome, occurrence when supine or during exercise, and association with palpitations or chest pain.[12] It is associated with higher morbidity and mortality.[5] The prevalence of cardiac disease, including structural heart disease and arrhythmias, rises dramatically with age.[5] Cardiac syncope should be considered in the presence of known structural heart disease, a history of coronary artery disease, or an abnormal ECG.[12]

Diagnosis

The gold standard for the diagnosis of cardiac syncope is symptom rhythm correlation—contemporaneous HR and rhythm recording during syncope.[12] Structural heart disease and an abnormal electrocardiogram are associated with a higher risk of arrhythmias and a higher mortality at one year.[36] Cardiac monitoring may identify diagnostic abnormalities, such as asystole longer than 3 seconds, rapid supraventricular tachycardia (SVT), or ventricular tachycardia (VT).[37]

Cardiac Monitoring

External loop recorders may be useful, but older patients often have difficulty operating the devices,[38] and they do not capture events unless the episodes occur during the monitoring period. Implantable loop recorders (ILR) can aid diagnosis during intermittent symptoms in up to 50% and are recommended for patients with recurrent unexplained syncope or falls.[12]

Patients with slow HR and cardiac pauses detected by implantable monitoring devices have excellent symptom control with cardiac pacing.[39]

Echocardiography

Echocardiography should be performed in patients in whom a structural abnormality is suspected. Cardiac arrhythmias are evident in up to 50% of patients with an ejection fraction of less than 40%.[40]

Electrophysiologic Study

Electrophysiologic study is indicated in older patients with syncope when a cardiac arrhythmia is suspected. Diagnosis is based on confirmation of an inducible arrhythmia or conduction disturbance.[41]

Management

Pacemaker insertion is often indicated for older adults who suffer from cardiac syncope and, if indicated, should be considered in all patients, including those with underlying frailty. Empirical cardiac pacing may be indicated in lieu of protracted diagnostic investigations if the older patient is at risk of injurious events, particularly fractured femurs, which can have high morbidity and mortality and after which almost half of older patients never regain baseline functional independence.[42]

FALLS IN THE OLDER PATIENT

Non-Syncopal Falls

The prevalence of non-syncopal falls increases with age, and they are the most common cause of injury in older adults.[33] They carry significant morbidity and mortality, while injuries and the resulting fear of falling accelerate functional decline and hasten admission to residential care.[33] The recent World Falls Guidelines recommend stratification of fall risk in older adults based on the following: presentation with fall, history of falls in the past 12 months, and/or the presence of gait impairment (gait speed <0.8 m/second or timed up and go >15 seconds).[43]

Those at high risk of falls should receive a multifactorial falls risk assessment, including a review of mobility, sensory function, cognition, functional ability, autonomic function, nutrition, environmental issues, medications, medical comorbidities (including screening for cardiovascular diseases, Parkinson's disease, and other neurological or depressive disorders).[43] Targeted, multi-domain interventions should be implemented based on the outcome of this assessment, with a particular focus on the patient's perspective of their falls.

Overlap between Unexplained Falls and Syncope

In TILDA, 25% of older adults who had unexplained falls experienced a syncopal episode. Unexplained falls rose with age, suggesting that syncope was more likely to present as falls with advancing years.[44] Given this significant overlap, a combined approach to assessment, based on dedicated syncope units, is recommended.

CHALLENGES IN THE OLDER PATIENT

Frailty

For older adults with frailty, individualized decisions need to be made that consider the potential benefits against any risk of harm. Injurious events such as fractures and head injuries are also more common due to a lack of awareness of prodromal symptoms and co-occurrence of osteoporosis and other comorbidities.[7]

Polypharmacy

Polypharmacy is common in older adults. Falls risk increasing drugs (FRIDS) include antihypertensives, antianginals, antihistamines, antipsychotics, tricyclic antidepressants, and diuretics.[45] Drug interactions can also cause syncope, particularly in older patients with multiple comorbidities and polypharmacy.[46] Even with long-standing established medications, the progression of age-related physiologic changes may precipitate syncope.[47]

Cognition

Cognitive issues are more common in older adults, with impaired recall making history-taking challenging.[7] Impaired executive function is associated with an increased prevalence of falls in older adults, while dementia has been shown to be an independent risk factor for falls in older adults.[48] Additionally, patients with Lewy body or Alzheimer's dementia have a higher prevalence of syncope, OH, and CSH.[7]

Focal Neurology with Syncope

One in 20 patients experience focal neurologic events at the time of syncope or presyncope.[49] Awareness of this phenomenon is important to prevent misdiagnosis of stroke and overtreatment of hypertension (given that the events are due to hypotension-induced hypoperfusion).

SUMMARY

- Syncope is experienced by up to 30% of adults in their lifetime with a rising incidence in those older than 70 years.

- Syncope may present atypically in older adults, with the absence of prodrome and amnesia for LOC more common.

- Vasovagal syncope, OH, and carotid sinus syndrome are the most common causes of syncope in older adults.

- Cardiac causes of syncope, including structural heart disease and arrhythmia, occur with higher frequency in older patients.

- More than one cause of syncope may be present, and significant overlap exists between unexplained falls and syncope.

- Injurious events such as fractures and head injuries are also more common due to a lack of awareness of prodromal symptoms and co-occurrence of osteoporosis and other morbidities.

REFERENCES

1. Romme JJ, van Dijk N, Boer KR, et al. Influence of age and gender on the occurrence and presentation of reflex syncope. *Clin Auton Res*. 2008;18(3):127–133. https://doi.org/10.1007/s10286-008-0465-0

2. Ruwald MH, Hansen ML, Lamberts M, et al. The relation between age, sex, comorbidity, and pharmacotherapy and the risk of syncope: A Danish nationwide study. *Europace*. 2012;14(10):1506–1514. https://doi.org/10.1093/europace/eus154

3. Chen LY, Shen W-K, Mahoney DW, Jacobsen SJ, Rodeheffer RJ. Prevalence of syncope in a population aged more than 45 years. *Am J Med*. 2006;119(12). https://doi.org/10.1016/j.amjmed.2006.01.029

4. Del Rosso A, Alboni P, Brignole M, Menozzi C, Raviele A. Relation of clinical presentation of syncope to the age of patients. *Am J Cardiol*. 2005;96(10):1431–1435. https://doi.org/10.1016/j.amjcard.2005.07.047

5. Parry SW, Tan MP. An approach to the evaluation and management of syncope in adults. *BMJ*. 2010;340(1):c880–c880. https://doi.org/10.1136/bmj.c880

6. Chen LY, Gersh BJ, Hodge DO, Wieling W, Hammill SC, Shen W-K. Prevalence and clinical outcomes of patients with multiple potential causes of syncope. *Mayo Clinic Proc*. 2003;78(4):414–420. https://doi.org/10.4065/78.4.414

7. O' Brien H, Kenny RA. Syncope in the elderly. *Eur Cardiol Rev*. 2014;9(1):28. https://doi.org/10.15420/ecr.2014.9.1.28

8. Aronow WS. Heart disease and aging. *Med Clin N Am*. 2006;90(5):849–862. https://doi.org/10.1016/j.mcna.2006.05.009

9. Verheyden B, Gisolf J, Beckers F, et al. Impact of age on the vasovagal response provoked by sublingual nitroglycerine in routine tilt testing. *Clin Sci*. 2007;113(7):329–337. https://doi.org/10.1042/cs20070042

10. Balestrini CS, Al-Khazraji BK, Suskin N, Shoemaker JK. Does vascular stiffness predict white matter hyperintensity burden in ischemic heart disease with preserved ejection fraction? *Am J Physiol Heart Circ Physiol*. 2020;318(6). https://doi.org/10.1152/ajpheart.00057.2020

11. Alboni P, Brignole M, Menozzi B. Diagnostic value of history in patients with syncope with or without heart disease. *ACC Curr J Rev*. 2001;10(6):72–73. https://doi.org/10.1016/s1062-1458(01)00502-5

12. Brignole M, Moya A, de Lange FJ, et al. ESC guidelines for the diagnosis and management of syncope. *Eur Heart J*. 2018; 39: 1883–1948.

13. O'Dwyer C, Bennett K, Langan Y, Fan CW, Kenny RA. Amnesia for loss of consciousness is common in vasovagal syncope. *Europace*. 2011;13(7):1040–1045. https://doi.org/10.1093/europace/eur069

14. Parry SW, Kenny RA. Drop attacks in older adults: Systematic assessment has a high diagnostic yield. *J Am Geriatr Soc*. 2005;53(1):74–78. https://doi.org/10.1111/j.1532-5415.2005.53013.x

15. Kenny RA, Rice C, Byrne L. The role of the Syncope Management Unit. *Cardiol Clin*. 2015;33(3):483–496. https://doi.org/10.1016/j.ccl.2015.04.016

16. Claffey P, Pérez-Denia L, Lavan A, Kenny RA, Finucane C, Briggs R. Asymptomatic orthostatic hypotension and risk of falls in community-dwelling older people. *Age Ageing*. 2022;51(12). https://doi.org/10.1093/ageing/afac295

17. Tan MP, Parry SW. Vasovagal syncope in the older patient. *J Am Coll Cardiol*. 2008;51(6):599–606. https://doi.org/10.1016/j.jacc.2007.11.025

18. Shmuely S, Bauer PR, van Zwet EW, van Dijk JG, Thijs RD. Differentiating motor phenomena in tilt-induced syncope and convulsive seizures. *Neurology*. 2018;90(15). https://doi.org/10.1212/wnl.0000000000005301

19. Bartoletti A. "The Italian protocol": A simplified head-up tilt testing potentiated with oral nitroglycerin to assess patients with unexplained syncope. *Europace*. 2000;2(4):339–342. https://doi.org/10.1053/eupc.2000.0125

20. Chrysant SG. The tilt table test is useful for the diagnosis of vasovagal syncope and should not be abolished. *J Clin Hypertension*. 2020;22(4):686–689. https://doi.org/10.1111/jch.13846

21. Brignole M, Moya A, Menozzi C, Garciacivera R, Sutton R. Proposed electrocardiographic classification of spontaneous syncope documented by an implantable loop recorder. *Europace*. 2005;7(1):14–18. https://doi.org/10.1016/j.eupc.2004.11.001

22. Brignole M, Donateo P, Tomaino M, et al. Benefit of pacemaker therapy in patients with presumed neurally mediated syncope and documented asystole is greater when tilt test is negative. *Circul Arrhyth Electrophysiol*. 2014;7(1):10–16. https://doi.org/10.1161/circep.113.001103

23. Kenny RA, Richardson DA, Steen N, Bexton RS, Shaw FE, Bond J. Carotid sinus syndrome: A modifiable risk factor for nonaccidental falls in older adults (safe pace). *J Am Coll Cardiol*. 2001;38(5):1491–1496. https://doi.org/10.1016/s0735-1097(01)01537-6

24. Puggioni E, Guiducci V, Brignole M, et al. Results and complications of the carotid sinus massage performed according to the "Method of symptoms." *Am J Cardiol*. 2002;89(5):599–601. https://doi.org/10.1016/s0002-9149(01)02303-7

25. Brignole M, Croci F, Solano A, et al. Reproducibility of carotid sinus massage. *Pacing Clin Electrophysiol*. 2020;43(10):1190–1193. https://doi.org/10.1111/pace.13934

26. da Costa D, McIntosh S, Kenny RA. Benefits of fludrocortisone in the treatment of symptomatic vasodepressor carotid sinus syndrome. *Heart*. 1993;69(4):308–310. https://doi.org/10.1136/hrt.69.4.308

27. Saedon NI, Pin Tan M, Frith J. The prevalence of orthostatic hypotension: A systematic review and meta-analysis. *J Gerontol Ser A*. 2018;75(1):117–122. https://doi.org/10.1093/gerona/gly188

28. Finucane C, O'Connell MDL, Fan CW, et al. Age-related normative changes in phasic orthostatic blood pressure in a large population study. *Circulation*. 2014;130(20):1780–1789. https://doi.org/10.1161/circulationaha.114.009831

29. Kenny RA, O'Shea D. Falls and syncope in elderly patients. *Clin Geriatr Med*. 2002;18(2):xiii–xiv.

30. Rivasi G, Rafanelli M, Mossello E, Brignole M, Ungar A. Drug-related orthostatic hypotension: Beyond anti-hypertensive medications. *Drugs Aging*. 2020;37(10):725–738. https://doi.org/10.1007/s40266-020-00796-5

31. Juraschek SP, Taylor AA, Wright JT, et al. Orthostatic hypotension, cardiovascular outcomes, and adverse events. *Hypertension*. 2020;75(3):660–667. https://doi.org/10.1161/hypertensionaha.119.14309

32. Benetos A, Petrovic M, Strandberg T. Hypertension management in older and frail older patients. *Circul Res*. 2019;124(7):1045–1060. https://doi.org/10.1161/circresaha.118.313236

33. Bourke R, Doody P, Pérez S, Moloney D, Lipsitz L, Kenny RA. Cardiovascular disorders and falls among older adults: A systematic review and meta-analysis. *J Gerontol Ser A*. 2023. https://doi.org/10.1093/gerona/glad221

34. Wieling W, Kaufmann H, Claydon VE, et al. Diagnosis and treatment of orthostatic hypotension. *Lancet Neurol*. 2022;21(8):735–746. https://doi.org/10.1016/s1474-4422(22)00169-7

35. Okamoto LE, Celedonio JE, Smith EC, et al. Continuous positive airway pressure for the treatment of supine hypertension and orthostatic hypotension in autonomic failure. *Hypertension*. 2023;80(3):650–658. https://doi.org/10.1161/hypertensionaha.122.2008

36. Blanc J, Janousek J. Specific causes of syncope: Their evaluation and treatment strategies. *Eval Treat Syncope*. 2006;205–212. https://doi.org/10.1002/9781444312812.ch20d

37. Moya A, Brignole M, Sutton R, et al. Reproducibility of electrocardiographic findings in patients with suspected reflex neurally-mediated syncope. *Am J Cardiol*. 2008;102(11):1518–1523. https://doi.org/10.1016/j.amjcard.2008.07.043

38. Rockx MA, Hoch JS, Klein GJ, et al. Is ambulatory monitoring for "community-acquired" syncope economically attractive? A cost-effectiveness analysis of a randomized trial of external loop recorders versus Holter Monitoring. *Am Heart J*. 2005;150(5). https://doi.org/10.1016/j.ahj.2005.08.003

39. Varosy PD, Chen LY, Miller AL, Noseworthy PA, Slotwiner DJ, Thiruganasambandamoorthy V. Pacing as a treatment for reflex-mediated (vasovagal, situational, or carotid sinus hypersensitivity) syncope: A systematic review for the 2017 ACC/AHA/HRS guideline for the Evaluation and management of patients with syncope: A report of the American College of Cardiology/American Heart Association Task Force on Clinical Practice Guidelines and the heart rhythm society. *Circulation*. 2017;136(5). https://doi.org/10.1161/cir.0000000000000500

40. Sarasin FP. Role of echocardiography in the evaluation of syncope: A prospective study. *Heart*. 2002;88(4):363–367. https://doi.org/10.1136/heart.88.4.363

41. Jiagao L, Zaiying L. Results of invasive electrophysiologic evaluation in 268 patients with unexplained syncope. *J Huazhong Univ Sci Technol [Medical Sciences]*. 2003;23(3):278–279. https://doi.org/10.1007/bf02829513

42. Tang VL, Sudore R, Cenzer IS, et al. Rates of recovery to pre-fracture function in older persons with hip fracture: An observational study. *J Gen Internal Med*. 2016;32(2):153–158. https://doi.org/10.1007/s11606-016-3848-2

43. Correction to: Guidelines for falls in older adults, medication reviews and deprescribing as a single intervention in falls prevention: A systematic review and meta-analysis, and, World Guidelines for Falls Prevention and Management for Older Adults: A global initiative. *Age Ageing*. 2023;52(9). https://doi.org/10.1093/ageing/afad188

44. Bhangu J, King-Kallimanis BL, Donoghue OA, Carroll L, Kenny RA. Falls, non-accidental falls and syncope in community-dwelling adults aged 50 years and older: Implications for cardiovascular assessment. *PLOS ONE*. 2017;12(7). https://doi.org/10.1371/journal.pone.0180997

45. Seppala LJ, Petrovic M, Ryg J, et al. STOPPFall (screening tool of older persons prescriptions in older adults with high fall risk): A Delphi study by the eugms task and finish group on fall-risk-increasing drugs. *Age Ageing*. 2020;50(4):1189–1199. https://doi.org/10.1093/ageing/afaa249

46. Gaeta TJ, Fiorini M, Ender K, Bove J, Diaz J. Potential drug-drug interactions in elderly patients presenting with syncope. *J Emerg Med*. 2002;22(2):159–162. https://doi.org/10.1016/s0736-4679(01)00471-1

47. Tan MP, Kenny RA. Cardiovascular assessment of falls in older people. *Clin Interven Aging*. 2006;1(1):57–66. https://doi.org/10.2147/ciia.2006.1.1.57

48. Buracchio TJ, Mattek NC, Dodge HH, et al. Executive function predicts risk of falls in older adults without balance impairment. *BMC Geriatr*. 2011;11(1). https://doi.org/10.1186/1471-2318-11-74

49. Ryan DJ, Harbison JA, Meaney JF, Rice CP, King-Kallimanis B, Kenny RA. Syncope causes transient focal neurological symptoms. *QJM*. 2015;108(9):711–718. https://doi.org/10.1093/qjmed/hcv005

Index

Note: **Bold** page numbers refer to tables and *italic* page numbers refer to figures.

For Product Safety Concerns and Information please contact our
EU representative GPSR@taylorandfrancis.com Taylor & Francis
Verlag GmbH, Kaufingerstraße 24, 80331 München, Germany